BTEC LEVEL 3 NATIONAL

HEALTH AND SOCIAL CARE (AAQ)

Student textbook

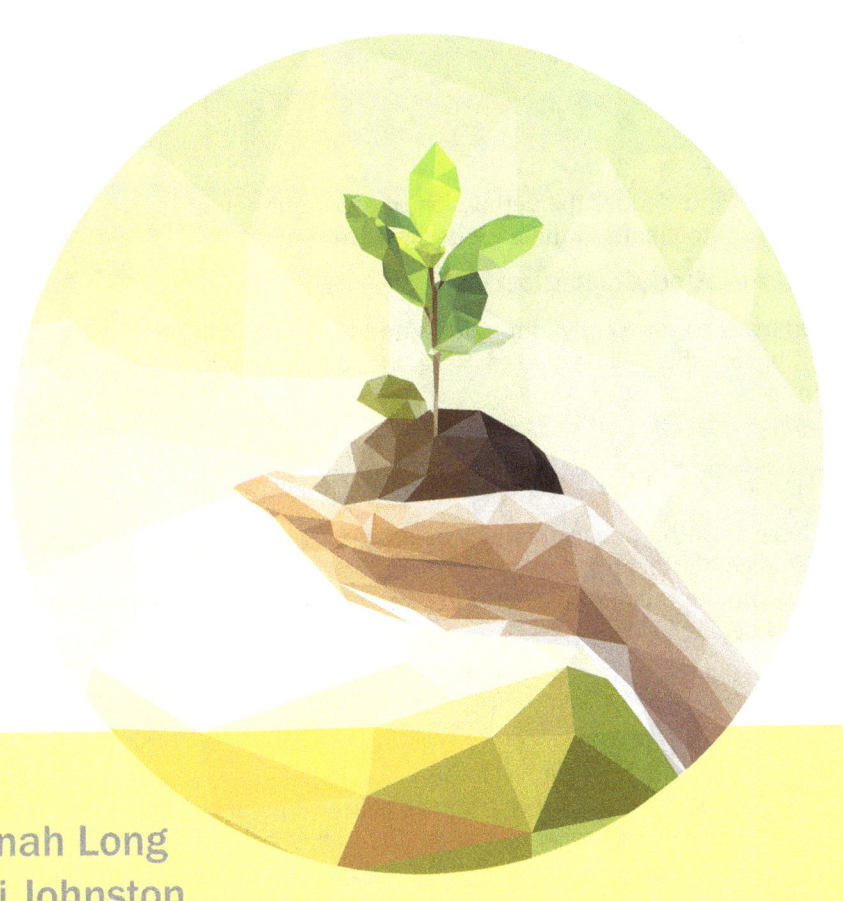

Hannah Long
Vicki Johnston
Niki Wilson
Jennifer Willis

eboru

The publisher gratefully acknowledges the permission of copyright holders to reproduce copyright material. Please see the photo credits at the back of the book.

Cover image: © LittlePerfectStock/Shutterstock

Every effort has been made to trace copyright holders and to obtain their permission for the use of copyright material. The publisher will be glad to make arrangements with any copyright holder it has not been possible to contact.

Copyright © 2025 Hannah Long, Vicki Johnston, Jennifer Willis, Niki Wilson

All rights reserved. No part of this publication may be reproduced, distributed, or transmitted in any form or by any means, including photocopying, recording, or other electronic or mechanical methods, without the prior written permission of the publisher, or under licence from the Copyright Licensing Agency. See www.cla.co.uk for more details.

First edition 2025. Impression 10 9 8 7 6 5 4 3 2 1

ISBN 978-1-917048-00-2

Whilst every effort has been made to ensure all information in this book is correct, the publisher shall not be liable for any loss of profit or any other commercial damages, including but not limited to special, incidental, consequential, personal, or other damages, due to any information or advice contained in this book.

If you do spot any errors in this book you can alert us at: enquiries@eboru.com

Ordering Information

Special discounts are available for class set purchases by schools, colleges and others. For details, contact the publisher at: orders@eboru.com

Trade orders: copies of this book are available through the normal wholesalers. For any queries please contact: orders@eboru.com

www.eboru.com

FEATURES IN THIS STUDENT BOOK

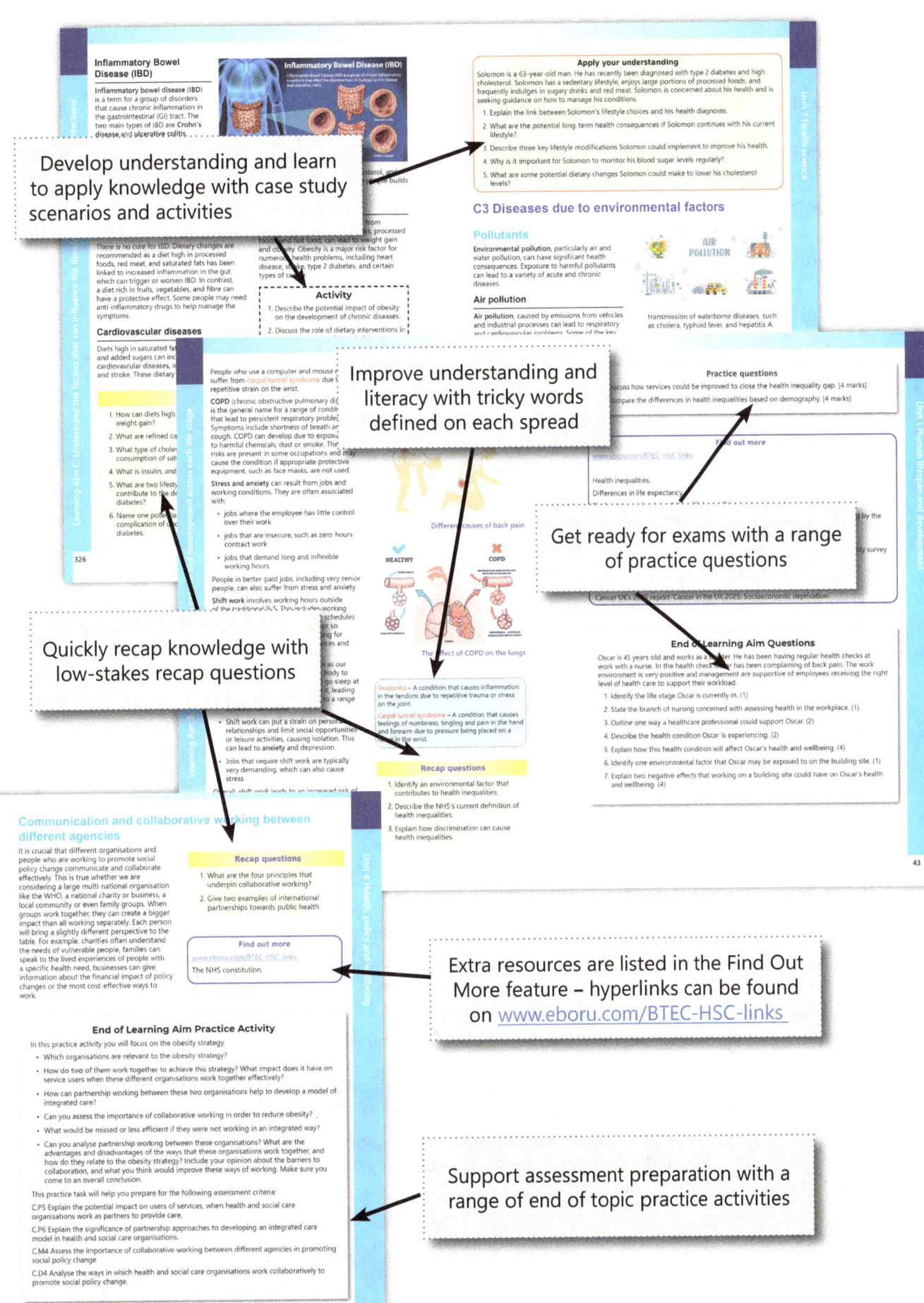

Develop understanding and learn to apply knowledge with case study scenarios and activities

Improve understanding and literacy with tricky words defined on each spread

Get ready for exams with a range of practice questions

Quickly recap knowledge with low-stakes recap questions

Extra resources are listed in the Find Out More feature – hyperlinks can be found on www.eboru.com/BTEC-HSC-links

Support assessment preparation with a range of end of topic practice activities

Contents

Unit 1 Human lifespan and development	5
Unit 2 Human biology and health	63
Unit 3 Principles of health and social care practice care	120
Unit 4 Health, policy and wellbeing	175
Unit 5 Promoting health education	202
Unit 6 Safe environments in health and social care	232
Unit 7 Health science	287

Answers are available online at:

www.eboru.com/BTEC-AAQ-HSC-answers

You can also check out our revision guide here:

www.eboru.com/BTEC-HSC-RG

BTEC Level 3 National in Health and Social Care (AAQ) Revision Guide

ISBN: 978-1-917048-05-7

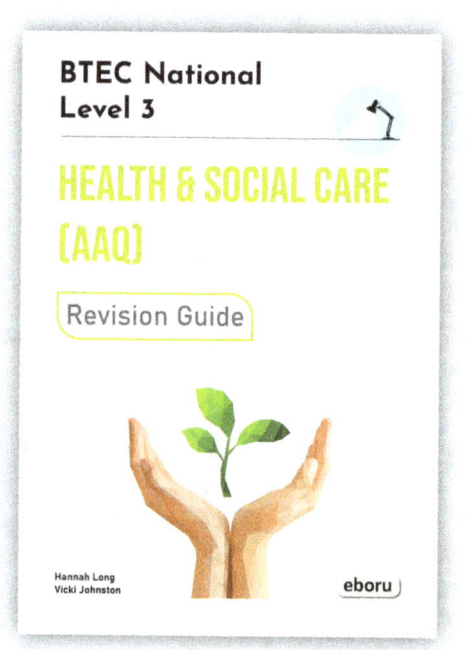

While this book is designed to help and support teachers and learners throughout the course the only official source of information about the qualification is the qualification specification and associated assessment guidance, published by the awarding organisation. Teachers and students should always refer to the specification and sample assessment material for definitive information about all aspects of this qualification. Specifications are also updated from time to time.

The practice questions, marks and answers included in this book are designed to help learners develop their knowledge, skills, understanding and technique but they do not replicate real examination papers, assessments or mark schemes.

Unit 1 Human lifespan and development

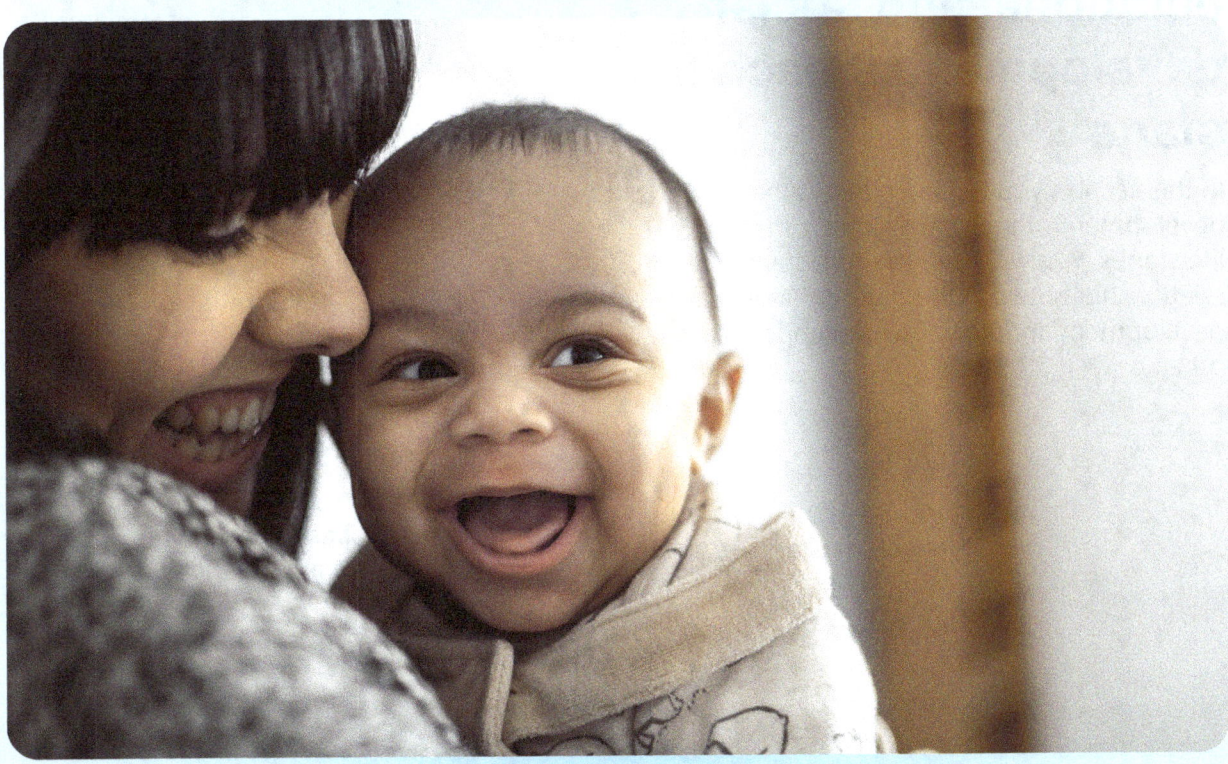

In this unit you will learn about how human lifespan develops across the life stages and the factors that can influence it.

You will learn about:

- Physical, intellectual, emotional and social development across human lifespan.
- The different factors that can affect human growth and development.
- The roles and responsibilities of those working in health and social care to meet the care and support needs of individuals.

How you will be assessed?

This unit has an exam worth 80 marks, lasting for 1 hour 30 minutes. The exam will have a mixture of multiple-choice questions, short and long answer questions.

Learning Aim A: Human growth and development through the life stages

Learning Aim B: Factors affecting human growth and development across each life stage

Learning Aim C: Health and social care promotion, prevention and treatment at different life stages

Learning Aim A: Human growth and development through the life stages

A1 Physical, intellectual, emotional and social development at each life stage

In this section you will learn about the holistic development of individuals across the six life stages. You will need to understand the relationship between the different areas of development and how they can impact each other.

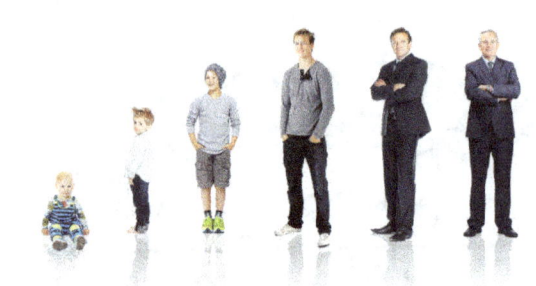

Physical
Anything to do with the body and how it grows. For example, height and weight.

Intellectual
Anything linked to the way an individual processes information. For example, language and memory.

PIES development

Emotional
Anything linked to the way an individual feels or expresses an emotion. For example, self-esteem and contentment.

Social
Anything to do the with the way individuals interact with others and build relationships. For example, peer pressure and friendships.

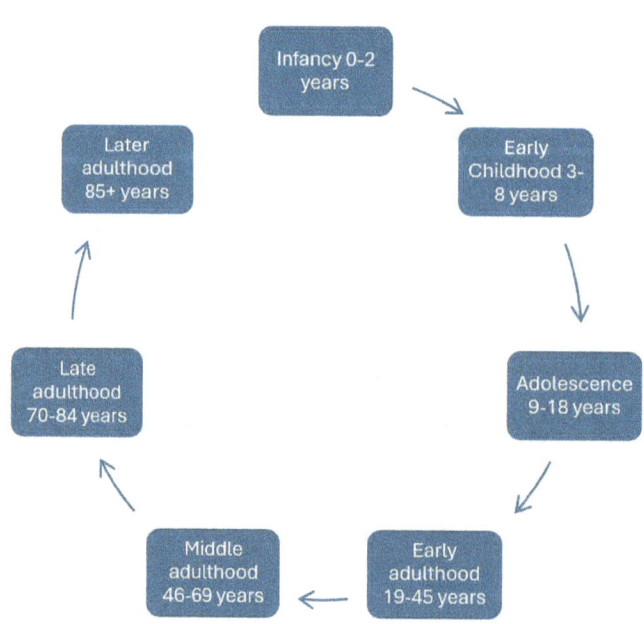

A1.1 Infancy (0-2 years)

During infancy, an individual will experience rapid growth and development where boys can reach half of their adult height by the age of two.

Physical

Physical growth refers to measurable quantities, such as height and weight. Children grow taller and heavier as they age. However, it is important to understand that an infant's growth is not a smooth process and is it not the same for each infant. We must recognise growth as a continuous process.

Growth in infancy is different for different parts of the body. For example, head circumference will grow most rapidly in the first few months of an infant's life. The average head circumference at birth for a girl is 34 cm and increases to just over 36 cm by the end of the first month. For a boy it is around 35 cm and increases to 37 cm by the end of the first month.

Babies gain **weight** very quickly during infancy. It is most rapid in the first six months of their lives. Healthy newborns will double their birth weight by the time they are five or six months old and by the end of their first year their birth weight will have almost tripled. The rate of weight development begins to slow once the infant enters early childhood because they are more active.

Babies also gain **height** rapidly during infancy. They can grow up to 50% in length in the first year, which is around 25 cm of growth on average.

> Holistic – Considering all aspects of something rather than individual parts.
>
> Rapid – When something happens at a quick rate.
>
> Head circumference – A measurement of a child's head around its widest part, which reflects brain size and is reviewed up until the age of 36 months.
>
> Paediatrician – A healthcare professional with a speciality in caring for the health needs of children.

An infant's growth will be recorded on a **centile chart**, which is completed during the infant's health and development review and recorded in their **personal child health record (PCHR)**. Boys and girls have slightly different charts as they tend to grow at a slightly different rate. Boys can be slightly heavier and taller. These charts allow health care professionals and parents/carers to be aware of the infant's pattern of growth. If there are any concerns, the infant is referred to a paediatrician.

Two more aspects of physical development in infancy are the development of gross and fine motor skills.

- **Gross motor skills** are the use of larger muscles and movements, such as the use of legs and arms to crawl, hold the head up, sit up and walk.

- **Fine motor skills** are the use of smaller muscles for more precise movements, such

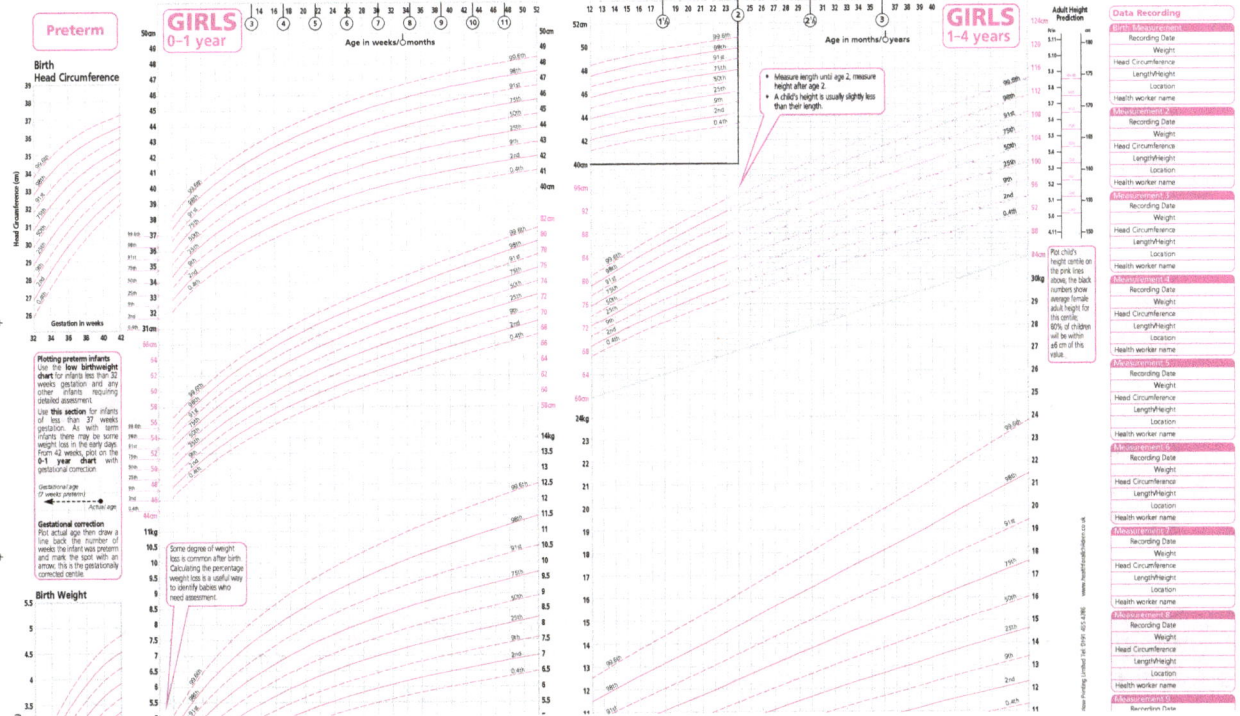

Growth charts. © 2009 Department of Health. Reproduced with permission of Royal College of Paediatrics and Child Health. These charts were developed by RCPCH / WHO / Department of Health.

as those in the hands, fingers and toes. For example, using the thumb and fingers (pincer grip) to pick up items, wriggling toes and holding a small toy.

Throughout the infancy life stage, a child is compared to **developmental milestones**, which are behaviours or skills that an infant displays as they grow. They are expected to reach different development milestones at certain life stages.

Age	Fine motor skills	Gross motor skills
Newborn	Tuck the thumb into the hand.	Primitive reflexes such as grasp.
1-3 months	Grasp a finger, which develops to grasping objects like a rattle.	Some control of the head, lifting the chin.
4-7 months	Shake a rattle, pick up objects and move them into the other hand.	Roll over, sit up with support and reach for objects with hands.
8-12 months	Use a pincer grip to pick up smaller objects such as pieces of food, place toys in particular places.	Sit up without support, crawl on the hands and knees and stand for a brief period.
18 months	Build a small tower block.	Climb using furniture.
2 years	Turn a page in a book, draw lines and circles with crayons.	Walk, squat to pick up toys, pull toys behind their back, throw a large ball.
2 and a half years	Use a spoon and fork to feed themselves, build a bigger tower.	Kick a ball, jump with two feet.

Gross and fine motor skills have their own set of developmental milestones

Intellectual

During infancy, the brain also experiences rapid growth and development. From a helpless newborn, a baby quickly acquires a large variety of skills and abilities. They learn the necessary skills and abilities through their interaction with their carers and the environment.

- Usually by two months old **interactions with carers** allows infants to **recognise familiar faces**, typically their primary carer(s).
- They will learn to imitate gestures from their carers.
- The environment provides an infant with opportunities to explore and **interact with their surroundings**, through the senses of touch, taste, smell, sight and sound. For example, an infant grabbing a toy is practicing co-ordination but also learning about spatial concepts, cause and effect, and how things feel. In this way they develop the ability to **manipulate objects**. Manipulating an object means controlling and interacting with it. Typical behaviours include grasping, shaking, moving, placing or transferring objects between hands.

Communication and **language** skills also develop rapidly.

- Newborn babies already show a preference for their mother's voice.
- From around two months, babies begin to recognise familiar voices and sounds through listening and imitation. They build schemas by associating people and objects with sounds, for example understanding that 'mama' and 'dada' are the names of their parents.
- The ability to talk also develops through stages. First, they communicate through vocalisations, such as cooing and gurgling. As they develop, they begin to understand words and develop their vocabulary. By the age of two, they can make 2-3 word sentences.

Emotional

Emotional development in infancy begins with **bonding** and **attachment**. Theorists highlight how important this is for later development and behaviour. By forming a strong bond and attachment with a carer, infants can begin to build their emotional literacy and empathy.

Bowlby's theory of attachment

John Bowlby (1953) states that an attachment is a deep and enduring emotional bond between a child and a primary carer. Bowlby's theory

Age	Language development
3 months	Babbling and cooing noises have a different cry for differing needs.
6 months	Gurgling sounds when playing, begins to make a range of sounds.
12 months	Copies sounds, develops single words like 'dada'.
18 months	Can say up to 20 words but know more, such as the names of people, objects and some body parts.
2 years	Say simple phrases such as 'more milk', ask one- or two-word questions, speak around 50 words. Although they can't say all of them, most will know between 200-500 words.

Language development milestones

originated in the 1930s, from his work as a child psychiatrist supporting emotionally disturbed children.

Bowlby argues that infants are biologically pre-programmed to form positive attachments with a primary carer who, he claimed, is predominantly the mother during the critical period of infancy. **Bowlby's attachment theory** outlines the possible consequences of poor early attachments on social, emotional and cognitive development, including the inability to form positive relationships later in life.

Bowlby observed that children would show signs of separation anxiety when their mother was not present, and that this level of distress would not reduce even with another carer present. This is because infants have an innate instinct to seek proximity to their primary carer when they feel stressed or threatened. Bowlby's theory means that the primary carer is the most important for forming positive attachments, as they are the ones to provide a high level of safety and security for the infant.

The impact of poor attachments during infancy can include:

- Less secure intimate relationships in the future.
- Reduced intellectual abilities.
- Low self-esteem.
- Feeling unsafe.

Ainsworth's theory of attachment

In the 1970s **Mary Ainsworth** expanded upon Bowlby's attachment theory. She explored the effects of attachment on behaviour, through her **Strange Situation** study. Ainsworth observed children between the ages of 12 and 18 months in the presence of their primary carer and a stranger. The experiment had eight steps, each with a duration of three minutes. In the original

Recap questions

1. Identify two fine motor skills experienced in infancy.
2. Give an example of growth in infancy.
3. Describe gross motor skills with an example.
4. What are the main point in Bowlby's attachment theory?
5. Describe how language development occurs in infancy.

Pincer grip – The use of the thumb and forefinger to pick up small objects.

Environment – The surroundings, such as the home or nursery.

Primary carer – The person that spends the most time with a child and meets most of their day-to-day needs.

Schema – The way in which our brains organise knowledge so we can understand the world. Schemas help a child learn about objects by making associations. For example, a schema for a bird is: 'It has feathers and can fly'.

Vocabulary – The number and range of words a person knows and uses.

Emotional literacy – The ability to express own emotions, and recognise and understand the emotions of others.

Empathy – Being able to put yourself into someone else's 'shoes' regarding their emotions or situation.

Biologically pre-programmed – Born with an ability to complete a particular task or behaviour.

Critical period – A time frame that is important for forming positive attachments.

Separation anxiety – A form of distress when an infant is parted from their primary carer.

Innate – Characteristics or abilities that are already present in a person from birth.

Proximity – Physical closeness to another.

experiment the primary carer was the child's mother, and the steps were:

1. The mother and child are left alone in the room.
2. The child is encouraged to explore the room.
3. A stranger enters the room and attempts to interact with the child.
4. The mother leaves the room. The child and stranger are now alone together.
5. The mother returns and the stranger leaves.
6. The mother leaves the room so the child is alone.
7. The stranger returns.
8. The mother returns and stranger leaves.

Ainsworth was able to identify three attachment types from this experiment:

- **Secure** – 70% of infants showed signs of trust and safety with the primary carer, when they were present or when they returned. This means an infant has likely experienced consistent, responsive and sensitive caregiving.
- **Anxious-resistant** – 15% of infants demonstrated conflicting behaviours towards the mother. For example, seeking proximity and closeness but then rejecting this on occasion. This means an infant has received inconsistent caregiving, where sometimes it may be responsive and other times inattentive.
- **Anxious-avoidant** – 15% of infants did not display signs of emotional closeness to the mother. These infants showed no signs of distress when the mother left and no interest in her when she returned. This means these infants may have experienced unresponsive or emotionally distant caregiving.

Ainsworth was able to conclude that the quality of caregiving can influence the type of attachment an infant displays. She had a particular focus on the responsiveness and sensitivity of the carer towards the infant, and how that shapes attachment and future emotional and social development.

Social

Social development refers to the way in which we learn to interact with all the different people in our lives.

In infancy, social development begins with the formation of **relationships with carers**. Carers create these relationships and bonds by showing love and affection through:

- holding and cuddling
- talking and singing
- looking into the baby's eyes and bringing their face close
- smiling
- responding to the baby's cries and comforting them
- making sure the baby is comfortable, safe and warm.

Babies quickly learn to interact with carers. For example:

- Babies aged 0-3 months begin to make eye contact with carers, recognise their faces, smile at them and imitate behaviour such as sticking out a tongue.
- At around 3-6 months babies can play peek-a-boo, and can respond to a carer's facial expression by laughing and smiling, and can hold their carers gaze.

Apply your understanding

Rachel is 18 months old. Rachel has been living with her grandmother since she was two months old as her mother has faced challenges with substance misuse and has spent some time in prison. Rachel is often placed into nursery for care, as her grandmother has a full-time job and lacks social support. Rachel often begins her day at nursery quite upset and distressed once her grandmother has dropped her off.

1. Who has Rachel developed a primary attachment to?
2. Explain this attachment using Bowlby's theory of attachment.
3. According to Bowlby, Rachel might be experiencing separation anxiety. Discuss this aspect of Bowlby's theory with reference to Rachel and possible future consequences.

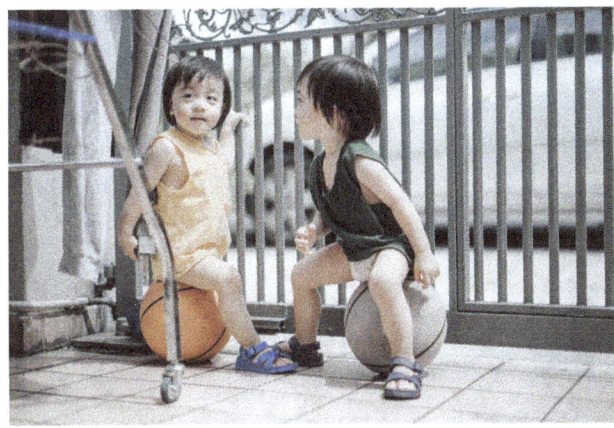

Responsiveness – The quality of a response to a person's needs in a positive and timely manner.

Sensitivity – The state of being considerate of another person's needs.

Solitary play – The period of play when a child only wants to play on their own.

Parallel play – Play alongside another child, but not quite together.

- From 6 months babies become more interactive, showing more interest in games and songs, such as clapping along.

In the later stages of infancy, an infant will **start to interact with others.** This can include other children through play, other adults as part of a wider family, or in a health or social care setting such as a nursery.

It is important that infants interact with other children, in order to develop relationships through the social skill of play. This is where infants develop a sense of self, learn how to make friends and how to role play.

The stages of play an infant will experience are:

- Solitary or 'solo' play (0-18 months) – an infant will have independence in their play and learning. This can involve exploring the environment through their senses, and play and chatting to themselves.

- Parallel play (18 months-2 years) – an infant may copy other children and adults, and enjoy playing alongside others, but they are not yet playing with others and there is little engagement between them. They have not yet established sharing and turn-taking skills.

Apply your understanding

Liam has just had his first birthday. Staff at the nursery have observed some distressing behaviour from Liam. He struggles to be apart from his mother, clinging to her and crying until they are separated by the staff. Throughout the day Liam struggles to engage with the other children and will often watch the door and say 'mummy'. When his mother does return to pick him up, he shows mixed emotions. He will cling to her leg but also hit her and cry.

1. Identify the attachment type Liam is displaying in Ainsworth's theory.

2. Explain how Ainsworth would interpret Liam's behaviour. What does this suggest about Liam's early caregiving experiences?

Recap questions

1. Give one example of physical development in infancy.

2. Identify an aspect of growth that can occur in infancy.

3. Briefly explain Bowlby's theory of attachment.

Practice questions

1. Describe how attachment and bonding can impact social development. [4 marks]

2. Describe how fine and gross motor skills can be influenced by social interactions with other children. [3]

3. Explain how the environment can influence an infant's holistic growth and development. [4]

A1.2 Early childhood (3-8 years)

In early childhood children continue to grow and develop at a steady pace. A child will begin to master and acquire new skills, such as problem solving and emotional regulation.

Physical

Throughout early childhood a child's growth continues but at a much slower rate than in infancy.

- **Height** increases by around 6–7 cm per year.
- **Weight** increases by around 2–3 kg per year.

These increases are influenced by factors such as genetics, nutrition and overall health.

Body proportions also change during this life stage. Body fat decreases as limbs get longer and muscles get stronger. These changes are supportive of other areas of physical development, such as balance, coordination and motor skills.

Fine and gross motor skills continue to develop, as children begin to master more complex movements.

Examples of gross motor skills:

- Walk on tiptoe by the age of three.
- Balance on one foot for a second by the age of three.
- Ride a small bike by the age of three.
- Kick and throw a large ball by the age of four.
- Hopping and skipping by the age of five.
- Participate in sports and activities by the age of eight, due to better strength and coordination.

Examples of fine motor skills:

- Use a pencil to trace letters and numbers by the age of three.
- Dress and undress self, including doing up and undoing buttons and laces by the age of five.
- Draw detailed pictures by the end of this life stage.

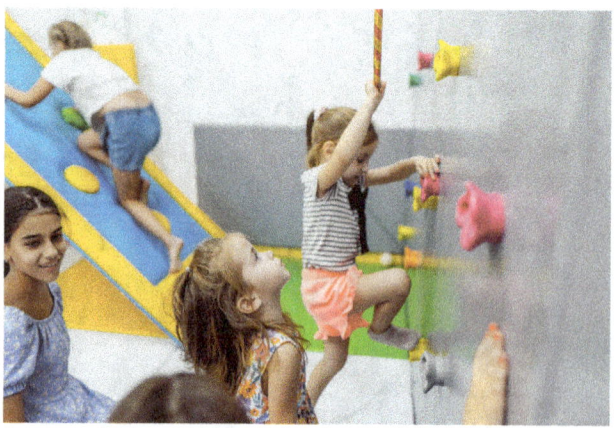

Intellectual

As a child encounters new environments that enable learning, there is a rapid growth in their language skills. As they are exposed to new words, from adults and other children, in nursery, pre-school and primary school, they will **increase their vocabulary**. This means children become able to **talk in full sentences**.

- By the age of four, children can begin to talk in clear sentences that anyone can understand but are still expected to make some mistakes with grammar.
- By the age of five, a child will be able to use adult grammar effectively, despite them still learning about grammar and vocabulary.

This increase in vocabulary means a child begins to **know basic information about themselves.** For example:

- When they are three or four they may be able to describe themselves as 'tall', know their age and their full name.
- As they get older they will know where they live, their birthday and other more complex details.

Children will develop new skills, such as **counting** and **problem solving**, through exposure to hands-on activities that encourage critical thinking.

- Counting skills are developed by exploring objects and using senses to organise and compare objects. For example, activities such as tower building with blocks, matching shapes and counting rhymes and songs all reinforce sequential learning.
- A child's problem-solving skills will adapt as they face challenges, such as completing a jigsaw puzzle and figuring out the correct pieces. This requires the use of different strategies and persistence to find the correct solution.

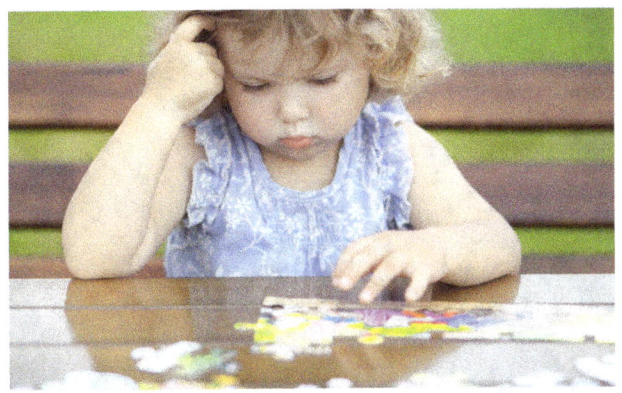

The activities that children can engage with in this life stage help the development of these skills. For example, providing activities based on real life, such as shopping scenarios where children need to work out how much money they can spend, further encouraging counting.

Numeracy and counting development milestones throughout early childhood include:

- **Ages 1-2** – A child will be able to count objects as they touch each object.
- **Ages 2-3** – A child will begin to recognise quantities such as 'more' or 'less'.
- **Ages 3-4** – A child can recite numbers up to 10 and begin basic problem solving.
- **Ages 4-5** – Counting accuracy improves. Children can count to 20 and can solve more complex problems, such as organising objects by shape or size.
- **Ages 5-6** – Children can count beyond 20 and begin to understand mathematical skills such as addition and subtraction. They can follow multi-step problems to solve complex problems.
- **Ages 6-7** – Children can now count to 100 and use strategic thinking such as trial and error to solve problems.
- **Ages 7-8** – **Children master basic arithmetic and can** begin to apply logic to scenarios, to be able to plan solutions and apply reasoning to solve problems.

Recap questions

1. What is the age range of early childhood?
2. Give an example of a gross motor skill that is mastered in early childhood.
3. Identify one example of intellectual development that occurs in early childhood.

Master – To become good at a skill or ability with practise.

Body proportions – The measurement of body parts in relation to each other. This helps to determine an individual's physique.

Sequential learning – The process a child goes through to learn something in a specific order.

Emotional

In early childhood, socialisation skills and the development of language help children to understand basic emotions and learn to **manage** their **own emotions**. A child should be supported in managing their emotions by a relevant adult. This can be done by:

- **Modelling emotional regulation** – Adults who talk openly about their emotions and show healthy coping mechanisms are likely to be imitated by a child.
- **Naming and validating emotions** – Helping a child to name their feelings, and teaching them that these emotions are okay, will support their understanding.
- **Teaching coping strategies** – Providing children with a range of techniques to regulate their emotions is important for building independence. Strategies can include taking deep breaths or counting to ten.

As a child begins to understand their own emotions, they also begin to **develop basic empathy skills**. Typically this begins at around the age of 4-5 years, and develops to a deeper level by the age of 8. This means they can **understand others' emotions** and respond in an appropriate way. For example, they will be able to recognise if another person is sad and try to understand why. They will also be able to respond by comforting that person.

At this life stage children begin the gradual process of forming a **development of self**.

- Between the ages of three to five, a child develops a more detailed self-concept and can define themselves based on observable traits, such as 'I am tall', or preferences such as 'I like cats', 'I don't like peas'.
- As a child enters the end of early childhood, their idea of self becomes more stable and complex as they reflect on their abilities in different areas, such as sports or subjects at school. This development is continually supported by relationships and experiences a child encounters.

Social

As children move through the stages of play, they **develop friendships with other children**. Between the ages of three and eight, children widen their social circle through co-operative play. This means they play with other children with a common goal in the same game, can share toys and take turns in activities. This stage of play is important for social development as it establishes friendships.

By the age of seven, a child will have established a few important friendships and may even have a 'best friend'.

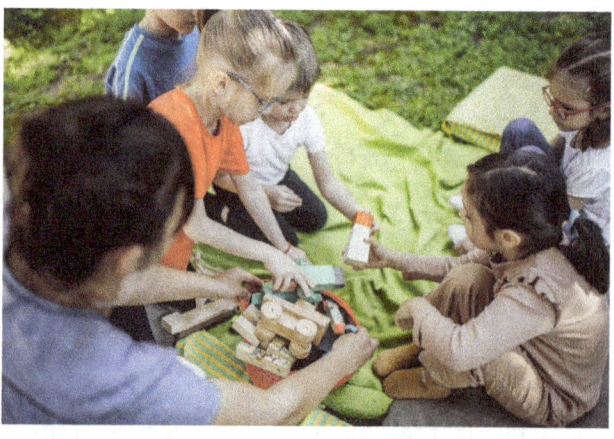

Co-operative play – A child plays with other children through the sharing of toys and turn taking.

Recap questions

1. Identify an example of a gross motor skill in early childhood.
2. Identify the age range of early childhood.
3. Describe how vocabulary develops in early childhood.

Practice questions

1. Describe how play can influence emotional development in early childhood. [4]
2. Explain how development changes between infancy and early childhood. [3]

A1.3 Adolescence (9-18 years)

Adolescence sees individuals experience growth spurts during puberty and develop more complex abilities intellectual, emotional and social skills. This life stage is considered to be the bridge from childhood into adulthood.

Physical

A big part of physical development during adolescence is the process of **puberty**. This is a period of rapid growth. The end of puberty sees individuals reach sexual maturity as they are biologically able to reproduce due to the development of **primary and secondary sexual characteristics**.

Puberty often begins between 11-13 years for girls and 13-15 years for boys. Sex hormones are responsible for the changes that occur in puberty. The pituitary gland located in the brain controls the release of **sex hormones** in both males and females.

- The main female hormones are oestrogen and progesterone, which are responsible for ovulation and menstruation.
- The main male hormone is testosterone, which stimulates the testes to produce sperm and causes the onset of physical changes.

Whilst they are sometimes thought of as 'female' and 'male' hormones, in fact all three sex hormones play a part in the development of fertility in both boys and girls.

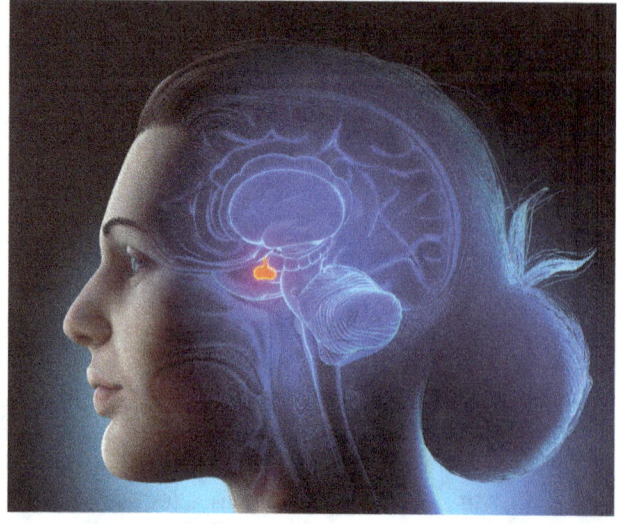

The location of the pituitary gland is marked in orange

	Primary sexual characteristics	Secondary sexual characteristics
Male	Enlargement of penis and testes. Sperm production and the beginning of ejaculation. Spontaneous erections can occur.	Voice deepens due to changes in the larynx. Pubic, facial and armpit hair. Fat and muscle tissues are redistributed.
Female	Uterus enlarges and vagina lengthens. Ovaries release eggs during ovulation. Menstrual cycle begins.	Breast buds develop. Pubic and armpit hair. Body fat redistributes to cause the hips to widen and waist narrows.

Table 1.3 Primary and secondary sexual characteristics

Sex hormones also support the **changes to primary and secondary sexual characteristics**.

- **Primary sexual characteristics** are associated with changes to reproductive organs that have been present from birth.
- **Secondary sexual characteristics** are the outward physical signs of development that develop during puberty, indicating adulthood.

Intellectual

Adolescents develop a greater capacity for **abstract thinking**. This means an individual can understand concepts that are not directly linked to an object, event or experience. It is a type of higher-order thinking that allow us to think about ideas, concepts and patterns.

For example:

- Concepts such as fairness, justice and love are abstract rather than tangible.
- Whist we normally learn about numbers by counting real objects, maths at secondary school becomes more abstract.
- Any form of planning for the future, or thinking about alternative scenarios, requires some level of abstract thinking.
- Music, painting and poetry are expressions of abstract ideas.

Abstract thinking helps us to answer 'why?' questions. It is crucial for problem-solving and logical reasoning, as well as for creative and imaginative tasks.

Emotional

Adolescents continue to **develop own identity**. At this stage, due to influences from secondary

Sexual maturity – The ability for males and females to reproduce due to the development of primary and secondary sexual characteristics.

Sex hormones – Chemical substances in the body that are responsible for the development of primary and secondary sexual characteristics and the onset of puberty in both males and females.

Oestrogen – A female sex hormone released by the ovaries to stimulate menstruation and ovulation.

Progesterone – A female sex hormone with the responsibility of regulating menstruation and supporting the female body to prepare for pregnancy.

Testosterone – A male sex hormone that affects the development of male secondary sexual characteristics produced in the testes.

Recap questions

1. Describe primary sexual characteristics.
2. Give two examples of secondary sexual characteristics.
3. Define abstract thinking.

school and peer relationships, individuals can explore and define themselves in various ways.

This stage sees the emergence of personal beliefs, values, interests and social roles. This **self-concept** then shapes a person's behaviour, relationships and life choices. It is linked to the way an individual thinks and feels about themselves. Self-concept encompasses self-image and self-esteem.

- **Self-image** is the view we have of ourselves. This can include our physical appearance but also includes more abstract ideas of how we think we are. For example, an individual may hold views about themselves such as 'plain', 'beautiful', 'clever', 'witty', or 'moral'. Self-image influences our self-esteem.

- **Self-esteem** is an individual's view of their self-worth and value. It has a big impact on confidence and how capable someone feels to achieve things.

It is important to understand that self-esteem, self-concept and self-image are not fixed but fluid. They can and do change throughout the life stages.

Adolescence is a difficult time to navigate emotions, because changes in hormone levels due to puberty can lead to changes in mood. Adolescents are also presented with new challenges that can confuse and alter their self-concept and self-esteem. For example, fitting in with peers, establishing new friendship groups and other people's ideas about body image can all influence how positively or negatively an individual views themselves.

Another part of adolescence is the development of new relationships, including intimate relationships. An **intimate relationship** is a deeper connection between two people, based upon feelings of attraction and emotional closeness that go beyond the typical family and friend relationships.

Intimate relationships develop as individuals begin to explore romantic attraction and develop the desire for a deep and loving bond. This is when adolescents might start to experience a crush, go on dates or initiate relationships with another person and be labelled as 'boyfriend', 'girlfriend' or 'partner'.

- These relationships are based upon shared thoughts, values and emotions, and a feeling of attachment.
- There involve deeper levels of trust, security and empathy.
- These relationships can alter self-image and self-esteem, due to the way the other person makes them feel.

Dealing with the end of an intimate relationship can also be very hard, at this life stage and in later stages, and can also affect self-image and self-esteem.

Social

Throughout adolescence, an individual often establishes a series of **friendships** and have

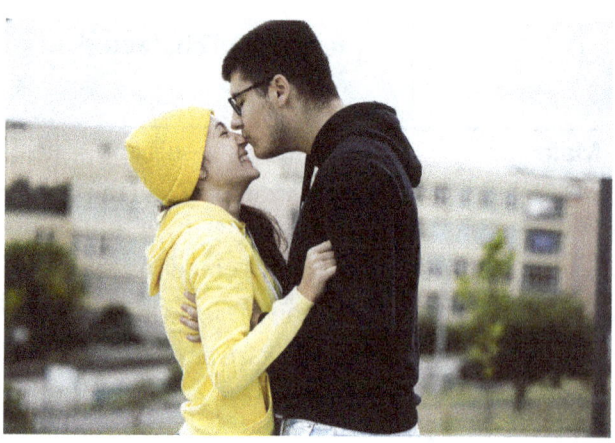

First romantic relationships often begin in the adolescent life stage

a circle of people they regularly engage with. Friendships can bring a range of benefits, including:

- Supporting each other through difficult life events.
- Supporting each other to maintain a healthy lifestyle.
- Providing a sense of belonging, in order to avoid loneliness.
- Encouraging positive self-esteem and self-image.
- Reducing stress.
- Increasing happiness and contentment.

However, friendships can also pose challenges, such as when individuals argue or if friends part ways due to a change in circumstance, such as moving school or house.

Peer pressure is common in an adolescent's life. Peer groups can have a large influence on an adolescent's views, values, behaviour and lifestyle choices. Peer pressure can involve the encouragement of negative and positive behaviours such as smoking, taking drugs or regular exercising. The way in which an adolescent cope with peer influences can vary depending on their own vulnerabilities. For example, neurodivergent adolescents, or those with learning disabilities, may be more susceptible to peer pressure or influence than neurotypical individuals.

This life stage also sees people begin to become more **independent**.

- Some adolescents begin working in part-time jobs, establishing some financial independence.
- Adolescents have more autonomy over

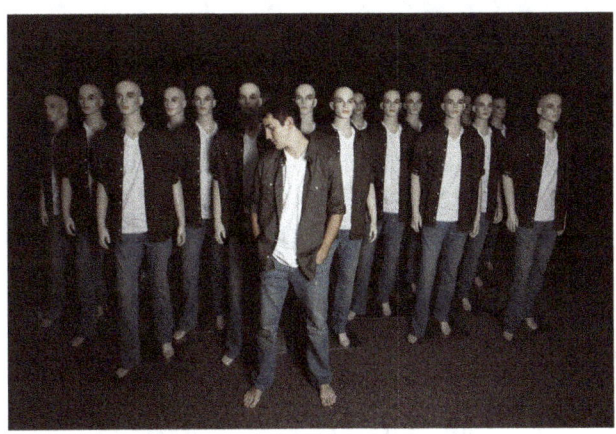

It can be hard to resist peer pressure at any life stage but particularly during adolescence

Peer groups – People in the same general situation as yourself, such as your classmates at school or college.

Neurodivergent – A term that describes people whose brain develops and works differently from a 'typical' brain. This can result in conditions such as autism.

Autonomy – Doing things independently and making your own decisions.

decision making, readying them for the future responsibilities they will have in adulthood.

- They begin to rely less on parental guidance and support, and begin to use their own initiative and abstract thinking to solve problems on their own.

- They also have a level of emotional independence that allows them to regulate and cope with differing emotions, again with less support from carers than they had in early childhood.

Independence is a critical element of social development in adolescence as it allows individuals to build confidence and resilience, and control their own lives.

Recap questions

1. Define the term 'self-concept'.
2. Identify two examples of social development experienced in adolescence.
3. Describe the difference between primary and secondary sexual characteristics.

Practice questions

1. Explain how intimacy links to emotional development. [3]
2. Explain why friendships in adolescence may be important than family. [3]

A1.4 Early adulthood (19-45 years)

In this life stage, individuals move towards complete independence, often accompanied by changes in self-concept. This life stage will also see the ending of some types of development.

Physical

People reach **physical maturity** in this life stage. Individuals reach peak physical condition, which means that an individual's height, strength and physical abilities are at their best and will not develop any further. Peak physical development typically occurs between the ages of 19 and 28 years.

Physical strength peaks because hormones which support muscle growth and repair, and which contribute to the development of muscle fibres, are at their optimal levels. These hormones include testosterone in men, oestrogen in women, and growth hormone.

Peak – Development is at its highest level and will not improve further.

Ovulation – The release of an egg from an ovary.

Conception – The process where a child is conceived.

Motility – The ability of something to move.

Fertility is also at its peak during this life stage.

- A woman in her 20s is at her most fertile, as both the quantity and quality of eggs are at its highest. This is because oestrogen and progesterone levels are now at optimal levels and well-balanced, which support regular ovulation, creating the conditions necessary for conception to occur. A woman's fertility declines from her mid-30s.

- A man's fertility remains stable throughout early adulthood and beyond, due to the continual reproduction of sperm. However, sperm quality, including motility and shape, is at its highest level in early adulthood, because testosterone levels are optimal. So, although men are able to produce sperm into later adulthood, its quality declines with age, so their ability to father children decreases with age.

A key physical development for many women in this life stage is **pregnancy** and **lactation**.

- The changes a woman experiences during puberty in adolescence are supportive of pregnancy. For example, secondary sexual characteristics, such as hips widening, support the woman's ability to conceive and labour a child.
- Changes to progesterone levels during early pregnancy ensure a woman maintains her pregnancy and oestrogen rises are responsible for the sickness ('morning sickness') some women experience.
- Once pregnant, women experience hormonal changes that impact the shape and appearance of their breasts. For example, the nipples and areolas darken, and breasts can become more sensitive to the touch. This is because blood supply increases to deliver more nutrients and oxygen, to support the development of milk glands for lactation.
- When pregnant, women produce high levels of a hormone called **prolactin** that stimulates milk production. **Oxytocin** is another hormone, that allows milk to be ejected from the breasts.

Brain growth continues until the early 20s. After that, individuals' brains begin to optimise their functions through a process called **synaptic pruning**. This is where synapses that are not being used are removed. This allows the remaining connections to become more efficient, so the brain becomes more adapted to each person's experiences. This means that processes such as emotion regulation and impulse control become more refined. However it also means that learning completely new skills, such as a new language, becomes harder. Synaptic pruning occurs until the mid-20s.

Intellectual

In early adulthood, individuals may continue studying in **further education** or **higher education**, or begin **work and careers**. As well as learning new things, they will also use knowledge and skills they have previously learnt. For example:

- They will acquire new knowledge as part of their studies or work.
- They may be required to think logically to solve problems and make appropriate decisions.
- They may also need to develop **new intellectual skills** to support their progress in work or education. This can include reflective thinking, where they consider their behaviour or thoughts after an event so they can alter behaviour in the future.
- They may also need to consider multiple perspectives and use more refined abstract thinking skills to generate solutions that are not at first obvious.

Emotional

Early adulthood also typically sees the beginning of **long-term intimate relationships**, or the continuation of those that began during adolescence. Typically, this means people have a partner that they have a deep and enduring connection to. This connection can be physical, emotional or both.

Intimacy can be defined as a connection between people that is based upon mutual trust, understanding and an emotional closeness. Those in an intimate relationship are more open to sharing thoughts and feelings with each other without fear of judgment or rejection. Intimacy can occur in different forms as well. For example, close friendships, romantic or familial.

An individual in early adulthood may also experience **changes to their self-concept**,

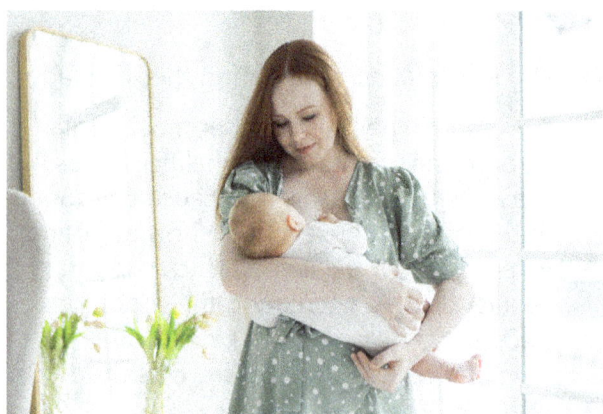

self-esteem and self-image based upon their lifestyles, including their experiences at work and with their family. These changes can be both positive and negative and can fluctuate throughout this life stage. This is because an individual's circumstances relating to work and family can change dramatically through early adulthood. This can be due to bereavements, redundancy, changes of career or promotions at work.

For example, an individual who began working in their early 20s in a junior position in a company can become very senior by the time they are 40. They may have increased self-esteem compared to when they were 18, due to their success and responsibility at work.

Bonding and attachment. People who choose to become parents typically have children during this life stage. They develop deep and enduring connections to their own child/children.

In adulthood, individuals have an increased understanding of the world and may develop a new appreciation for their family members, including parents/guardians. This can strengthen bonds that were not as strong. However, these bonds can also weaken in this life stage if individuals become more distant from family members, for example if they move a long way from family.

Social

As people progress through early adulthood they can become completely **independent**, depending on the individuals' circumstances. Independence is about a person's ability to function and complete tasks on their own without the support of others. For example:

- Adults often move out of their family home and look after themselves.
- Adults have financial responsibilities, which means they must manage money and bills.
- Adults have jobs which have lots of responsibilities, including basic ones such as turning up on time.

Early adulthood often also sees a shift in **friend groups**. This can be because of life circumstances. For example, moving away from home, starting a new career and going to university can all cause existing friendship groups to change or strengthen, and can lead to new friends. Typically in early adulthood, an individual will have an established group of

Areola – The circular area around the nipple.

Synapses – Connections between neurons (nerve cells). All thoughts, feeling and emotions, as well as memory and the capacity to learn, are a result of signals travelling between neurons.

Intimacy – A close or personal bond that occurs between individuals that are familiar with each other. This can be seen in relationships or friendships.

Bereavement – The death of a close relation or friend.

Redundancy – The loss of a job.

Generational and cultural differences – Differences in ideas or behaviour due to when a person was born, how they were raised or based upon their cultural norms and values.

Recap questions

1. What is the age range of early adulthood?
2. Identify two types of physical development experienced in early adulthood.
3. Describe how occupation impacts intellectual development in early adulthood.
4. Identify one example of physical development in early adulthood.
5. Give two examples of how an individual in early adulthood might improve their intellectual skills.
6. Describe how self-concept changes in early adulthood.

Practice questions

1. Explain how independence changes from adolescence to early adulthood. [3]
2. Discuss the impact of bonding and attachment on an individual's emotional wellbeing in early adulthood. [4]

friends that lasts throughout the remaining life stages.

Whilst we have discussed social development throughout the life stages so far, it is important to remember that not all individuals develop social relationships in the same way, due to generational and cultural differences.

A1.5 Middle adulthood (46-69 years)

Middle adulthood sees the beginning of reflection over an individual's life and the decline of certain physical functions.

Physical

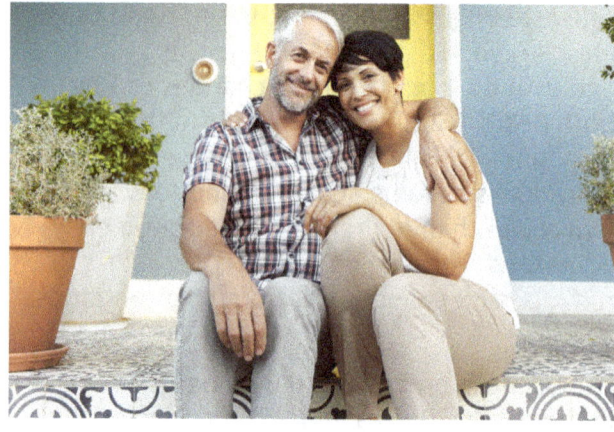

Between the ages of 45 and 55 years, women experience a decline in fertility.

- The **perimenopause** is the transition stage before full menopause. It is marked by a reduction in oestrogen levels, which causes the ovaries to produce fewer eggs. This effects the pattern and regularity of a woman's period.
- Once a woman has not had a period for 12 months, menstruation is considered to have stopped. They are deemed to have experienced **menopause**. This signifies the end of fertility.

The menopause can also cause a rise in the production of **gonadotropins**, which are hormones that contribute towards **hot flushes** and **night sweats**. These hormones try to stimulate egg production, without success.

Other common symptoms of the perimenopause and menopause include:

- Headaches
- Dizziness
- **Vaginal dryness**
- Weight gain
- Difficulty sleeping
- Feeling depressed
- Mood swings
- Loss of libido

Towards the end of middle adulthood, people's **physical strength** begins to **decline**. This is because they begin to lose muscle mass, in a process known as sarcopenia.

As individuals age, they also begin to experience **vision and hearing loss**.

- Vision can decline due to a hardening of the lens in the eye, a condition known as presbyopia. It leads to issues with reading small print, causing headaches and eyestrain. Most people need reading glasses as they move through this life stage.
- Vision can also decline due to other eye health issues, such as floaters in the eye, dry eyes and developing a greater sensitivity to light.
- Individuals gradually lose the ability to hear higher frequencies as they age. This is a natural part of ageing but can be accelerated in people who have been exposed to high noise levels over the years, such as working in noisy environments without ear protection.

People in this life stage can also experience physical health changes in **relation to lifestyle factors**. This includes smoking, diet, alcohol consumption, substance misuse and physical activity. These lifestyle factors can contribute to the following physical health changes:

- **Weight gain** – As individuals age metabolism can slow. This means that the body needs fewer calories to perform its normal functions. Continuing to eat a diet high in calories can lead to an increase in weight, because excess calories are stored as body fat.
- **Joint pain related to wear and tear** – This can occur as cartilage in joints breaks down, causing joint pain and conditions such as osteoarthritis.

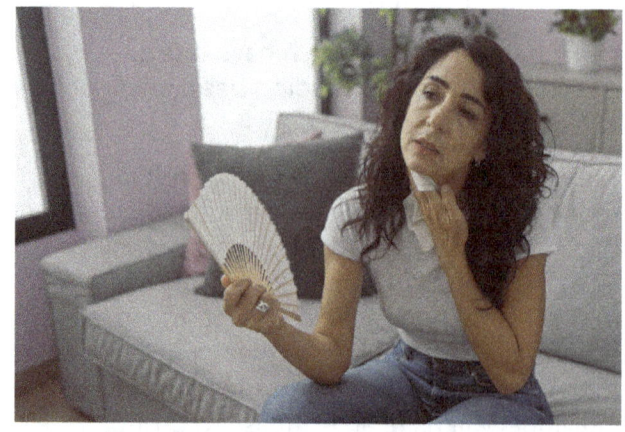

> **Recap questions**
>
> 1. Identify two life stages before middle adulthood.
> 2. Give two symptoms of the perimenopause.
> 3. Describe how verbal skills are developed in middle adulthood.

Intellectual

During this life stage, individuals can experience improvements in their intellectual capabilities, including in **verbal and reasoning skills**. They benefit from **applied learning**, where people can use their past experience to solve future problems.

- They have a larger vocabulary and comprehension skills. This means adults in this life stage are better equipped to tackle complex pieces of information to address a question or to develop further knowledge around a subject.
- Reasoning skills are also at their highest in this life stage. People have experience of challenging situations and problems, and the emotional maturity to think things through clearly and rationally.

Emotional

As individuals age, they can better regulate and control their emotions. They are also at a point in their lives where they can **re-evaluate** their **priorities**. This means they assess their life circumstances and consider whether they need to alter their priorities and commitments.

- A common re-evaluation relates to work/life balance. Some people spend a lot of time working in early adulthood, and decide that they need to spend more time with family and friends as they are getting older.
- A re-evaluation might be due to a change in circumstance, for example, the arrival or loss of family members, or relationship changes. Or it might simply be because of the passing of time.

People with children, who are now growing up, may feel proud of the part they have had in **contributing to the next generation**. However, as children grow up and leave the family home, it can lead to a **sense of emptiness** – also known as empty nest syndrome.

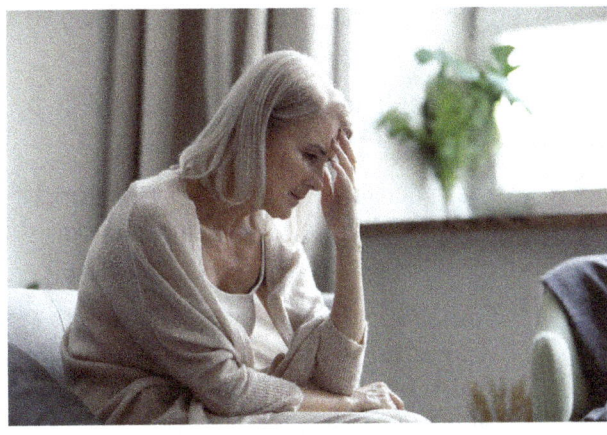

> Libido – Sexual desire.
>
> Sarcopenia – The loss of muscle mass that is related specifically to aging.
>
> Presbyopia – The loss of an individual's ability to see objects close due to aging.
>
> Metabolism – The rate at which the body consumes calories.
>
> Vocabulary – The number of words someone knows.
>
> Empty nest syndrome – A phrase that describes the process of children leaving the family home.

Individuals can also experience emotional upheaval during the menopause process. For example, it can cause **changes to mood** and loss of libido. This is due to the decrease in the sex hormone oestrogen which contributes to mood swings and loss of sexual drive. As well as hormonal changes, there is an emotional context to the change in fertility and associated self-image.

Social

This life stage can see individuals build and develop new relationships.

- They can develop connections with **peers at work** that can develop into friendships beyond the workplace. This can develop because of shared interests and work patterns.
- There can be a rise in an individual's **social lifestyle** because they have more free time for hobbies and activities they like. Reasons for having more social time include:
  * Children are less dependent, or no longer dependent, on their parents/carers.
  * Retirement or early retirement from work.

However, other people in this life stage may have limited social activities because:

- The are unable to retire yet, or simply do not want to.
- If they are actively working in a job, work pressures can **limit an individual's social life.**
    * Some jobs often involve additional work outside of traditional working hours, leaving little time left to socialise with friends and family.
    * Some people may now have very senior jobs, which require them to spend a lot of time working or thinking about work.

Both of these can contribute to breakdowns in relationships, leading to isolation.

Middle adulthood can also see an individual's **role change** if they become **grandparents**. They may often be leaned upon for support and babysitting duties. It also means that new relationships with grandchildren are formed and continue to grow, throughout the grandchild's and grandparent's lives.

> Isolation – When an individual is not around other people and is often alone.

Recap questions

1. Identify two physical effects of the perimenopause and menopause.
2. Outline one reason why verbal skills improve during middle adulthood.
3. Explain two impacts upon social development in middle adulthood.

Practice questions

1. Explain why an individual may begin to re-evaluate their priorities in middle adulthood. [2 marks]
2. Discuss the impact of menopause upon emotional development in middle adulthood. [4 marks]

A1.6 Late adulthood (70-84 years)

A decline of physical and intellectual functions begins in this life stage, that can intensify as an individual approaches later adulthood.

Physical

A number of physical functions begin to noticeably decline in this life stage:

Reduction of lung capacity. Physiological changes due to aging reduce the body's ability to take oxygen into the blood. The main reasons for this are:

- A loss of elasticity in the lungs, which makes it harder for them to expand and contract fully during breathing.
- A weakening of the respiratory muscles, used for breathing.

Thickening of the arteries and heart muscle. Artery walls become thicker and less elastic due to arteriosclerosis. This causes the arteries to become stiff and resist blood flow, leading to hypertension. As a result, the heart must work harder to pump blood around the body.

As well as the increased risks associated with

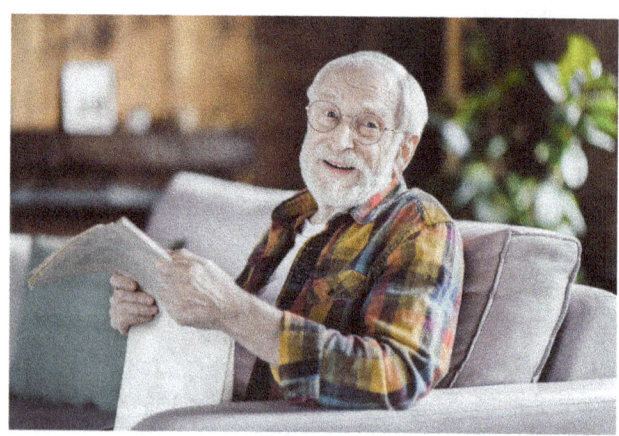

high blood pressure, such as a stroke or heart attack, the heart's additional workload causes the heart muscle to thicken. This reduces flexibility in the heart, reducing its ability to fill with blood during the relaxation phase (diastole). This means the heart becomes less functional.

Brain cells can also lose some function. In this life stage, neurons (nerve cells) can begin to die or shrink, or lose connections to each other. This can lead to reduced brain functions. For example, if brain cells in the hippocampus shrink, this can result in memory loss. However, this process is gradual and the brain can adapt to these changes, meaning that there is no noticeable change in brain function for lots of people.

Reduced mobility is caused by a continued decline in muscle mass along with weaker and stiffer joints. This increases the risk of **falls** which can lead to broken bones, cuts and bruising.

Intellectual

Intellect in late adulthood generally remains intact. People's ability to learn remains the same, however **the learning process may take longer** than before. This is due to slower processing speed, resulting in adults taking longer to absorb, interpret and respond to new information. This can also be impacted by a decline in hearing and vision.

An adult in this life stage may also experience a **decline in their short-term memory**, meaning they are **less able to recall** recent information. This is due to the loss of neurons (nerve cells in the brain) as we have already discussed.

However, despite this, late adults still retain wisdom and creativity.

- **Wisdom** means using knowledge and experience to make clear and sensible judgements. A late adult has lots of learning, work and life experiences to draw upon.
- **Creativity** is when someone uses their imagination to create something new, or apply their original ideas to a situation.

Emotional

Individuals in late adulthood can enter a state of **calm**. They may be more at peace with themselves and their lives, with feelings of contentment about their past and current circumstances. This often occurs during this life stage as individuals become more reflective and accepting of their lives. However, some people may begin to feel more anxious as they face their own mortality in the later years of their life.

Feelings of loneliness are quite common in this life stage, because they are more likely to experience bereavements of close family and friends. As well as causing grief, this also reduces their social network.

Later adults can also **feel younger than their age**. Individuals may be in denial about their

> Arteriosclerosis – A blockage in blood vessels due to a build-up of fat.
>
> Hypertension – The medical term for high blood pressure.
>
> Diastole – The phase where the heart relaxes and fills with blood.
>
> Mortality – The fact that none of us will live forever.

age and, if they are in good physical shape, they do not feel 'old'. However, other individuals may start to feel **frail** and more vulnerable. Daily tasks of life may begin to feel overwhelming.

Social

Almost everyone in this age group has now retired from working.

This provides benefits for some, as there are more **opportunities to meet friends** and to **meet new people when taking on new activities** or hobbies. Retirement often sparks new interests for individuals to take up, such as hiking and crafting.

However, more bereavements mean a **reduction in** their **social circle of peers**. This can lead to isolation and loneliness.

Recap questions

1. Outline one reason why there is an increased risk of cardiovascular disease in late adulthood.
2. Identify two types of intellectual development experienced in late adulthood.
3. Identify the correct age range for late adulthood.
4. Define the term 'wisdom'.
5. Explain two types of physical development experienced in late adulthood.

Practice questions

1. Describe one difference between the emotional development experienced in middle and late adulthood. [2 marks]
2. Explain why an individual's ability to learn new skills will take longer in late adulthood. [3 marks]

A1.7 Later adulthood (85+ years)

The final life stage an individual will experience is later adulthood. This will see a decline in many distinct functions

Physical

Organs

A gradual **reduction in organ function** is a natural part of this life stage. It is caused by changes to cells and tissues around the body. Examples of changes include:

- The **heart pumps less blood** around the body due to the thickening of the heart and artery walls.
- **Kidneys reduce their filtering efficiency**, meaning the ability to remove waste declines.
- **Lungs lose elasticity**, which means less oxygen enters the body during breathing.
- The **liver is less able to metabolise medication and toxins**.

Mobility

Mobility continues to decline due to a **loss of bone density**, known as osteoporosis. This leads to weak bones that can easily break. Women are particularly susceptible to osteoporosis:

- Oestrogen plays an important role in maintaining healthy bones in women
- During the menopause oestrogen levels decrease.
- The decline in oestrogen causes a decrease in bone density.

There are also factors that can also contribute to the onset of osteoporosis for all genders, such as:

- Reduced hormone levels (oestrogen and testosterone).
- Genetic inheritance.
- Long-term use of steroid tablets.
- Smoking and excessive alcohol use.
- Rheumatoid arthritis.
- Low physical activity for extended periods of time.

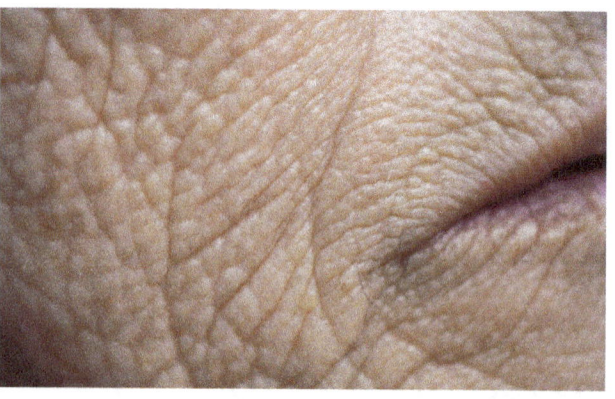

Ligaments and tendons

Ligaments connect bones to bones, and **tendons** connect bones to muscles. Ligaments and tendons **lose elasticity** as we age due to changes in the amount of elastin. The loss of elasticity means individuals are **less flexible** and are prone to **stiffness in their movements**.

The skin

The skin also undergoes changes:

- The thickest layer of skin, the **dermis**, loses collagen and elastin over time, which means the skin's strength and elasticity declines. This can be seen when individuals develop wrinkles.
- The **skin becomes thinner**.
- There is less fat in the body, providing padding underneath the skin. It also becomes drier as sebaceous glands produce less oil. This leads to the skin becoming more fragile, and more likely to tear.
- Other factors that can also contribute to the thinning of skin including exposure to UV rays without protection, menopause, and smoking.

Chronic health conditions

Individuals in later adulthood are **more prone to chronic and long-term health conditions**. The term 'chronic' refers to conditions that have a long duration and progress slowly, such as cardiovascular disease, and respiratory diseases.

- As individuals age, the body loses its ability to repair damaged tissues in organs. This leads to loss of organ function.
- People's immune system becomes less effective in old age. There are two aspects to this:
  * Low level inflammation increases. Inflammation contributes to many diseases.

* The immune response to pathogens is less effective, making it more likely that infections will take hold and damage organs. The immune system also becomes less effective at tackling cancerous cells.

Vision and hearing

Vision and hearing continue to deteriorate into later adulthood. The structures linked to vision and hearing are unable to repair themselves as easily as they could in early adulthood.

- Individuals can experience health conditions associated with sight such as glaucoma, a condition that is quite common in this life stage and can result in severe visual impairment or even blindness. This is due to a build-up of pressure around the eye's drainage pathway, causing it to become blocked.

- Hearing also deteriorates due to the stiffening of the eardrum, which means the amount of noise being transmitted to the middle ear is lessened.

Intellectual

There is the **potential for lapses in memory function** in later adulthood. This means people start to forget key information or some memories. This can be due to changes in brain structures and hormone levels.

- The hippocampus deteriorates as brain cells are lost. This part of the brain is responsible for forming and retrieving memories.

- The brain overall loses volume, which means slower processing and communication between different parts of the brain. All of this affects memory functions.

Conditions such as a **stroke** also cause **cognitive decline**. A stroke is caused when blood flow and oxygen to the brain has been disrupted, causing neurons (brain cells) to die in the affected areas. This can cause issues with memory, attention, problem-solving and language. The level of cognitive decline depends on which areas of the brain have been affected.

Dementia is a progressive disease that causes damage to neurons over time. It causes issues with the brain's ability to process, store and retrieve information and memories. The hippocampus is normally the first part of the

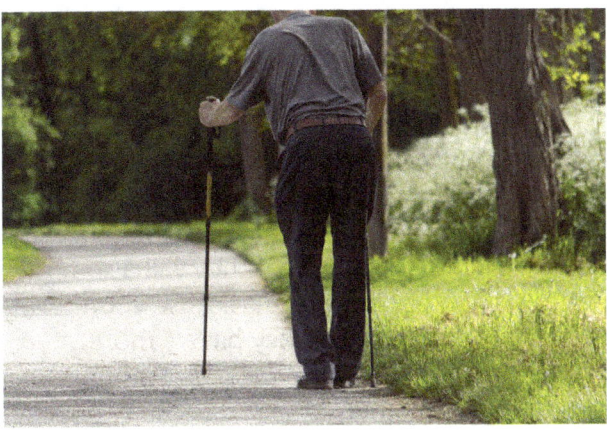

Osteoporosis – A disease that causes the bones to weaken due to a loss of bone density.

Elastin – A protein that helps keep skin and other tissues elastic and stretchy.

Glaucoma – A condition that causes damage to the optic nerve, caused by a build-up of pressure in the eye. It can lead to vision loss.

Recap questions

1. Describe why elasticity of the skin declines in later adulthood
2. Outline the cause of dementia.
3. Identify a physical health condition that can develop in later adulthood.

brain affected by dementia, leading to memory issues. It then branches into other areas of the brain responsible for language, attention and problem solving. Dementia is a progressive disease that gets worse over time and always results in severe cognitive decline.

Whilst many people experience cognitive decline in this age, there are exceptions known as **cognitive super-agers**. These people have maintained their cognitive abilities, including memory, attention and critical thinking skills, with no signs of a decline in performance. There are a wide range of reasons as to why this can occur, including:

- regular exercise
- balanced diet
- genetics
- good emotional regulation
- good brain structures.

Emotional

Emotional regulation is an individual's ability to cope and adapt to the emotions they feel. In this life stage an individual tends to have **improved emotional regulation** as individuals typically have had a great deal of experience in dealing with their emotions. They will also tend not to worry about things that cause younger people anxiety, because they have a more rounded perspective on what is truly important in life.

On the other hand, some individuals can experience **depression relating to loss**. There are different types of loss:

- **Loss of people** – In later, adulthood people experience bereavements of those closest to them, such as their peers or family members. Individuals may have to navigate new circumstances such as loneliness, isolation or a reduction in their ability to socialise
- **Loss of independence** – It can be very hard to come to terms with losing independence and having to rely on family, friends or carers.
- **Loss of skills** – It is hard for people not to be able to do the things they used, for example drive a car.

Depression can also be a side effect from medications for certain health conditions

As we age through later adulthood individuals become **more aware of their own mortality and frailty**. This means individuals become very aware of death and that their physical and intellectual state makes them more vulnerable. This can negatively impact upon an individual's self-esteem, as they become worried about their health and reduced capabilities.

Social

As individuals progress into later adulthood there is a **significant reduction in social activity**. This is because of reduced physical capabilities and reduced social circles due to loss.

- What a person can and cannot do influences the types of activities and socialising in which they can partake.
- If an individual has experienced significant loss of peers or family members, they may have fewer people left to socialise

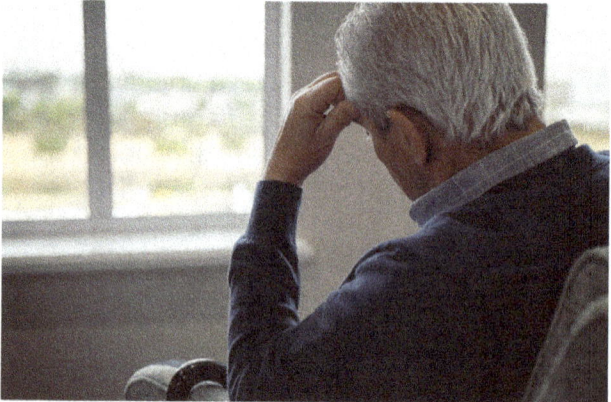

with, further decreasing their social opportunities.

Individuals may need **support to be able to meet friends and family outside of their home** because of their physical and intellectual condition. This includes practical help such as being driven to someone's house. This means that socialising becomes harder to organise and requires the consent of other people.

There are some theories about what happens to social development for the late adulthood stage:

- In 1961 Cummings and Henry proposed **disengagement theory**. This argues individuals in later adulthood voluntarily choose to disengage or step away from their social roles and socialising, to have a more relaxed lifestyle. Cummings and Henry argued that as individuals approach death, their ability and desire to engage decreases. By disengaging in social activities, they become freed from social norms and can behave as they want to. Ultimately, disengaging from others loosens the social ties that individuals have, making it easier to face death. It also allows family and friends to restructure and take over the active role that the individual used to play.

- In response to disengagement theory, Havighurst (1968) developed **activity theory** which contradicts disengagement theory. It states that older adults are at their happiest and most fulfilled when they participate in social interactions, and when their social role remains active throughout later adulthood. Havighurst believed an individual's social roles could be adapted for their lifestyle and circumstances, in order to meet their current physical and intellectual needs. For example, new roles during retirement, such as charity work, or taking up a new hobby, both of which can involve socialising with new people.

Find out more

www.eboru.com/BTEC-HSC-links

An infant's growth.

Osteoporosis.

Glaucoma.

Disengagement theory.

Activity theory.

Practice questions

1. Describe one difference between disengagement theory and activity theory. [2 marks]

2. Discuss the impact dependency on others can have upon an individual's overall development in later adulthood. [6 marks]

Recap questions

1. Describe the term cognitive super-agers.
2. Describe one difference between the intellectual development in late adulthood and later adulthood.
3. Identify two examples of emotional development in later adulthood.

End of Learning Aim Questions

Simone is a 37-year-old female who has recently taken a career break from her job as a marketing executive to focus on raising her two year old daughter Suki. Simone is currently struggling to maintain a balanced diet with her busy schedule and often finds herself feeling overwhelmed with the day-to-day care of her daughter.

1. Identify the life stages Simone and Suki are in. (2)
2. Give one example of social development Simone might be experiencing. (1)
3. Explain two types of physical development Suki may experience. (4)
4. Explain two types of emotional development Simone may experience. (4)
5. Explain two ways an unhealthy balanced diet could affect Simone's physical development. (4)
6. Identify the name of the factor that depends on people's own choices and behaviour. (1)

Learning Aim B: Factors affecting human growth and development across each life stage

In this section you will learn about a range of factors that can have both positive and negative effects upon an individual's growth and development across the life stages. You will need to understand each category of factor and the effects they can have upon physical, intellectual, emotional and social development.

B1 Genetic factors

There are three main genetic structures: DNA, genes and chromosomes.

- **DNA** (deoxyribonucleic acid) is a complex molecule. It contains all of the instructions that our body needs to carry out all of its functions over its entire life.

- **Genes** are made up of sections of DNA, that carry instructions on how to produce proteins. There are many different types of proteins but they are essential to the structure and function of every aspect of the body.

- **Chromosomes** are collections of genes packaged together in every cell in your body. Humans have 46 chromosomes which are organised into 23 pairs. One chromosome in each pair comes from the father and the other chromosome in each pair comes from the mother. When a cell divides all of the chromosomes are replicated in the new cell.

- Each set of chromosomes carries unique genes that make each person. For example, genes can determine hair colour, shoe size and height.

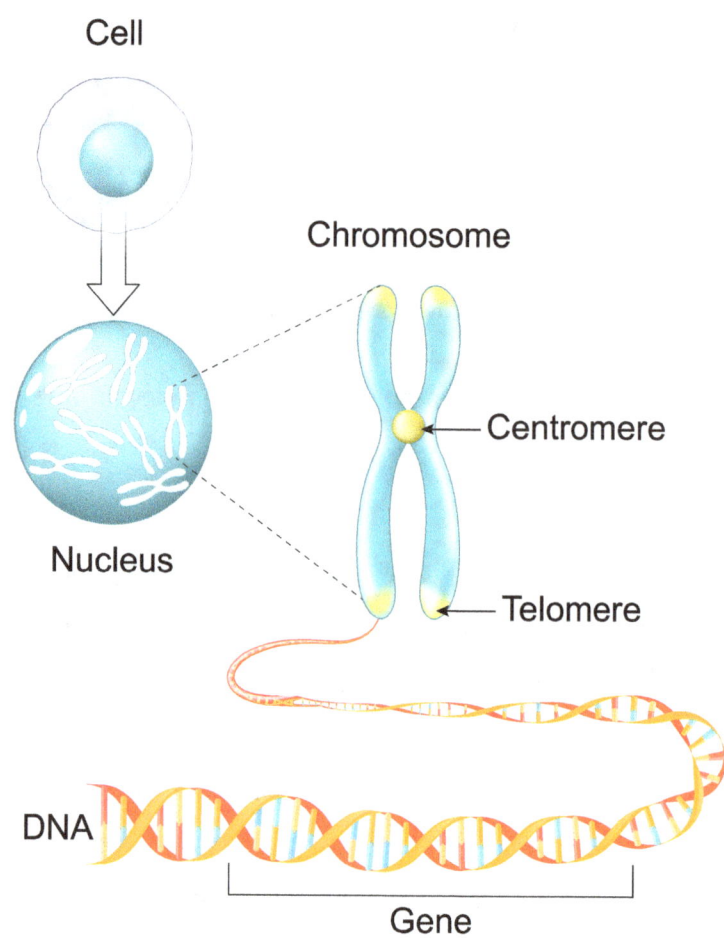

The structure of cells, chromosomes and DNA

B1.1 Genetic predisposition

A **genetic predisposition** is the likelihood that an individual will develop either a **health or ill health condition** from inheriting a condition from either or both biological parents.

- A genetic predisposition does not guarantee the development of a health condition

- There is nothing anyone can do about a genetic predisposition.

- There are many different types of conditions that hold a genetic predisposition, such as cancer, obesity, diabetes, mental illness and heart disease.

However, environment and lifestyle also influence whether individuals develop these conditions. Individuals can influence these factors through living a healthy life.

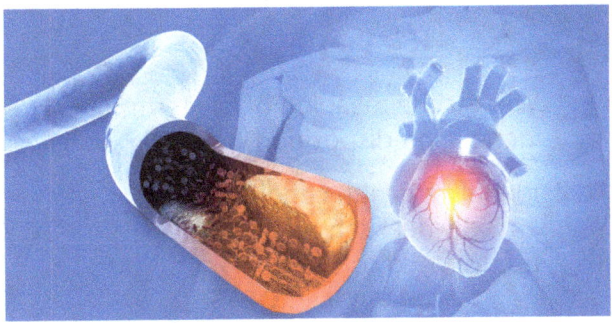

Fatty deposits in blood vessels

> Stroke – A life-threatening condition that happens when the blood supply to parts of the brain has been disrupted due to a blocked or burst artery.
>
> Heart attack – The body's response when one or more arteries becomes blocked due to a build-up of fatty deposits, narrowing the arteries and restricting blood flow.
>
> Tumours – An abnormal growth of tissue in certain parts of the body. Tumours can be benign (non-cancerous) or malignant (cancerous).

Cardiovascular disease

Cardiovascular disease or heart disease is a condition that affects the heart and blood vessels.

- It is caused by a build-up of fatty deposits in the arteries, narrowing the space and making it harder for blood to travel through.
- As blood struggles to flow around the body, the heart will try to pump blood harder, causing an increased heart rate and blood pressure.
- This then puts a strain on the cardiovascular system which can then lead to more serious health consequences such as a stroke or heart attack, both of which can have life-changing implications.

Some people have a genetic variation on chromosome 9p21, which means blood vessels are more susceptible to **inflammation**. Inflammation is a key contributor to the build-up of fatty deposits in arteries.

Breast and prostate cancer

Breast cancer can affect both males and females but is most common in females. It is a disease where abnormal breast cells grow to form tumours.

Causes of breast cancer are not clear but the following are risk factors:

- Genetic predisposition or family history.
- Age – people over 50 are at higher risk.
- Having had certain other breast conditions.
- Having higher levels of oestrogen, progesterone or testosterone. There are a number of reasons for this, including starting periods early, taking the contraceptive pill or having hormone

SYMPTOMS OF BREAST CANCER

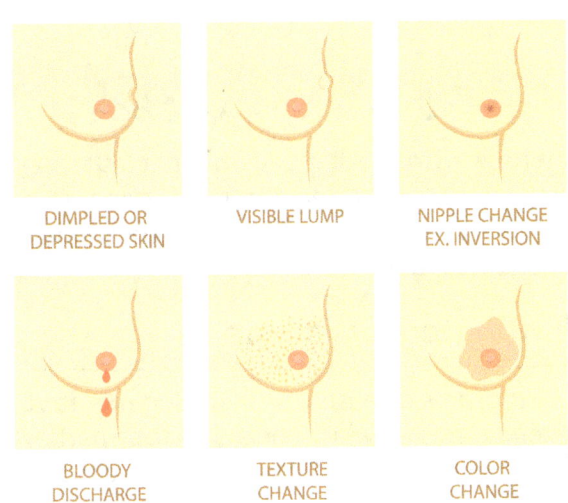

Symptoms of breast cancer

replacement therapy. However there is only a slight increase in risk.

Symptoms of breast cancer include:

- A lump or swelling in breast, chest or armpit.
- A change in the skin of the breast such as dimpling or redness.
- A change in size to breasts.
- Nipple discharge.
- Nipple appearance changes.
- Pain that does not go away in the breast or armpit.

Prostate cancer. The prostate is a small gland located just below the bladder in males. It makes up part of the male reproductive system. It can take many years for signs of prostate cancer to show. It is not usually noticed until the cancer causes the prostate to enlarge, affecting

Prostate Cancer

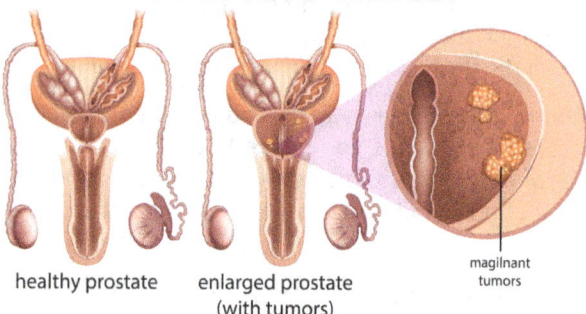

healthy prostate | enlarged prostate (with tumors) | magilnant tumors

the urethra. This then causes symptoms such as straining when urinating, an increased need to urinate and a feeling that the bladder is not fully emptied.

Recap questions

1. What is the meaning of the term 'genetic predisposition'?
2. Identify a health condition that an individual can be genetically predisposed to.

There can be a genetic basis for both breast and prostate cancer. People with mutations to the BRCA1 and BRCA2 genes are more likely to develop these cancers. Tests can now determine if people possess the BRCA1 or BRCA2 gene mutations. This allows for monitoring, early treatment and changes to be made to an individual's lifestyle or environment.

B1.2 Genetic disorders

A **genetic disorder** happens when a mutation occurs in genes. Having a mutated gene does not always mean an individual will develop a genetic disorder.

Huntington's Disease

Huntington's disease is a **neurodegenerative** genetic disorder, which means it stops parts of the brain from functioning adequately over time. It is inherited from a biological parent who has the condition. Each person has two copies of the HTT gene. If one of them is faulty then you will develop the condition.

- If one parent has the affected gene then the child has a 50% chance of inheriting a faulty gene and developing the condition.
- If both parents have the affected gene the child has a 75% chance of inheriting a faulty gene and developing the condition.

The symptoms for the condition typically begin between the ages of 30 and 50 but can happen at any age. Early symptoms can sometimes go unnoticed and can be mistaken for other health conditions, such as mood swings including irritability, and becoming fidgety. Other symptoms include:

- Lack of concentration and memory lapses.
- Issues swallowing, breathing and speaking.
- Mobility issues.
- Personality and mood changes.

There is currently no cure for the disease and

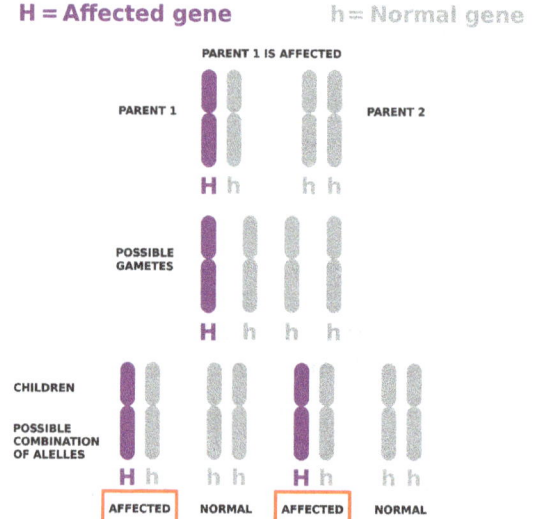

The chances of inheriting Huntington's disease if one parent has the affected gene

symptoms get slowly worse. Eventually it requires continuous management and support, such as:

- Medication for depression, medicine to control and reduce involuntary movements, and medicine to stabilise moods.
- Relevant professionals, such as occupational therapists to support adjustments in the home to encourage independent living, speech and language therapists to enable communication and a physiotherapist to help with movement issues.

In the later stages of Huntington's disease an individual's movement and cognitive abilities are affected considerably. An individual will need to rely on others for care and support. This can include full-time nursing care in a

F = Normal gene   f = Cystic fibrosis gene

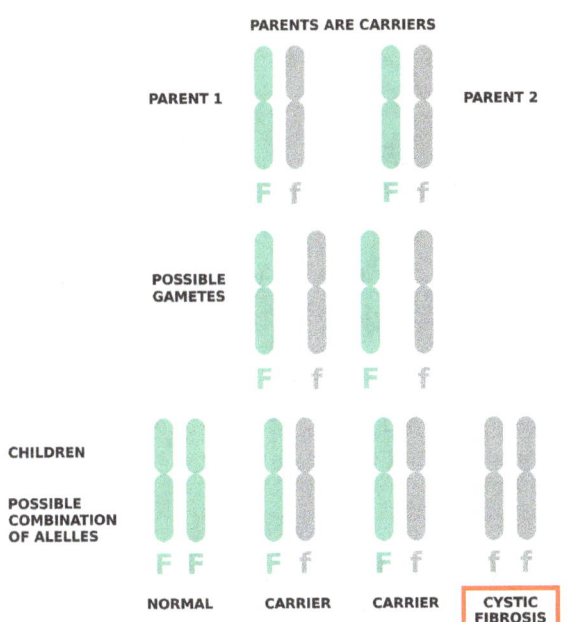

There is a 25% chance of developing CF if both parents have the affected gene

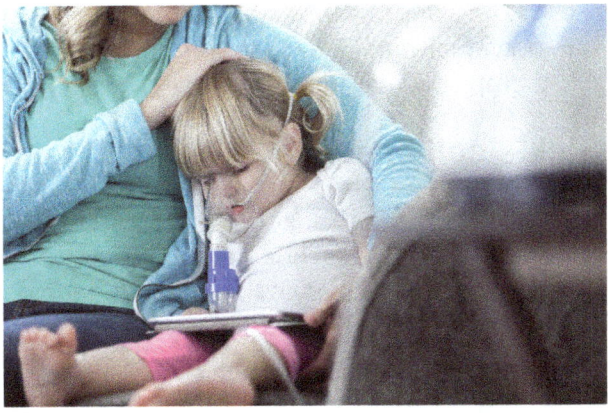

A child with CF receiving help to breathe

nursing home or in the home, with options for respite care.

Cystic fibrosis

Cystic fibrosis (CF) is a condition that is inherited due to a mutation in **both** copies of the CFTR gene. This is known as a recessive condition. Each copy is passed down from a different biological parent.

If a person only has one copy of the faulty gene then they cannot develop the condition but they can be a **carrier** of faulty gene, and pass it on to their children.

- If only one parent is a carrier there is 0% chance of their children developing the condition, but a 50% chance that each child becomes a carrier themselves.

- If both parents are carriers there is a 25% chance of each child developing the condition, and a 50% chance that each child becomes a carrier themselves.

This disorder is usually diagnosed in newborns using the **heel prick test**. Symptoms begin in early childhood and is a progressive disorder which will get worse over time.

The main symptom of CF is a thick sticky mucus in the lungs that causes breathing difficulties and an increased risk of lung infections. Other symptoms include:

- Recurring chest infections.

Urethra – A tube that passes through the prostate and into the penis, allowing urine to leave the bladder and semen to be released from the testes.

Occupational therapist – A professional that aims to improve an individual's daily abilities by supporting adaptations in the home or advising on new ways on how to complete certain tasks.

Speech and language therapist – A professional that conducts assessments and treats individuals with varying levels of communication needs.

Physiotherapist – A professional that aims to support individuals with mobility difficulties so that they can regain some level of independence in their movements.

Respite care – A place where individuals with illness or disability can go, to give their daily carer a break.

Recessive – A gene which someone needs two copies of before its effects are expressed.

Jaundice – A condition that causes yellowing of the skin, eyes and urine, caused by a build-up of bilirubin in the blood.

- Coughing or wheezing.
- Shortness of breath.
- Weight and growth issues.
- Jaundice.
- Constipation or diarrhoea.

Cystic fibrosis has no cure, only treatments to try and manage symptoms.

- Medication such as antibiotics and steroids help treat and prevent lung problems.

- Professionals will also advise regular exercise, to keep the lungs clear from mucus. Suitable exercises will differ from person to person and will need to be agreed with a physiotherapist.

- A range of professionals will support an individual with CF such as a respiratory therapist, dietician and pulmonologist.

Sickle cell anaemia

Just like CF, **sickle cell anaemia** is a recessive condition – one that is inherited due to a mutation in both copies of the affected gene. Each copy is passed down from a different biological parent. The mutated gene is called the **sickle cell gene**.

Just as with CF, if a person only has one copy of the sickle cell gene they cannot develop the condition, but they can be a **carrier** of the faulty gene, and pass it on to their children.

- If only one parent is a carrier of the sickle cell gene there is 0% chance of their children developing the condition, but a 50% chance that each child becomes a carrier themselves.
- If both parents are carriers of the sickle cell gene there is a 25% chance of their children developing the condition, but a 50% chance that each child becomes a carrier themselves.
- If one parent has the disorder, and the other is a carrier of the sickle cell gene, then there is a 50% chance of a child developing the condition, and a 50% chance that they become a carrier.

Red blood cells are responsible for carrying oxygen around the body by using the substance haemoglobin. Sickle cell anaemia is a disorder which affects haemoglobin, and results in unusually shaped red blood cells. The red blood cells can clump together and block blood vessels, and do not live as long as healthy red blood cells.

The blockages in vessels causes severe pain that can last for long periods of time (days or weeks). This commonly affects the limbs and back but can happen anywhere in the body.

Sickle cell anaemia is most common amongst individuals of African and Caribbean backgrounds as they are at an increased risk of mutations in the gene responsible.

Other symptoms include:

- Infections such as a cold or meningitis.
- Anaemia, which causes headaches, dizziness and fainting.

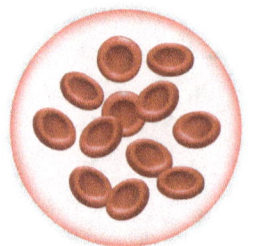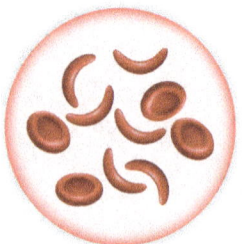

Normal blood cells (left) and affected blood cells of someone with sickle cell anaemia (right)

> Pulmonologist – A doctor that specialises in the diagnosis and treatment of lung diseases and disorders.

- Delayed growth and development including problems during puberty.
- Bone and joint pain.
- Leg ulcers.
- Blurred vision.
- Hypertension (high blood pressure).

This disorder will require ongoing treatment by a multi-disciplinary team that has the primary aim of preventing and reducing painful attacks. This can be done through medication and lifestyle advice such as drinking fluids to avoid dehydration, wearing warm clothes, avoiding quick temperature changes and dietary supplements such as folic acid to support the production of red blood cells.

Recap questions

1. Identify two physical symptoms of cystic fibrosis.
2. Identify a professional who can support an individual with Huntington's disease.
3. Describe how a genetic disorder is inherited.
4. Identify the correct term that means you are more likely to develop a disease due to your biological parents.
5. Identify two lifestyle factors that can influence the development of cardiovascular disease.
6. What is cystic fibrosis?

Find out more

www.eboru.com/BTEC-HSC-links

Gene variation.

Cardiovascular disease.

Genetic testing.

Breast cancer.

Huntington's disease.

Cystic Fibrosis.

Sickle Cell Anaemia.

Apply your understanding

Nikola is 54 years old. She has recently been diagnosed with breast cancer and has started having chemotherapy to treat it. Nikola's mum is also having treatment for breast cancer.

1. Identify the life stage Nikola is in.
2. Give the term that describes an increased likelihood of developing a disease because of genetics.
3. Identify two symptoms of breast cancer.

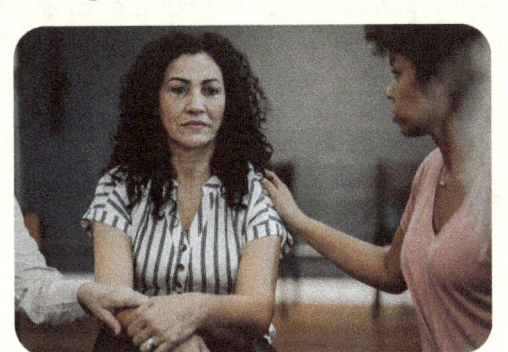

Practice questions

1. Explain the main features of the genetic disorder Huntington's disease, including how it is inherited. [4 marks]
2. Discuss the difference between a genetic disorder and being genetically predisposed to a condition. [3 marks]

B2 Lifestyle factors

A **lifestyle factor** is something an individual can choose to do, for example, eat a healthy balanced diet or brush their teeth. People's choices are influenced by income, culture and the people around them.

B2.1 Diet and weight management

A **healthy balanced diet** should follow the UK government's **Eatwell Guide**. The guide explains how to consume the right amounts and types of fats, carbohydrates, protein, vitamins and minerals. The guide recommends that healthy adult men consume 2500 kcal per day, and women 2000 kcal per day, to provide enough energy whilst maintaining a consistent and **healthy weight**.

The benefits of maintaining a healthy weight from a balanced diet are:

- Healthy skin, teeth and eyes.

- Strengthens bones and supports muscle development.
- Supports brain development.
- Maintains a strong immune system.
- Good digestive functions.
- Positive self-image/esteem.
- Good cognitive abilities.

Weight management

If someone consumes more than the recommended number of calories this can cause a calorie surplus. The excess calories are stored in the body as body fat, and lead towards weight gain and, in extreme cases, obesity.

Weight gain can lead to a number of issues, such as:

- Type 2 diabetes.
- Poor mobility or joint problems.
- Respiratory issues such as shortness of breath.
- Fatigue.
- Lethargy.
- Cardiovascular issues such as heart disease.
- Mental health issues such as depression.
- Low self-esteem and poor self-image.

An individual can also be in a calorie deficit which means they are not consuming enough calories, leading to weight loss. In extreme cases this can lead to, or be caused by, an eating disorder.

Under-eating can lead to malnutrition, which is a condition caused by a lack of key nutrients in the body. Weight loss and being underweight can lead to serious health risks and symptoms such as:

- Fatigue.
- Dizziness.
- Fainting.
- Anaemia.
- Infertility.
- Osteoporosis.
- Heart failure.
- Weakened immunity.

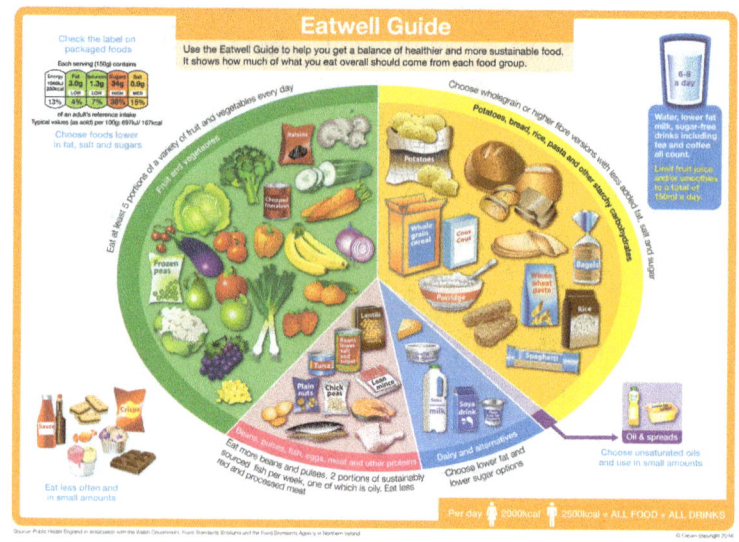

The Eatwell Guide

> **Recap questions**
>
> 1. Give two examples of lifestyle factors.
> 2. Identify one genetic factor.
> 3. Identify two physical effects of an unhealthy diet.

B2.2 Level of exercise

Exercise is a very important lifestyle factor for may different health conditions. It has many health benefits and also plays an important role in the management of weight.

Modern life means that many people do not exercise enough, because we don't move as much as we used to:

- Lots of people have jobs which involve sitting at a desk.
- Leisure activities, such as playing computer games or watching TV, also involve sitting down and staying still.
- More people drive cars or use public transport rather than walk or cycle.

All of these contribute to a sedentary lifestyle. Inactivity, such as sitting down and not moving for long periods of time, is actually very bad for our health.

The UK's Chief Medical Officer's Physical Activity Guidelines state that the average healthy adult should aim to

- Do at least 150 minutes of moderate physical activity, or 75 minutes of vigorous physical activity, every week.
- Be active every day.
- Do muscle-strengthening exercises at least twice per week.
- Minimise periods of inactivity and sitting down.

Following this advice reduces the risk of the following conditions:

- Type 2 diabetes.
- Hypertension.
- Cardiovascular disease.
- Certain types of cancers.
- Joint and back pain.

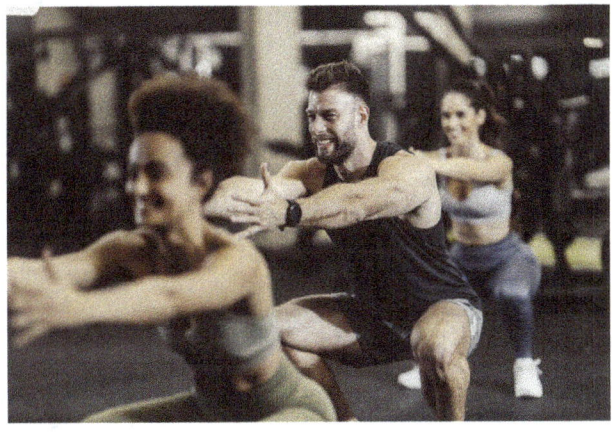

Exercise has many physical and mental health benefits

- Depression.
- Osteoporosis.

There are also other benefits:

- Better sleep.
- Reduced stress.
- Maintains a healthy weight.

B2.3 Alcohol and tobacco

The Department of Health recommends that:

- Adults should consume no more than 14 units of alcohol a week.
- People who drink as much as this should spread it out over three or more days.
- People should aim to have several drink-free days a week.
- People should never binge drink.

There are health risks for those who do not follow these guidelines. Higher levels of alcohol intake are associated with:

- Heart disease.
- Hypertension.
- Strokes.
- Liver disease.
- Various types of cancer, including the mouth, throat, breast and bowel.

Alcohol abuse can also cause temporary cognitive impairment leading to:

- Accidents and injuries.
- Violence.
- Taking excessive risks (such as drink driving or unprotected sex).

In addition, pregnant women should never drink alcohol. It can stunt physical development of the foetus, damage the foetus' brain, cause birth defects, and lead to foetal alcohol spectrum disorder. This causes life-long problems for the baby, including issues with learning, memory, movement and balance, emotions, speech and major organs.

Calorie surplus – When you consume over the recommended number of calories a day.

Obesity – The state of being overweight due to excessive fat around the body.

Calorie deficit – Consuming less than the recommended number of calories a day.

Malnutrition – A condition caused by not eating enough of the right nutrients causing issues such as fatigue and dizziness.

Osteoporosis – A disease that causes bone weakness, which means bones are more likely to break or fracture.

Sedentary lifestyle – A lifestyle with little to no exercise and that mostly involves a lot of inactivity and sitting.

Foetal alcohol spectrum disorder – A disorder that causes babies to be born with physical and intellectual disabilities, due to alcohol consumption during pregnancy.

Tobacco use is attributed to around 74,600 deaths in the UK per year. Tobacco can affect all the vital organs in the body but does poses a specific threat to the lungs. Most cases of lung cancer are due to smoking.

Lung cancer develops because carcinogens in cigarette smoke cause cells in the lung to mutate and become cancerous, leading to tumours.

Smoking is also responsible for other ill health conditions such as heart disease, strokes and emphysema.

Passive smoking is when people around smokers inhale second-hand smoke. This also increases the likelihood of developing health conditions such as cancer.

Smoking during pregnancy also poses dangers to the foetus. It can:

- Increase the chance of premature birth.
- Lead to a low birth weight, as the foetus does not receive enough oxygen and nutrients in the blood due to the presence of carbon monoxide and nicotine.

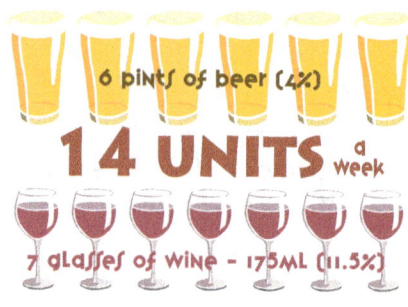

The UK government recommend that people drink fewer than 14 units of alcohol in a week

To prevent individuals from smoking, cigarette manufacturers must place health warnings on cigarette packaging.

> **Recap questions**
>
> 1. Identify two physical effects of smoking.
> 2. Identify an emotional effect of alcohol misuse.
> 3. Describe how exercise can impact social health and wellbeing.

B2.4 Quality of sleep

For adults an adequate amount of **sleep** is around 7-9 hours per night, but this can vary depending on a person's age. Sleep is essential for the following reasons:

- It restores the body's energy levels and repairs damage to cells.
- It helps maintain a positive mood during waking hours.
- It improves cognitive abilities.
- It can support cardiac health and reduces the risk of hypertension.

However, consistently poor sleep, due to lifestyle, sleep deprivation from disturbances or suffering from conditions such as insomnia can lead to:

- A weakened immune system, leaving the body more vulnerable to infections.
- Difficulty in concentrating, recalling information and making appropriate decisions.
- Irritability.
- Physical health problems such as type 2 diabetes, obesity and hypertension.

B2.5 Oral health

Oral health refers to how clean a person keeps their mouth through regular teeth and gum cleaning, to avoid disease or decay.

Good oral health means

- brushing their teeth twice daily
- flossing between teeth
- using mouthwash to remove bacteria and food.

Those who don't maintain good oral health are at risk of infections, pain, tooth decay and tooth loss, which can then have further negative impacts upon eating and speaking.

Some more serious conditions, such as gum disease, are linked to further health issues including heart disease and diabetes.

B2.6 Pregnancy

For a healthy **pregnancy** women must ensure they follow the advice and guidance of health care professionals, such as their GP and midwife. Foetal development is significantly impacted by factors including, **prenatal substance use** and **misuse** and **diet**.

- **Prenatal vitamins** are important for a healthy pregnancy. For example, **folic acid** is advised prior to conception up until 12 weeks of pregnancy. This supports early development of the foetus and helps prevent serious birth defects of the neural tube. Other supplements such as vitamin D, vitamin C, iron and calcium may also be recommended.
- **Tobacco**, **alcohol** and **drugs** pose serious health risks to an unborn baby. The dangers of smoking and alcohol for an unborn child have been discussed in the previous sections. Illegal drug use, such as cannabis, cocaine and ecstasy, can also contribute to premature birth, a low birth weight, developmental problems, and problems with feeding and breathing.

A healthy balanced diet is vital for supporting a healthy pregnancy and ensuring the growth and development of the foetus.

The recommended healthy diet for pregnancy is very similar to any adult. However there are a few differences.

- **Calcium and vitamin D**. Calcium is important for bone formation and vitamin D helps the body absorb calcium. Both are found in dairy products such as milk.
- **Iron**. Iron is important during pregnancy for its role in delivering oxygen in the blood to the foetus. Sources of iron include lean meat, beans and nuts.
- **Protein**. Pregnant women should eat more protein because it important for the growth of new tissue. Protein can be found in lean meat and fish, dairy, beans and pulses, seeds and nuts, and meat-alternatives such as tofu.

Food to avoid in pregnancy:

- Liver.
- All pâtés, including vegetarian versions.
- Game, such as goose or partridge.
- Cured meats (e.g. chorizo) and fish (e.g. smoked salmon). All meat should be thoroughly cooked.
- Raw fish should not be eaten.
- Two portions of fish are recommended each week, with at least one of them an oily fish. However, no more than two portions of oily fish should be eaten each week.
- Tuna does not count as on oily fish, but should also be limited to four cans in a week.
- Shark, swordfish and marlin.
- Raw or partially cooked eggs that do not have the British Lion mark.
- More than 200mg of caffeine. A cup of filter coffee has 140mg.
- Vitamin A supplements.

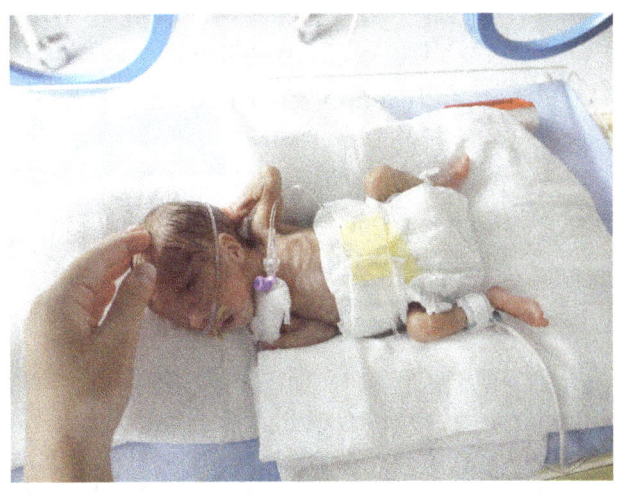

Carcinogens – Chemicals that cause cancer.

Insomnia – A condition that causes difficulty falling or staying asleep, often caused by anxiety, stress or some level of trauma.

Recap questions

1. Identify one negative effect of a sedentary lifestyle on growth and development.
2. Identify one lifestyle factor that can influence the risk of a premature birth.
3. Explain two ways that poor oral health can impact physical development.

> **Practice questions**
>
> 1. Discuss the importance of a healthy diet on pregnancy. [6 marks]
> 2. Explain how quality of sleep can influence the level of exercise a person does. [4 marks]

> **Find out more**
>
> www.eboru.com/BTEC-HSC-links
>
> The Eatwell Guide.

Apply your understanding

Benjamin is 19 years old and has recently joined his local gym. He goes to the gym five times a week to try to lose weight. Benjamin has also been working out at home. As a result of all this exercise he has not been getting enough sleep and his grades at college have started to slip.

1. Identify the category of factor 'quality of sleep' belongs to.
2. Outline one positive effect of exercise on Benjamin's health and wellbeing.
3. Explain two negative effects of Benjamin's quality of sleep on health and wellbeing.

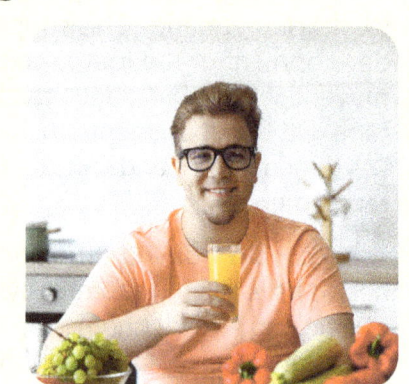

B3 Health Inequalities

B3.1 Current NHS definition of health inequalities.

The NHS describes **health inequalities** as:

'Unfair and avoidable differences in health across the population, and between different groups within society.'

They recognise that certain demographic groups can be treated differently to others. This leads to widespread differences in services and health outcomes, depending on the groups you belong to.

(Students should note that this definition can be updated and should check the NHS website for the current definition.)

B3.2 Health inequality examples

Difference in life expectancy across different socioeconomic groups

Life expectancy refers to the average number of years a group of people are expected to live for, on average. For example, in 2022 the life expectancy for:

- Males in the UK was 78.6 years
- Females in the UK was 82.6 years.

However, this differs depending on the area of the UK a person lives in. Those who live in more deprived areas live shorter lives than those in more affluent areas.

These differences are driven by limited resources and limited access to health care services in deprived areas. When access is to services depend on where you live, this is known as a postcode lottery.

Deprived areas are more likely to experience more significant health conditions at a higher rate, contributing towards an overall lower life expectancy. For example, according to Office for National Statistics data, in 2021-2023:

- The local areas with the ten highest life expectancies in the UK were in the south of England.
- The local areas with the ten lowest life expectancies in the UK were in Scotland, the north of England and Wales.
- Male life expectancy in the south east of England was 3.0 years higher than in the north east of England.

These top-level figures are averages that hide some other details – for example, there are parts of Scotland, the north of England and Wales where life expectancy is higher than some parts of London and the south of England. However, in general, there is a geographical divide.

The reasons for these differences include levels of deprivation and levels of education, and how these both influence lifestyle factors.

Mental health prevalence

There are differences in the prevalence of mental health problems according to socioeconomic group, gender, race, and ethnic background.

- **Socioeconomic groups.** There are significantly higher rates of mental health issues amongst individuals from **deprived areas of the UK**. These develop due to factors such as financial strain, unemployment, poor housing and lack of access to services.
- **Gender.** There are disparities between mental health support for males and females. Females are more likely to experience issues such as depression and anxiety but are more likely to seek support compared to males. This means there is then a high proportion of mental health issues amongst males that go unreported and undiagnosed, contributing to the high suicide rates amongst males. According to government statistics, men in the UK are three times more likely to commit suicide than women.
- People in different **racial and ethnic groups** also experience inequalities in mental health care and support:
- According to Mind, almost one in three people from racialised communities reported that they had experienced stigma and/or discrimination from a healthcare professional when getting support for their mental health.

> Demographic groups – Individuals that are grouped based on a characteristic such as age, race, gender, religion and income.
>
> Postcode lottery – Describes the inequalities in the provision of health care services based upon location.

- Black people were 3.5 times more likely to detained under the Mental Health Act in 2022-2023, according to government statistics.
- 23% of Black or Black British people experience a mental health condition compared to 17% of white British people, according to research by NHS Digital in 2016 'Mental health and wellbeing in England: Adult psychiatric morbidity survey 2014.')

Access to health services

Health inequalities can develop because **access to health services** are not equal, leading to **different experiences in healthcare** for different groups of people.

Learning disabilities

- Individuals with **learning disabilities** have worse physical and mental health than those without a learning disability.
- The 2022 Learning Disabilities Mortality Review found that women with a learning disability die on average 23 years earlier than women without a learning disability. For men, the figure was 19 years. Many of these deaths would have been avoidable through 'good quality healthcare'.

The barriers to accessing appropriate health services that people with learning disabilities face include:

- A lack of accessible transport.
- Lack of understanding from healthcare professionals about learning disabilities.
- A failure of professionals to recognise when someone has a learning disability.
- Not being given the right diagnosis.
- Inadequate follow-up care.

Gender

Gender refers to a person's identity as female, male, non-binary or transgender. Access to health services can depend on gender and are not always equal.

- Research into treatment and medicine has traditionally focused on men with little consideration of how they might translate to women. This means that diagnosis and treatment of some conditions may not have been suitable for women. For example, it has recently been discovered that women respond differently to treatments for cardiovascular disease than men.
- Women's symptoms are more likely to be dismissed, increasing the number of misdiagnoses and leading to poorer health outcomes.
- There has been less research and interest in conditions that affect only women. For example, **endometriosis** is a common gynaecological condition which has a severe impact, but which takes a long time to receive a correct diagnosis for.
- Transgender and non-binary individuals may find that services are not fully equipped to understand or meet their needs.
- Men may be less likely to seek support for mental health problems.

Discrimination

Discrimination is defined as treating an individual or groups of individuals differently or unfairly because of a certain characteristic, such as gender, sexual orientation, pregnancy or disability. There are nine characteristics that are

> Discrimination – Treating a person or group of people unfairly because of a particular characteristic they possess, such as gender, sexual orientation and pregnancy.

protected under the Equality Act 2010, making such discrimination illegal.

However, despite this, discrimination and stigma still occur, and significantly affect an individual's access to services.

- According to the report 'Patient Experience and Trust in Primary Care', published by the NHS Race & Health Observatory, over half of Black, Asian and ethnic minority patients have experienced discrimination by a healthcare professional.
- A 2018 British Medical Association survey reported that 45% of Black, Asian and minority ethnic doctors reported they didn't feel there was a respect for diversity, or a culture of inclusion, where they worked.

Discrimination leads to **lower levels of trust** in health and social care services and **lower rates of access to services**. This leads to health inequalities.

Recap questions

1. Identify two examples of health inequalities.
2. Describe one reason for health inequalities occurring.

B3.3 Environmental inequalities

Environmental inequalities accumulate due to things like pollution or poor-quality housing. The fundamental reasons for these inequalities are often socioeconomic or geographical factors.

- For example, those who live in poverty are more likely to live in areas with high **exposure to** air **pollution**. Exposure to air pollution increases the risk of developing health conditions such as respiratory diseases (including asthma), cardiovascular disease and cancer.
- **Unsafe housing conditions** includes overcrowding, damp or mould, and exposure to cold or noise. This can lead to a range of physical and mental health conditions, such as respiratory diseases, cardiovascular, the spread of infections, anxiety and depression.

Asthma

Asthma is a chronic respiratory condition that affects one in five households in the UK. It can result from poor environmental conditions. Air pollution, mould, dust and pet hair can all increase the risk of developing asthma.

Asthma occurs when inflammation and narrowing of the airways begin to make it difficult to breathe. Key findings from the organisation Asthma + Lung UK found that asthma rates are more prevalent in more deprived areas with individuals from disadvantaged backgrounds.

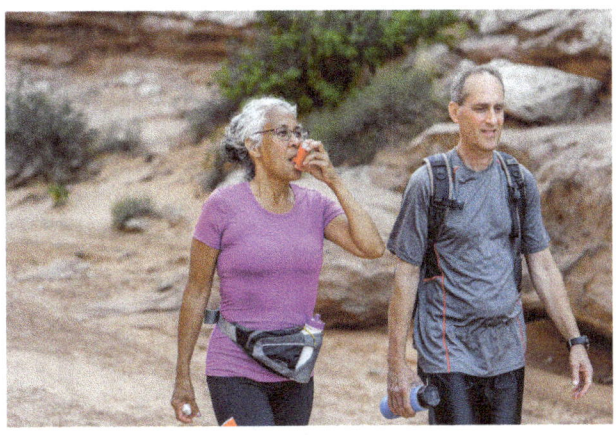

Asthma sufferers often require inhalers to help them breathe

Asthma

Tuberculosis

Tuberculosis (TB) is an infectious disease that is easily spread. It affects the lungs but can also impact other areas of the body. TB is commonly spread through coughs and sneezes and is easily transmitted in poor housing conditions that are unclean or overcrowded. TB rates in the UK remain low but are the highest in large urban areas such as London.

B3.4 Economic inequalities

A person's **level of income** and **employment status** has a big impact on health inequalities. These economic factors influence an individual's access to resources, living conditions and overall health and wellbeing.

For example, a low income or unemployment can mean that:

- People cannot afford fresh food in order to maintain a healthy balanced diet.
- It is hard to get to health care appointments. This is because travel may be expensive, or inconvenient if people do not own a car.
- People are less likely to be able to miss work to attend appointments. Lower-paid work is also likely to be more insecure, more physically demanding and more hazardous.
- People are more likely to live in poorer-quality houses, in more polluted areas.
- People can't afford some costs associated with health. Whilst the NHS is free at the point of contact, there are still costs for prescriptions, dental services and eye care.

Those with poorer economic factors are more susceptible to ill health conditions such as obesity, type 2 diabetes and asthma. Cancer UK's 2025 report 'Cancer in the UK 2025: Socioeconomic Deprivation' states that death rates from cancer are 60% higher for people living in deprived areas.

B3.5 Occupational related health inequalities

Health inequalities that result from the jobs that people have.

These inequalities can be because of the nature of the work, the workplace conditions and a lack of access to adequate health protection.

Inequalities due to occupation are themselves often due to other inequalities. The type of job an individual can access is influenced by their socio-economic status, their level of education and the availability of different types of jobs where they live. For example, individuals in more deprived areas are more likely to work in lower-paid jobs that are more physically demanding, with more hazardous working conditions.

Health inequalities due to occupation can result in the following conditions.

Musculoskeletal problems can result from manual work, such as construction, warehousing and delivery, and care. This can include conditions such as joint pain, tendonitis or chronic back pain.

People who use a computer and mouse can suffer from carpal tunnel syndrome due to the repetitive strain on the wrist.

COPD (chronic obstructive pulmonary disorder) is the general name for a range of conditions that lead to persistent respiratory problems. Symptoms include shortness of breath and a cough. COPD can develop due to exposure to harmful chemicals, dust or smoke. These risks are present in some occupations and may cause the condition if appropriate protective equipment, such as face masks, are not used.

Stress and anxiety can result from jobs and working conditions. They are often associated with:

- jobs where the employee has little control over their work
- jobs that are insecure, such as zero-hours contract work
- jobs that demand long and inflexible working hours.

People in better-paid jobs, including very senior people, can also suffer from stress and anxiety.

Shift work involves working hours outside of the traditional 9-5. This includes working evenings, nights or having to rotate schedules between night and day every week or so. It is often the standard way of working for those in healthcare, emergency services and transportation.

- Our natural body clock is known as our **circadian rhythm**. This tells our body to wake up during daylight and to go sleep at night. Shift work interferes with it, leading to sleep deprivation. This leads to a range of health conditions.
- Shift work can put a strain on personal relationships and limit social opportunities or leisure activities, causing isolation. This can lead to **anxiety** and depression.
- Jobs that require shift work are typically very demanding, which can also cause stress.

Overall, shift work leads to an increased risk of cardiovascular disease, type 2 diabetes, anxiety and depression. The International Agency for Research on Cancer classified night shift work as 'probably carcinogenic'.

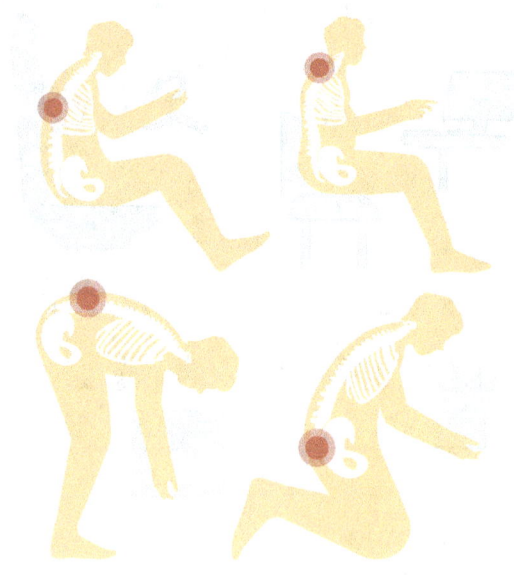

Different causes of back pain

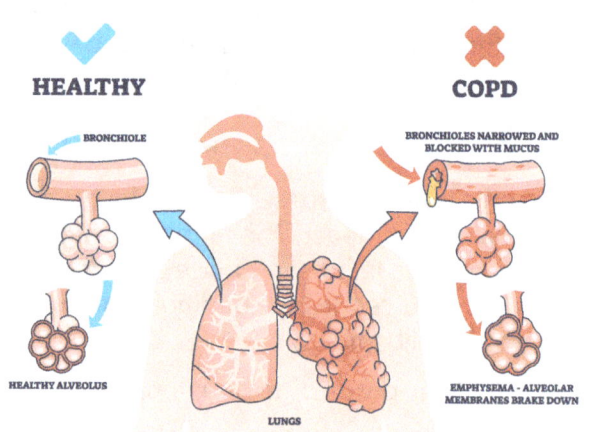

The effect of COPD on the lungs

Tendonitis – A condition that causes inflammation in the tendons due to repetitive trauma or stress on the joint.

Carpal tunnel syndrome – A condition that causes feelings of numbness, tingling and pain in the hand and forearm due to pressure being placed on a nerve in the wrist.

Recap questions

1. Identify an environmental factor that contributes to health inequalities.
2. Describe the NHS's current definition of health inequalities.
3. Explain how discrimination can cause health inequalities.

Practice questions

1. Discuss how services could be improved to close the health inequality gap. [4 marks]
2. Compare the differences in health inequalities based on demography. [4 marks]

Find out more

www.eboru.com/BTEC-HSC-links

Health inequalities.

Differences in life expectancy.

Find out more about mental health inequalities.

Find out more about the Patient Experience and Trust in Primary Care report, published by the NHS Race & Health Observatory.

Barriers that people with learning disabilities face.

NHS Digital in 2016 'Mental health and wellbeing in England: Adult psychiatric morbidity survey 2014.

Find out more about asthma rates.

Find out more about TB rates.

Cancer UK's 2025 report 'Cancer in the UK 2025: Socioeconomic deprivation'.

End of Learning Aim Questions

Oscar is 45 years old and works as a builder. He has been having regular health checks at work with a nurse. In the health check Oscar has been complaining of back pain. The work environment is very positive and management are supportive of employees receiving the right level of health care to support their workload.

1. Identify the life stage Oscar is currently in. (1)
2. State the branch of nursing concerned with assessing health in the workplace. (1)
3. Outline one way a healthcare professional could support Oscar. (2)
4. Describe the health condition Oscar is experiencing. (2)
5. Explain how this health condition will affect Oscar's health and wellbeing. (4)
6. Identify one environmental factor that Oscar may be exposed to on the building site. (1)
7. Explain two negative effects that working on a building site could have on Oscar's health and wellbeing. (4)

Learning Aim C: Health and social care promotion, prevention and treatment at different life stages

In this section you will learn about a range of health conditions that are common in each life stage. You will learn how these conditions can be prevented and the professionals that support individuals with these conditions. You will need to understand how these professionals can work together as part of a multi-disciplinary team.

C1 Prevalent health conditions

Each life stage is witness to certain health conditions. You need an understanding of these conditions and the life stages in which they typically occur.

C1.1 Infancy and early childhood

A newborn relies upon the immunity gained from their mother but, over time, this immunity reduces and the baby's own immune system develops. While their immune system matures, they are more susceptible to infections. In early childhood children are exposed to new pathogens all the time, due to interactions with other children, adults and new environments. These pathogens can lead to common illnesses such as **flu**, **chicken pox**, **ear infections**, **meningitis** and **conjunctivitis.**

As well as infections, children in early childhood can also experience **speech development problems** and **tooth decay.**

Flu

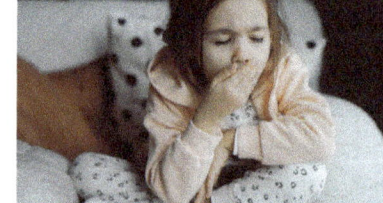

Age most prevalent: Children under the age of five.

Description of condition: An infection caused by a virus. It causes symptoms such as a high temperature, tiredness, dry cough, runny nose and ear pain.

Chicken pox (varicella)

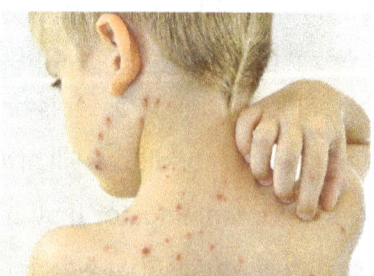

Age most prevalent: Children under the age of 10.

Description of condition: A viral infection that spreads through contact with another infected person. Commonly associated with red spots or blisters all over the body.

Ear infections

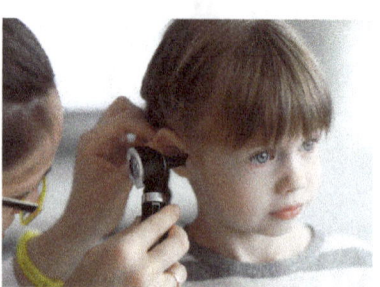

Age most prevalent: Common in children aged six months to three years.

Description of condition: Caused by bacteria or a virus in the middle ear, often linked to other illnesses such as a cold or flu. Symptoms include pain inside the ear, sickness, high temperature, low energy levels and difficulty hearing.

Meningitis

Age most prevalent: Infants and children under the age of 5.

It is important to note that meningitis can affect adolescents and young adults as well.

Description of condition: An inflammation of the protective membrane around the brain and spinal cord, caused by a viral or bacterial infection. Bacterial meningitis is rarer but even more serious.

Symptoms include a high temperature and fever, headaches, nausea and vomiting, a stiff neck, seizures, and a rash that will not go away when a glass is rolled over it.

Meningitis can become very serious and result in death. Suspected cases should be treated as an emergency.

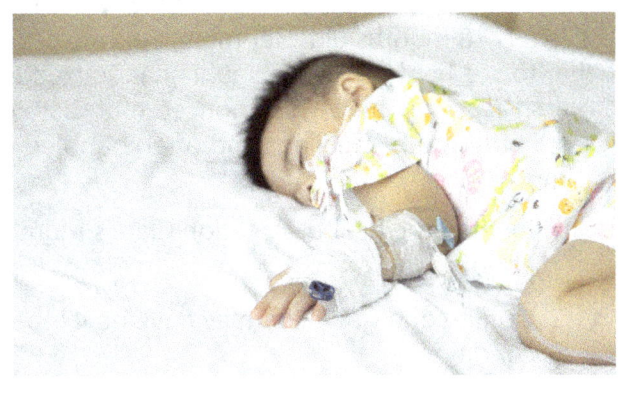

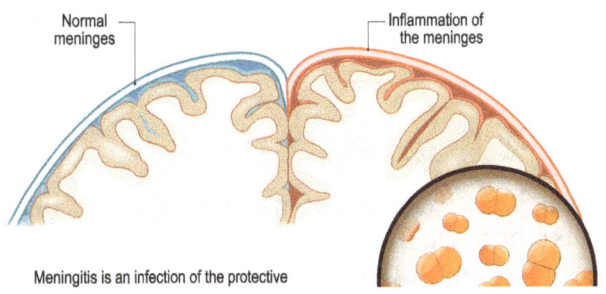

Meningitis is an infection of the protective

Conjunctivitis

Age most prevalent: Any age.

Description of condition: A highly contagious condition linked to secretions from the eye or eyes. It can make the eyes red, burn, produce pus and itch.

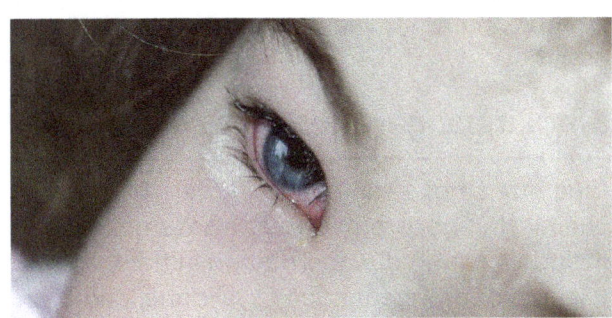

Speech development problems

Age most prevalent: Typically identified around the age of 12 months, if a child is not yet communicating.

Description of condition: Develop for a variety of reasons including a hearing impairment and conditions such as autism and ADHD.

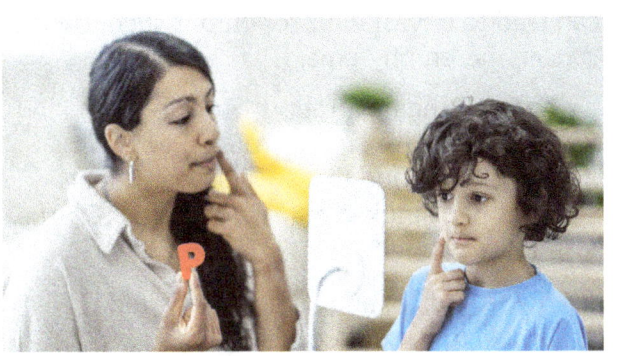

Tooth cavities and decay

Age most prevalent: Can happen at any age but cavities are more common in children.

Description of condition: A cavity is a small hole or area of decay in tooth enamel. The enamel is damaged due to plaque build-up through poor oral hygiene or by eating too many sugary foods and drinks.

A cavity leads to tooth pain, sensitivity and spots on the teeth.

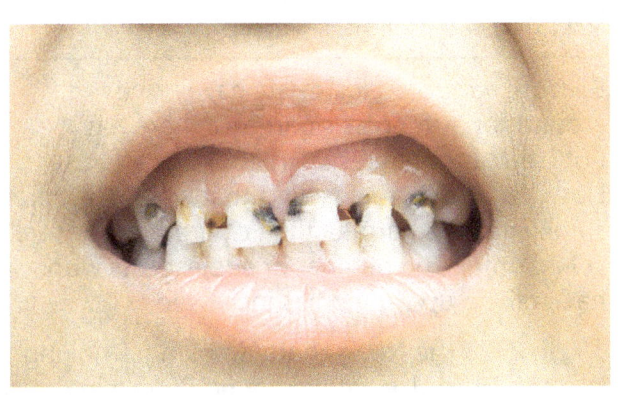

Apply your understanding

Clara is 18 months old. Her mum, Sophia, has recently taken her to see her local GP as Sophia has started to develop spots and itchy skin. The GP also noticed that Clara was unable to communicate her feelings and often babbled instead of saying simple words.

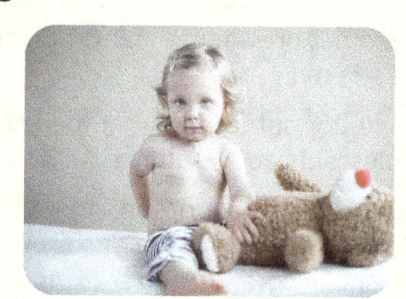

1. Identify the health condition Clara's mum is concerned about.
2. Outline one way Clara may have developed this health condition.
3. Explain which health condition the GP is concerned about.

C1.2 Adolescence

Adolescence can lead to riskier lifestyle choices, often because they are more heavily influenced by peers and social media. However, the following lifestyle choices can lead to serious health conditions, and habits that last well into adulthood.

Smoking cigarettes

Cigarette smoke contains many very harmful chemicals. Short-term effects from smoking include a cough due to irritation in the throat, a rise in blood pressure due to nicotine, and bad breath. Smoking over a longer period of time can lead to devastating conditions such as lung cancer and emphysema.

- In 2023 the NHS report 'Smoking, Drinking and Drug Use among Young People in England, found that 11% of 11-15 year olds had smoked at least once. In 1996 the figure was 49%.
- Two-thirds of adult smokers started smoking in adolescence.

Vaping

Because vapes (e-cigarettes) have not been around for as long as cigarettes, there has not been as much research about its effects. However, the current view is that whilst they are somewhat less harmful than cigarettes, they are still harmful. The number of adolescents who have taking up vaping has increased.

- In 2023 the NHS report 'Smoking, Drinking and Drug Use among Young People in England, found that around 25% of 11-15 year olds had tried vaping. It is illegal to sell vapes containing nicotine to under-18s. The extent of the long-term effects of vaping is still being assessed.

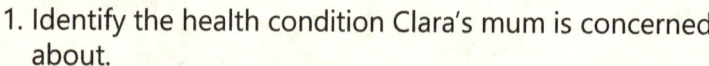

The percentage of 11-15 year olds reporting by year if they had ever taken drugs (Source: NHS, 2023)

Recreational drugs

Drugs such as cannabis, ecstasy and cocaine pose a number of short-term and long-term health risks. There are particular health risks for adolescents as the brain continues to develop in this life stage.

- In 2023, the NHS report 'Smoking, Drinking and Drug Use among Young People in England, 13% of 11-15 year olds reported that they had taken drugs at least once. This trend is shown in the chart above.

Alcohol

Alcohol has many longer-term health consequences. Specifically for adolescents, there is evidence that drinking alcohol can result in physical or mental health conditions and affect brain development. There is also a greater risk of injury and accidents caused by alcohol. Alcohol can also interfere with school, causing people to fall behind, which can have consequences for the rest of people's lives. There is also a greater risk of violence and unsafe sexual behaviour.

- In the 2023 NHS report, 37% of 11-15 year olds said they had tried alcohol at least once.
- This was down from 44% in 2016.

Sexual health

Sexual health is driven by hormonal changes during puberty that lead to sexual curiosity. This can also be fuelled by social pressures from peers and social media. This can cause some adolescents to carry out sexual activities without the adequate knowledge or access to sexual health advice, leading to an increase in sexually transmitted infections (STIs) or an unplanned pregnancy.

- The WHO 'Health Behaviour in School-aged Children' international report from the 2021/2022 survey found that 21% of girls and 18% of boys in England had sexual intercourse by the age of 15.

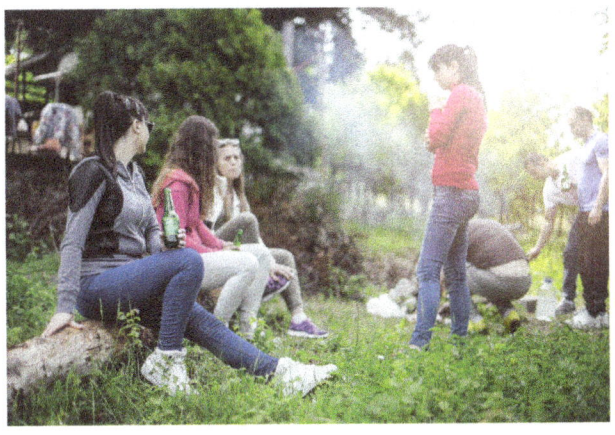

- The same report found that, of those 15 year olds who had sex, 48% of the girls and 61% of the boys had used a condom the last time they had sex. Which means a significant number of them did not.

Recap questions

1. State the age range of adolescence.
2. Explain how lifestyle choices in adolescence can be negative upon health and wellbeing.
3. Give an example of two health conditions prevalent in early childhood.

C1.3 Early and middle adulthood (19-69)

Mental health

Mental health issues are prevalent in early and middle adulthood due to the pressures of daily life. For example, individuals may have additional responsibilities at work or home including childcare that can contribute to issues such as **stress**, **depression** and **anxiety**. Each of these health issues can lead to symptoms such as:

- Increased heart rate.
- Headaches.
- Fatigue.
- Lethargy.
- Difficulty concentrating or making decisions.
- Irritability.
- Panic attacks.

Accidents

Individuals in these life stages have the freedom to make their own decisions and lifestyle choices. This can result in accidents due to risk-taking behaviour. For example, taking part in extreme sports, reckless driving, experimenting with drugs or alcohol, and ignoring safety regulations. This increases the likelihood of individuals **acquiring brain injuries** and life-changing injuries such as the loss of limbs.

- For example, government statistics show that car drivers aged 17-24 are proportionally involved in far more serious road accidents (where someone is killed or seriously injured) than any other age group, apart from people aged 86 and over.

Inactivity

Individuals are also more likely to become less active as they move through this life stage. This means they spend less time exercising and more time sitting down, particularly if they have a sedentary job. This poses a serious risk to health and can contribute to health issues such as:

- Obesity.
- Cardiovascular disease.
- Type 2 diabetes.
- Depression and anxiety.

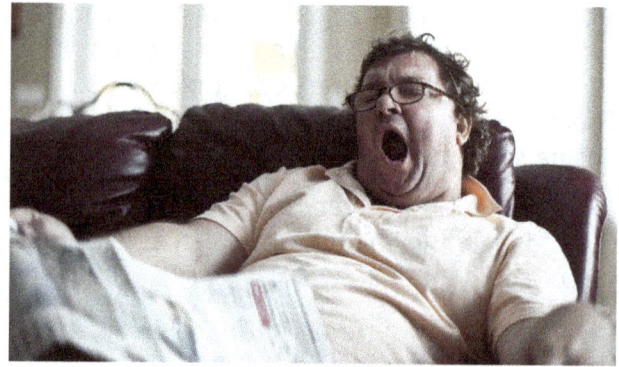

C1.4 Late and later (old age) adulthood (70+ years)

As we age the risk of developing health conditions such as **dementia, heart disease and oral health** conditions also increases.

This table describes some health conditions associated with late and later adulthood.

Health condition	Description	Causes
Dementia	A degenerative condition of the brain which causes symptoms such as amnesia, decreased thinking speed, difficulty speaking and mood swings.	There are different types of dementia. The most common cause is the build-up of proteins in the brain which causes nerve cells to stop functioning properly and eventually die.
Heart disease	A condition that affects the heart, blood vessels and arteries. Common symptoms of heart disease include, angina, breathlessness, fainting, nausea and pain the neck, shoulders, jaw or arms.	The heart's blood supply is blocked or disrupted by fatty deposits in the coronary arteries known as atherosclerosis.
Oral health conditions	Natural ageing can lead to natural wear and tear of teeth and gums. This can increase the chance of infections, inflammation, tooth loss and dentures. All of which can also contribute to conditions such as heart disease.	This is a natural part of ageing but dental treatment can help prolong tooth health. Medications can also cause a dry mouth which reduces saliva that is essential for protecting teeth and gums. Some individuals may find oral health difficult to manage because of other health conditions.

As individuals age the risk of **injury from falls** also increases, due to a loss of muscle mass and strength, balance and co-ordination issues, and slower reaction times.

- Falls are even more dangerous if an individual has a condition such as osteoporosis that causes weakened bones and joints. This makes an individual more susceptible to breaks or fractures.
- The environment a person lives in can also increase the risk and severity of falls, for example slippery surfaces or poor lighting.

A fall poses some extreme health risks including hip fractures, head traumas and cuts that have an increased risk of infection if not treated.

- A hip fracture is a very serious injury for an older person. The National Hip Fracture Database 2024 Report states that 6% of people die in the UK within 30 days of a hip fracture. Various sources suggest that 20-30% die within a year. This is because of the risks of infections after surgery and conditions associated with lack of mobility, such as blood clots.

A **weakened immune system** is a natural part of ageing. This is known as immunosenescence, where there is a gradual decline in immune function as the body's T-cells decline in numbers. This makes it harder for the body to fight infections, increasing the risk of illness and infection. Contracting infections in this life stage can lead to further, secondary infections or conditions such as pneumonia.

C1.5 Obesity

Obesity can develop in any life stage for a variety of reasons: a genetic, inherited reason, lifestyle choices or metabolic factors. Obesity develops because excess fat is stored in the body. Obesity leads to a number of symptoms and increased risk of a number of conditions:

- Shortness of breath
- Fatigue
- Poor mobility and joint pain
- Type 2 diabetes
- Cardiovascular disease
- Hypertension
- Osteoarthritis
- Cancer.

Older adults are at increasing risk of heart disease

Degenerative – The progressive deterioration or loss of function of a particular organ or group of organs.

Amnesia – The inability to recall information either partially or fully.

Angina – Chest pain that occurs when the heart is not getting enough oxygenated blood.

Atherosclerosis – Build-up of fatty deposits in the artery walls that causes narrowed arteries meaning blood flow is restricted to the heart.

Immunosenescence – Gradual deterioration of the immune system that is part of the ageing process.

Find out more

www.eboru.com/BTEC-HSC-links

NHS report 'Smoking, Drinking and Drug Use among Young People in England' (2023).

The WHO report Health Behaviour in School-aged Children international report (2021/2022).

Government car driving casualties statistics

Find out more here about dementia.

Find out more here about heart disease:

National Hip Fracture Database Report 2024

Recap questions

1. Identify the life stage that is particularly susceptible to ear infections.
2. Describe the health condition dementia.
3. Explain which health conditions are more likely to develop in adolescence.

Practice questions

1. Discuss reasons why individuals in early adulthood are more likely to experience health issues linked to taking risks. [4 marks]
2. Explain why obesity can happen in any life stage. [3 marks]

C2 Health and social care promotion and prevention

You will explore ways to promote and prevent certain health issues.

C2.1 Vaccinations

Vaccines are a type of medicine that encourages the body's immune system to create antibodies to protect against a particular disease. They help prevent deaths for a range of diseases and have saved millions of lives.

Herd immunity is when a large percentage of individuals in a population have developed immunity against an infectious disease, making it hard for the disease to spread. This provides protection for those people who do not have immunity.

Vaccines begin at the age of 8 weeks old, and we can continue to have vaccines into later adulthood.

Individuals at any age can opt in for the flu vaccine. Pregnant women are also offered additional vaccines to protect themselves and the foetus from diseases such as whooping cough.

Individuals who are more vulnerable to disease may also be offered additional vaccines, such as the flu or hepatitis A or B vaccine.

Age	Vaccine
8 weeks – 16 weeks	6-in-1 vaccine (spread across 3 doses) – to protect against hepatitis B, polio, tetanus, diphtheria, Hib and whooping cough
1 year	MMR vaccine – to protect against measles, mumps and rubella
3 years	MMR second dose
2- 15 years	Flu vaccine every year until the end of secondary school
12 – 13 years	HPV vaccine – to protect against human papillomavirus (HPV)
	MenACWY vaccine – to protect against meningitis and sepsis
65 + years	Flu vaccine Shingles vaccine

Table to show the range of vaccines and ages.

C2.2 Age-related health checks and screening

Screening and **age-related health checks** are a way of discovering if individuals have already developed certain health issues. They are also used to check people who are more susceptible to developing conditions due to a predisposition. They allow health care professionals to intervene early.

Newborn and infant checks

Newborns are offered **hearing screening** to identify if they have any hearing loss or impairment. This ensure that babies and parents/carers can receive the right level of support from as early as possible. The test is known as the **automated otoacoustic emission (AOAE) test**. Soft earpieces are placed in the ears and play a gentle clicking sound, to determine if there are any hearing issues. The results are immediately available after the test and support is provided as necessary.

A health visitor will continue to monitor and review an infant's **growth and development** until they are around two years old. This is done by completing a **personal child health record (PCHR)** so that health professionals can easily monitor and review any changes. It is used to record the height and weight of the child as they grow. This allows for any issues to be identified early, and the right support given to the infant. For example, poor weight gain could be due to a metabolic disorder which would then require intervention such as medication or a change in diet.

Developmental milestones also checked regularly to ensure an infant's physical, intellectual and social skills are developing as expected. For example, by nine months old an average infant can sit up without support. However, it can be perfectly normal for these milestones to be achieved at slower or faster rates. Healthcare professionals are more concerned if skills do not develop at all.

Developmental delays are identified from these checks and further screening services can determine the seriousness of the delay.

See Learning Aim A of Unit 6 for more information on health care professionals.

Hearing and eyesight checks

Hearing and eyesight checks are conducted across all the life stages.

NHS services promote hearing and sight tests to certain groups of individuals, such as people under 16, those aged 60 or over, people diagnosed with certain health conditions such as diabetes and those on certain benefits such as universal credit.

NHS health checks

The NHS offers health checks for everyone aged 40-74 who do not already have existing conditions, such as diabetes or heart disease. (People who have these conditions will already have checks in place). The NHS health check is so people can identify if they have a condition, or are at risk of developing one. The tests are for:

- **Diabetes** – These are blood tests which tests for blood sugar levels.
- **Blood pressure** – This is to check for hypertension, using a sphygmomanometer.
- **Height/weight** – These measurements are used to calculate body mass index, BMI, which can indicate if someone is overweight or obese.
- **Cholesterol** – This is measured through a finger-prick test or through a blood test. High cholesterol does not normally cause any immediate symptoms but can cause serious health problems if left untreated.

Once results of the tests are in, health professionals discuss them with service users, suggesting adjustments to lifestyle choices if necessary, and carrying out further investigations as required.

Cancer screening

Treating cancer early improves positive outcomes. Cancer screening helps detect cancer before it shows any symptoms. **Early cancer screening** programmes are in place for cervical, bowel and breast cancer.

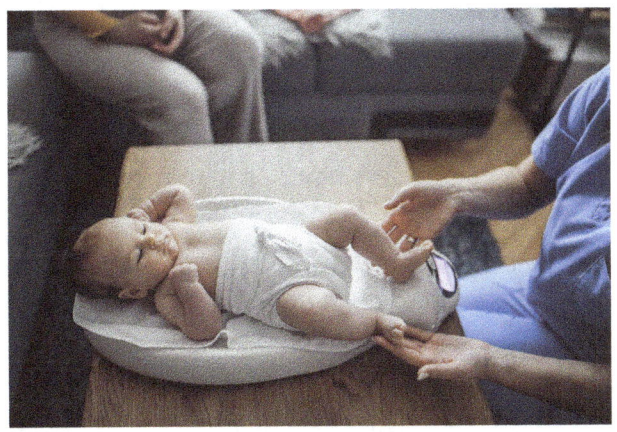

Weight checks are carried for all newborns

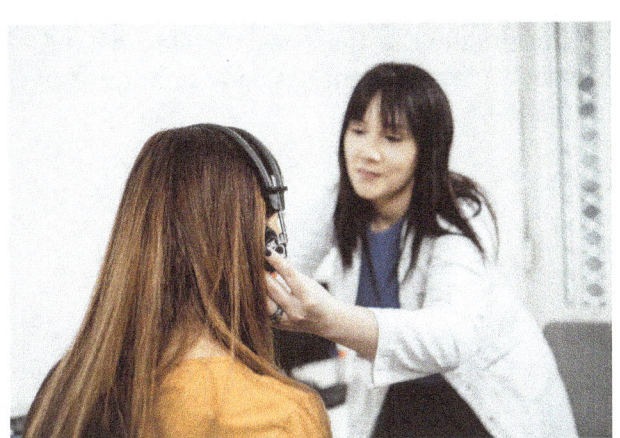

A hearing test

Sphygmomanometer – A device used to measure blood pressure.

- **Cervical cancer screening** is available for 25 to 64-year-olds. It is offered every three years for those under 49, and every five years between 50–64.
- **Bowel cancer screening** is offered to everyone between the ages of 54–74. Everyone registered with a GP receives a home testing kit through the post. People take a stool sample and send it for testing through the post. Bowel cancer does not show any symptoms until later stages.
- **Breast screenings** are called mammograms. They use X-rays to examine the breast. They are offered to people between the ages of 50–71. People who are at greater risk of breast cancer may be offered screening at an earlier age.

Health promotion campaigns, such as cancer awareness months, have generated significant increases in the number of early diagnoses and treatments.

Dementia screening tests

Dementia can also be tested prior to diagnosis through a combination of screening tests:

- Cognitive assessments to test memory and thinking
- Blood tests, which are used to see if there are any other conditions which may present similar symptoms to dementia.
- Brain scans, such as fMRI (functional MRI). These are taken after the other two types of test.

There is no standardised screening programme in place in the UK. These tests are taken if a GP suspects that a patient has early symptoms of dementia.

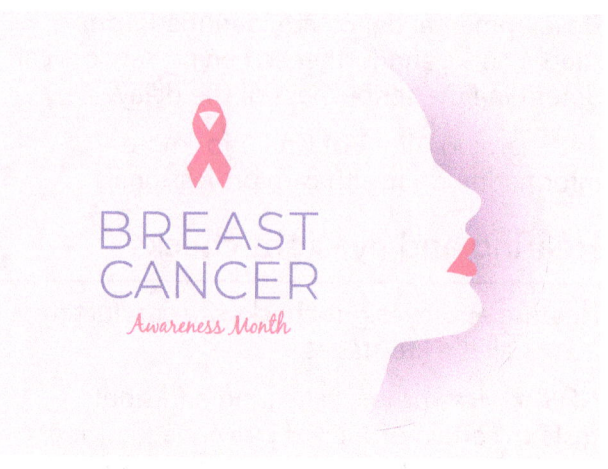

Recap questions

1. Identify a health condition that can have screening.
2. Describe the importance of conducting health checks on newborns.
3. Describe the term herd immunity.

Apply your understanding

Maja has just given birth to a baby boy, Ionut. The midwife needs to complete her routine checks of Ionut. Maja suffers with hearing loss and is concerned this may have been passed down to Ionut.

1. Identify and outline one health screening check the midwife will conduct with Ionut.
2. Outline two vaccinations Ionut will need to have.
3. Explain why Maja is concerned about Ionut's hearing.

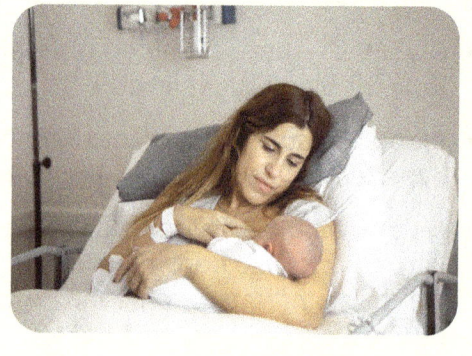

C2.3 Mental health education

NHS mental health education is critical in promoting understanding and helping to prevent or lessen the impact of mental health conditions.

Mental health education helps individuals to understand different conditions, and empowers them to make choices to positively impact their own mental health.

Mental health education helps:

- Reduce the stigma around mental health.
- Individuals to recognise symptoms of common mental health conditions, and learn about the support that is available to help them.
- Individuals to learn about strategies for managing conditions, such as stress management through breathing techniques.
- Encourage the active discussion of mental health in wider society, promoting helping to raise further awareness and ultimately prevent conditions from escalating.

Mental health education can be in the form of:

- National campaigns, such as Every Mind Matters and Mental Health Awareness Week.
- Coverage in the media, such as on TV programmes, YouTube or TikTok.
- Discussion by celebrities and role models, such as Billie Eilish and Selena Gomez.
- Coverage in lessons in school or college.
- Resources such as leaflets and posters in public spaces such as libraries and doctor's surgeries.

C2.4 Dental checks

Regular dental checks and the promotion of good oral hygiene are essential.

- Like other health conditions, regular dental checks allow for early detection and intervention, to treat problems such as tooth decay, infections and gum disease, before they get out of hand. People who leave these conditions until they cause pain are likely to need teeth removing.
- Good oral health starts when children grow their first teeth. Education campaigns are important so that parents understand that brushing teeth twice a day, and limiting sugary food and drink, has a big impact on their child's health.

Oral health is vitally important as disease in the teeth or gums also contributes to conditions such as heart disease and diabetes.

C2.5 Health education

A large number of people become seriously ill or die from preventable conditions caused by **unhealthy lifestyles**, such as smoking, alcohol, drug use and risky sexual health. Providing information about health consequences ensures people are informed about the lifestyle choices they make, and hopefully choose healthier options.

- **Education can begin in schools**. For example, by discussing the high risk of lung cancer for smokers and the dangers of overdose with certain drugs.
- **Support groups**. For example, the NHS runs 'stop smoking groups' to help smokers to quit and to highlight the risks linked to smoking, such as emphysema.
- The annual **Stoptober** day is the UK Department of Health's annual stop smoking day, which attracts plenty of media and online coverage.
- **Dry January** is a national campaign to encourage people to stop drinking alcohol in January, and Alcohol Awareness Week aims to put alcohol and its consequences in the national conversation. Both are run by the charity Alcohol Change UK.
- **Taking Action on Addiction** is a campaign to educate on the nature of addiction, primarily alcohol and drug addiction, as ultimately a mental health condition that

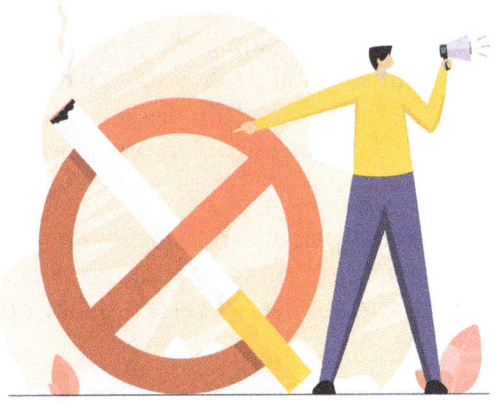

requires support like any other health condition.

- **Sexual Health Week** is run by the charity Brook, which focuses on a range of issues related to sex and sexual health. In addition, World Sexual Health Day is celebrated every September, by the World Association for Sexual Health.

Overall, health education is a vital source of health promotion to build healthier communities through better informed choices.

C2.6 Accident prevention

Accidents can be caused by a variety of things. Various campaigns have tackled issues such as falls, road traffic accidents, workplace injuries and home safety risks.

- The Royal Society for the Prevention of Accidents runs campaigns such as the Safer Stairs Change Campaign and the Falls Prevention Campaign.
- The Child Accident Prevention Trust run **Child Safety Week**, to highlight the main accidents that endanger children and how to avoid them. For example, burns, choking risks, dogs, button batteries and poisoning.
- Brake, the road safety charity, runs **Road Safety Week**, involving lots of schools and communities to educate all road users about road safety and the impact of accidents.
- THINK!, the UK government's official road safety campaign body, runs lots of campaigns to make roads safer, including **Is Pushing it Worth It?** which aims to raise awareness of the impact of breaking the speed limit.

Educational campaigns, often including advertisements, encourage people to understand the dangers of certain behaviour.

> **Find out more**
> www.eboru.com/BTEC-HSC-links
> Find out more about vaccines.

> **Recap questions**
> 1. Explain one way in which vaccinations can protect the community.
> 2. Identify two health conditions for which the NHS may conduct screenings.
> 3. Give an example of a health education campaign.

> **Practice questions**
> 1. Discuss the overall importance of health promotion and prevention campaigns. [4 marks]
> 2. Explain the difference between health promotion and prevention. [3 marks]

There have been some particularly hard-hitting adverts showing the devastation caused by car accidents.

C3 Health and social care professionals

In this section you will learn to identify and outline the role of professionals that care and support individuals with health conditions from section C1

C3.1 Nurses

Nurses are an integral part of the health and social care workforce. They are the largest group of professionals working in the healthcare sector. 2023 saw around 750,000 nurses registered in the UK, with nearly half of these being employed by the NHS.

There are four main branches of nursing: **mental health, learning disability, adult** and **children and young people (CYP) nurse**. There are also community-based roles for nurses including **health visitors, children's practice nurse, school nurses** and **occupational health nursing**.

The table overleaf outlines the role of each type of nurse.

Nurse	Description of role
Mental health	Nurses who work in a variety of settings such as psychiatry units in hospitals, community healthcare centres, day care settings, residential settings and prisons. They promote and support recovery.
Adult	Supports adults of all ages with a wide range of health conditions in settings such as hospitals, GP surgeries and clinics. They can also make up part of a domiciliary care team, supporting patients in their home. They are responsible for assessing and monitoring patients, administering medication, administrative tasks and assisting with day-to-day tasks.
Learning disability	Support patients with a learning disability, often in the community such as in schools and workplace, or in their own homes. They aim to support patients towards achieving as much independence as possible.
Children and young people	Nursed who support children and young people (0-18) with a range of health conditions. They also support parents/carers. They aim to not only support the physical health of the child but also the mental and emotional health of the child and family.

A **specialist community public health nurse's** role is to support and improve health outcomes and also reduce health inequalities across communities and populations. These nurses have differing roles in the community such as those outlined below.

Public health nurse	Description of role
Health visitor	Supports families and infants by carrying out regular assessments on the growth and development of young children to ensure developmental milestones are met. They will liaise with other professionals in the sector, such as GPs, to ensure early intervention and appropriate support if issues occur.
Children's practice nurse	Nurses who work in GP surgeries and are responsible for tasks such as taking blood samples, child vaccination programmes and health screening of individuals with varying conditions.
School nurse (SN)	Typically employed by a school with direction from NHS services. They are responsible for vaccination programmes, monitoring and reviewing development and progression, and promoting health education.
Occupational health nursing (OHN)	Nurses that are based in the workplace to prevent work-related injuries and illnesses, as well as promoting positive mental health amongst company employees.

C3.2 Midwives

A **midwife's** main role is to provide care and support to women throughout pregnancy (antenatal), childbirth and the after birth (postpartum or postnatal period). This can include tasks such as:

- Monitoring of mother and baby.
- Providing health education.
- Giving information and advice on things such as birthing plans, aid in labour and delivery.
- Providing emotional support throughout pregnancy.

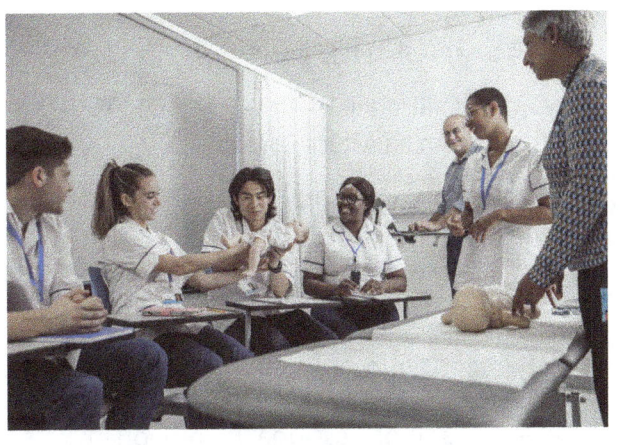

A midwife can be based in settings such as a hospital's maternity unit, local clinics, GP surgeries and in the home.

C3.3 Doctors

A **general practitioner** (**GP**) is typically the first point of contact for an individual experiencing ill health. GPs are providers of primary care and have many responsibilities, including:

- Health education and preventative care.
- Diagnosis of injury or illness.
- Prescribing medication.
- Professional referrals to secondary care or tertiary care services.
- Vaccination programmes.
- Monitoring of ill health conditions.

Surgeons have a pivotal role in diagnosing and treating medical conditions that need surgical intervention. A surgeon is responsible for performing an operation to repair or remove damaged tissues or organs, and treat disease or infection. They work with a variety of healthcare professionals to ensure the highest level of care before and after surgery. There are ten main specialities of a surgeon:

- **Cardiothoracic** – Heart, lungs and vital chest organs.
- **General** – Emergency and elective surgeries.
- **Neurosurgery** – Central and peripheral nervous system.
- **Paediatric** – Working exclusively with children.
- **Plastic** – Cosmetic surgery following trauma, illness or an elective surgery.
- **Trauma and orthopaedic** – Musculoskeletal system.
- **Urology** – Urinary system for both males and females.
- **Vascular** – Arteries and veins.
- **Oral maxillofacial** – Diseases that affects the mouth, jaw, face and neck.
- **Otorhinolaryngology** (**ENT**) – Ear, nose and throat.

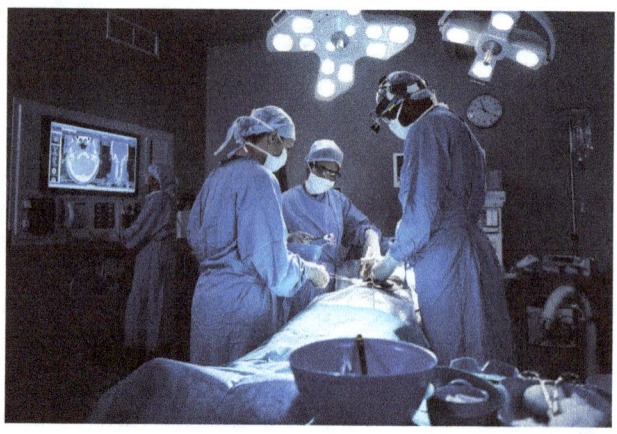

Primary care – The first point of contact for people in need of healthcare. GPs, pharmacies and dentists are all examples of primary care services.

Secondary care – Specialised medical care that requires a professional referral from a primary care service. Examples include cardiologists and dermatologists.

Tertiary care – Highly specialised care for individuals with complex or rare health conditions. For example, oncologists and neurosurgeons.

A **psychiatrist** is a doctor that specialises in diagnosing, treating and preventing mental health disorders such as depression, bipolar disorder, schizophrenia and anxiety. Psychiatrists assess patients through psychological evaluations by talking to their patients to determine an overall diagnosis and treatment plan. They liaise with a variety of health care professionals to provide appropriate support for an individual's holistic needs. For example, they may work with a social worker to ensure adequate support is provided at home. As with medical doctors, they can prescribe medicine or talking therapies to help people with mental health conditions.

Recap questions

1. Identify two branches of nursing.
2. Outline the role of a general practitioner.
3. Give an example of a lifestyle factor that individuals can receive health education on.

C3.4 Allied professions

An allied health professional is someone who specialises in the maintenance of an individual's daily life by promoting independence.

Allied professional	Description of role
Physiotherapist 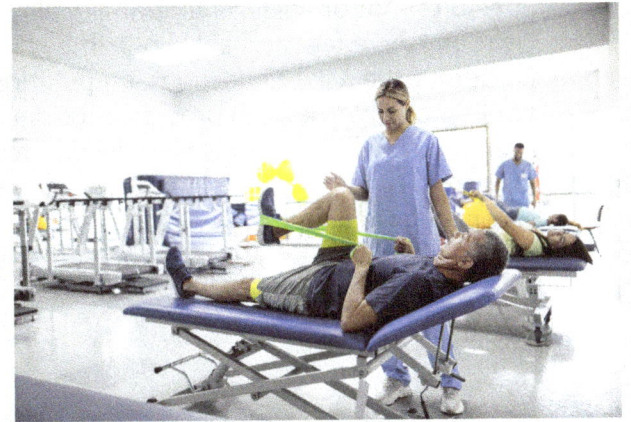	Assesses individuals with physical conditions that specifically impact mobility or movement. They can offer treatments through massage therapy or exercises, to promote movement and encourage independent moving.
Occupational therapist 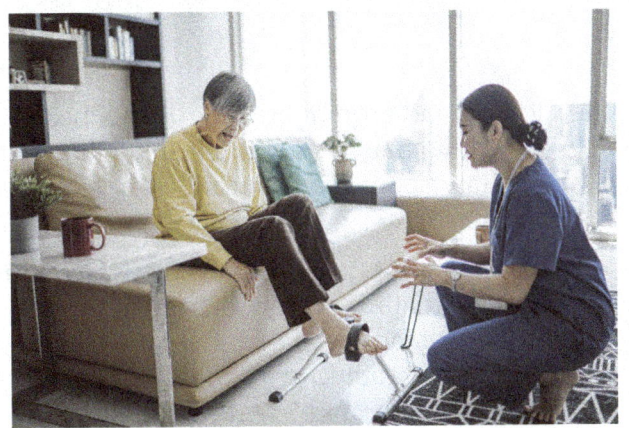	Supports people of all ages that have difficulty in completing day-to-day tasks, such as washing, cleaning, cooking and attending appointments. They will assess the individual and provide specific adjustments or activities to help increase their patients' independence.
Speech therapist 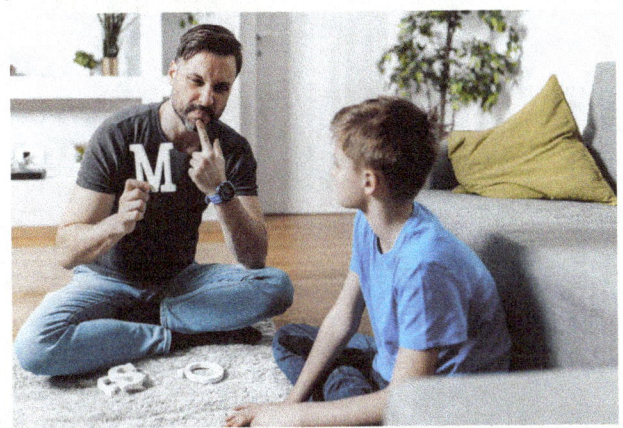	Responsible for assessing and treating issues with speech, language, communication and swallowing. They can be based in community health centres, hospitals, schools, prisons and day centres.
Radiographer 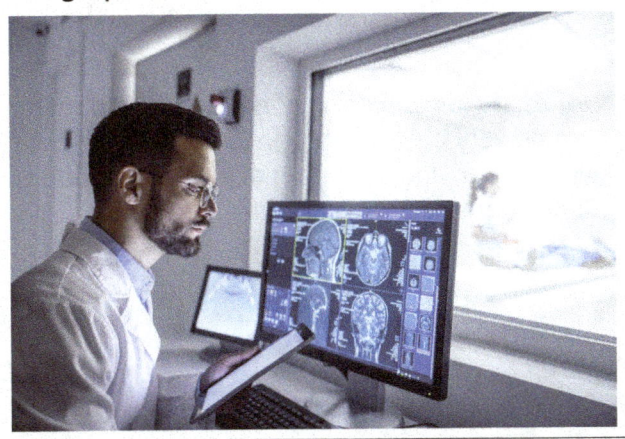	Typically based in hospitals, they are responsible for taking and interpreting medical images using for diagnosis. A radiographer will be accountable for operating high-tech equipment such as X-ray machines, PET scanners and MRI scanners.

Allied professional	Description of role
Podiatrist 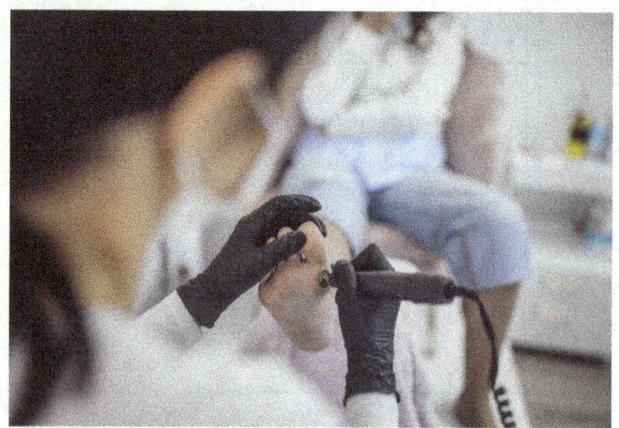	Responsible for treating problems with a person's foot or ankle. Their primary aim is to preserve feet and ankle health by reducing the risk of infections, amputation or immobility. They can provide individuals with exercises or custom-made insoles for shoes, in order to maintain movement and mobility of the feet.

C3.5 Dental care

A **dentist** is a primary care professional responsible for the maintenance of good oral health for the local community they practise in. They provide routine check-ups, diagnose and perform procedures to address dental issues such as cavities, tooth decay and gum disease. Treatments they can perform include fillings, root canals, dentures and cosmetic treatments, such as teeth whitening or veneers.

Dentists are also responsible for health education and promotion of good oral health by educating patients about brushing, flossing and dietary habits that can contribute to poor dental health.

Dental hygienists provide preventative oral care to patients that have been referred to them by a dentist. A hygienist can educate people on how best to brush teeth to prevent plaque and tartar from building up on the teeth. They can also carry out procedures such as polishing teeth.

C3.6 Social worker

Social workers aim to find solutions to social problems that individuals have, in order that they can have independent and safe lives. They support individuals of all ages who face a variety of issues. An important role they have is to safeguard vulnerable people, such as those with disabilities, older people and children.

A social worker is responsible for assessing an individual's circumstances to determine the best course of action for them. For example, they can support individuals and families in poverty, people who have experienced trauma or discrimination, or those at risk of abuse.

There are two main branches of social workers, one for adults and another for children. Both aim to ensure the health, wellbeing and safety

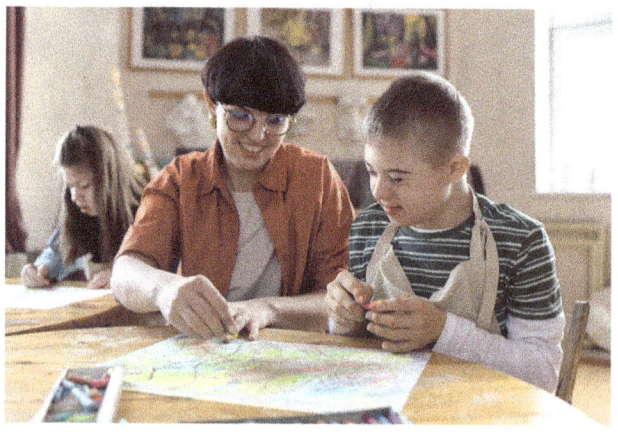

of their clients. Social workers can encounter some very challenging circumstances and behaviour, and have to make some difficult but important decisions at times.

C3.7 Dietician

A **dietician** supports individuals with nutrition-related issues, including dietary issues, obesity and malnutrition. They will assess a person's level of need, then develop and implement nutritional plans to support those needs. They can provide advice and information about diet and foods to empower individuals in their choices surrounding food.

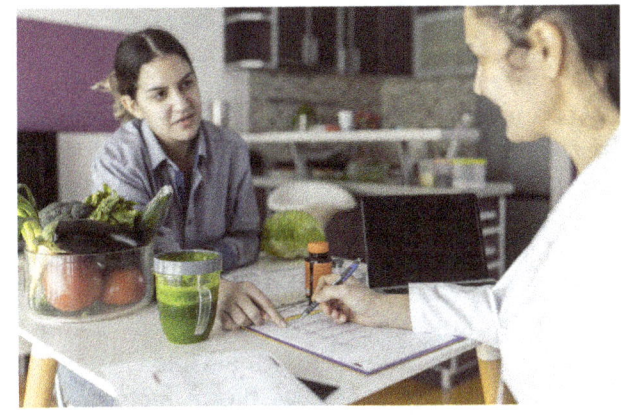

C3.8 Care and support workers

Care and support workers provide essential support to those struggling with daily living due to age, illness, injury or disability. Their main role is to help those with personal care tasks such as washing, dressing, eating and toileting. They can also provide companionship and emotional support as well as ensuring and maintaining an individual's dignity throughout the care process.

Domiciliary carers are based in a person's home and **residential carers** are based in residential settings such as care homes.

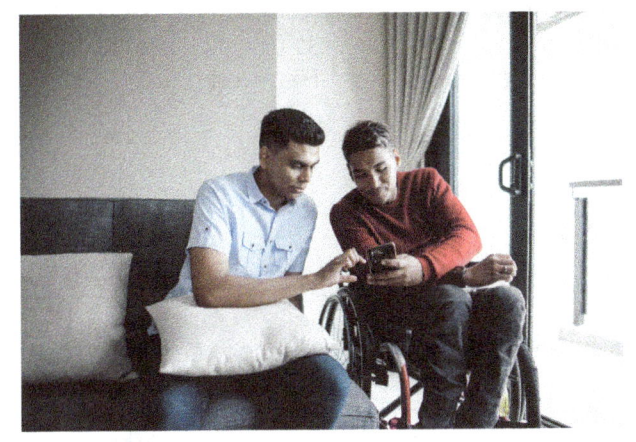

C3.9 Psychologist and counsellor

A **psychologist** is someone that has an advanced degree in psychology, with deep knowledge of mental health conditions such as schizophrenia, depression and bipolar, and their treatments. However, unlike psychiatrists, they are not medical doctors and cannot prescribe medication.

A **counsellor** supports individuals with specific challenges issue in their life, such as those relating to relationships, bereavement, stress or other problems someone may face. However, they are not qualified to diagnose more complex mental health conditions.

Both professionals will use a range of talking therapies to support individuals with their mental health, and provide them with coping techniques.

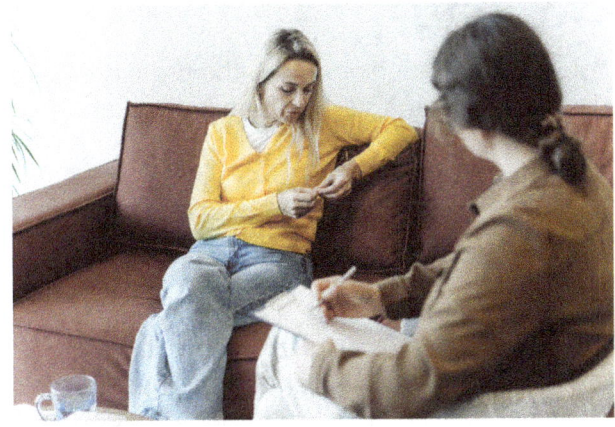

C3.10 Youth worker

A **youth worker** supports young people aged 11 to 25 years by acting as a mentor, to help them navigate the struggles and challenges of life. They provide resources and run support groups that help people build vital skills needed for daily life. For example, a youth worker may help with interview techniques to support individuals getting into employment.

Youth workers collaborate with other services, such as a social worker and teachers, to promote the health and wellbeing of young people through health education and the development of vital life skills.

C3.11 Social prescriber

Social prescribers provide personalised care by connecting individuals to activities, groups and services to meet their holistic needs. A social prescriber helps co-ordinate and co-produce a personal care and support plan, which links together different services and professionals. Co-production helps individuals take control of their own health and wellbeing. Social prescribing is useful for people who have complex social needs which affects their wellbeing.

The NHS have begun to implement social prescribers into primary care services, so that all individuals have access to social prescribing services through their GP surgery.

> **Find out more**
>
> www.eboru.com/BTEC-HSC-links
>
> Social prescribing
>
> Careers into nursing here:

> **Recap questions**
>
> 1. Identify a professional that can support an individual with depression.
> 2. Identify a professional that can support an individual with osteoarthritis.
> 3. Explain two ways a midwife can support women during pregnancy.

> **Practice questions**
>
> 1. Explain the difference between a psychiatrist and a counsellor. [3 marks]
> 2. Discuss which set of professionals are the most appropriate to support an individual in later adulthood with dementia. [4 marks]

C4 Personalised care and multi-disciplinary working

You need to understand how the professionals outlined in C3 can work together as part of a multi-disciplinary team to support an individual.

C4.1 Integrated care systems

See unit 3 section B3 for more information on integrated care systems.

An **integrated care system** is designed to allow different services to form partnerships to ensure an individual receives the best quality care. A well-run integrated care system means that all services are in constant communication with each other, and work to complement each other's service, to meet all of the service user's needs.

An integrated care system needs a **multi-disciplinary** and **multi-agency approach**.

- A **multi-disciplinary team** consists of several professionals from the same service but with differing roles. For example, they could all work within a hospital but occupy a different role, such as a nurse and psychiatrist.

- A **multi-agency approach** is when difference teams from different services work together. For example, the NHS might team up with a voluntary organisation to support an individual. Both approaches are responsible for providing co-ordinated and holistic care.

C4.2 Person-centred approach to care

See unit 3 section A2 for more information on person-centred care.

A **person-centred approach** considers the holistic needs of an individual by carrying out assessments on a person to determine:

- what kind of support is needed, such as services to support specific physical and emotional needs.
- the level of each of their different needs.

Roper and Tierney developed a holistic model of assessing individuals, called the **Activities of Daily Living**, in order to provide effective person-centred care. Typically, an activities of daily living assessment will determine how an individual's life has been affected by an illness or injury, so that plans can be made to support independence and quality of life.

Part of the model includes assessing an individual's ability to carry out activities of daily living, such as:

- Breathing.
- Maintaining a safe environment.
- Being able to communicate.
- Eating and drinking.
- Elimination of bodily waste.
- Washing and dressing.
- Controlling temperature.
- Getting around independently.
- Working and playing.
- Sleeping.
- Expressing sexuality.
- Death and dying.

C4.3 Features of multi-disciplinary team working

There are some key features of multi-disciplinary team working:

- **Shared decision making** – Professionals must ensure discussions about individuals' diagnoses and treatment plans involve the individual, in order to keep them at the heart of the care process. Professionals must also keep each other informed about the individual's health and wellbeing, and ensure any changes are communicated. Decisions should be made jointly, having been agreed upon by the individual and all professionals in the team. Failing to make decisions as a team means that misunderstandings are more likely, which can have severe consequences for an individual's health.

- **Different professionals** working together – A multi-disciplinary team means that several different professionals will be contributing towards the care of an individual. Each individual comes from a different department or team, who are likely to have their own systems and ways of working. To be effective, the multi-disciplinary team must establish a way of working together so that everyone can contribute and be aware of what is happening. For example:

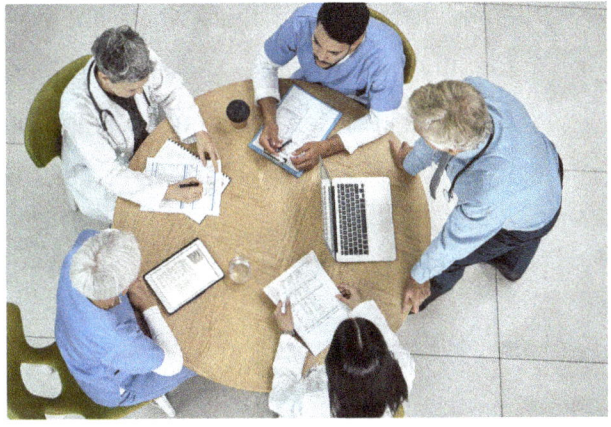

- In-person meetings might be set up at convenient times and locations for everyone once per week.

- There might be an agreement to share a summary of updates through a weekly email, so that people who are not in every meeting know what is happening.

- It is also important that professionals within a multi-disciplinary team understand each other's role so that they can best direct queries to that professional.

- Different professionals must find ways to compromise if one team's way of working is quite different to another's.

- Throughout a multi-disciplinary team professionals should ensure that **a person's family and significant others are also kept informed** about decisions or options for that person's care. It is important that a professional within the team is designated as the main contact for family and partners. This professional should be in regular communication with them. This might also depend on the wishes of the person or their age. For example, those under 16 years old will require family input before care is provided.

Recap questions

1. Describe one feature of a multi-disciplinary team.
2. Describe an integrated care system.
3. Identify two activities of daily living proposed by Roper and Tierney.

Practice questions

1. Discuss the importance of multi-disciplinary and multi-agency approaches. [4 marks]
2. Discuss the implications of professionals failing to work as part of a multi-disciplinary team. [6 marks]

End of Learning Aim Questions

Sandeep is a 36-year-old who has recently suffered an accident whilst out running. She has sustained a life-altering injury where she will now need to use a wheelchair.

1. Identify two life stages Sandeep has already gone through. (2)
2. Give one lifestyle factor that has contributed to Sandeep's injury. (1)
3. Explain one way a physiotherapist and a general practitioner can work together to support Sandeep. (4)
4. Assess how Sandeep's injury can affect her holistic health and wellbeing. (6)

Unit 2 Human biology and health

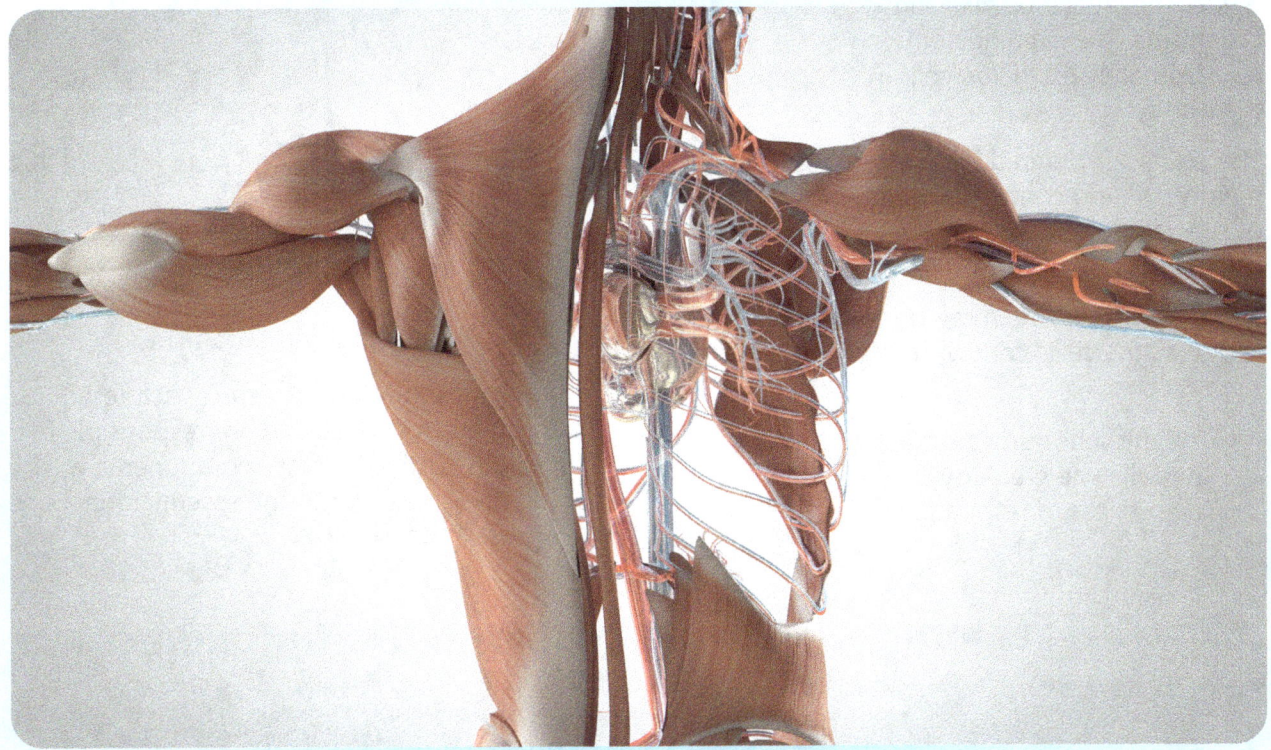

The human body is a marvel of organisation. It is a complex and intricate system where every part plays a crucial role in maintaining life.

In this unit you will learn about:

- The structures that make up the body.
- The main organs and body systems, including:
  * the cardiovascular system
  * the respiratory system
  * the nervous system
  * the endocrine and renal systems
  * the musculoskeletal system.
- Common disorders of these body systems, including:
  * coronary heart disease
  * strokes
  * COPD
  * diabetes
  * cancer.

How will I be assessed?

This unit has an exam worth 80 marks, lasting for 1 hour 30 minutes. The exam will have a mixture of multiple-choice questions, short and long answer questions.

Learning Aim A: Organisation of the human body

Learning Aim B: Body systems

Learning Aim C: Disorders of the body and effect on body systems

Learning Aim A: Organisation of the human body

A1 Cells

Cells are the basic building block of life. They make up all living organisms. The average adult has approximately 32 trillion cells in their body.

The cell is surrounded by a membrane and contains a variety of specialised structures called organelles.

- The **nucleus**, often referred to as the cell's control centre, contains the genes.
- The **mitochondria** are the 'powerhouses' of the cell, where energy is released through the process of respiration.

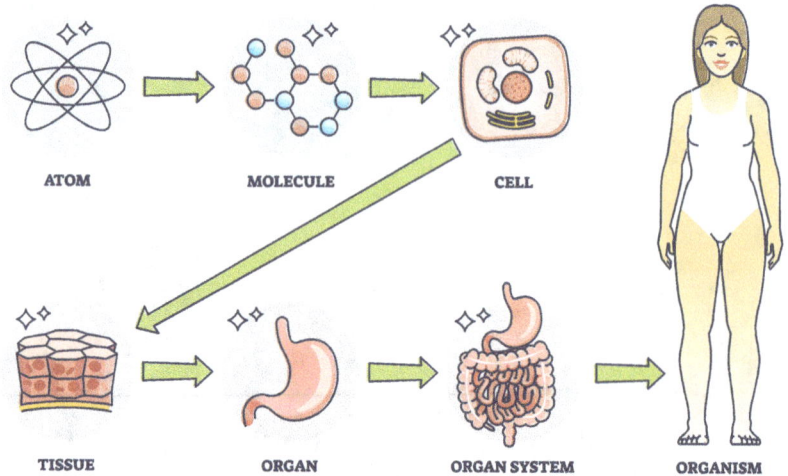

Organisation in organisms

- **Ribosomes** are tiny structures scattered throughout the cell and are responsible for protein synthesis. These components work together to carry out the essential functions necessary for life.

A1.1 The structure of animal cells and the function of organelles

Cell membrane

The **cell membrane** forms a flexible barrier that separates the cell's internal environment from the outside world. The membrane is **selectively permeable**, this means that it only allows certain substances to pass through, while stopping others. It allows gases (like oxygen) and nutrients (like glucose) to enter the cell. Waste products (like carbon dioxide) leave the cell via the membrane.

Nucleus

The nucleus is often referred to as the "control centre" of the cell. The nucleus is surrounded by a membrane, and contains the cell's genetic material, **DNA**.

- The DNA is organised into structures called **chromosomes**. Human body cells contain 23 pairs of chromosomes, which are made up of smaller units called genes.
- Each **gene** contains instructions for producing a particular protein. These proteins determine an individual's traits, from eye colour to height and susceptibility to diseases.

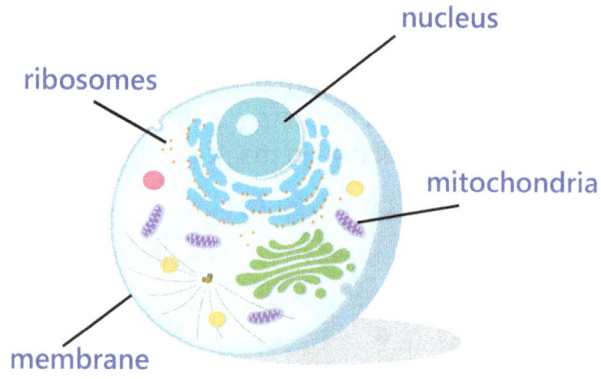

The structure of a cell

Ribosomes

Ribosomes are the smallest of the cell organelles. Their function is to produce proteins (protein synthesis).

- Ribosomes read the genetic code carried by messenger RNA (mRNA) molecules and link amino acids together in the specified order to form proteins.
- **Proteins** are the building blocks of many structures found in the cell and within the

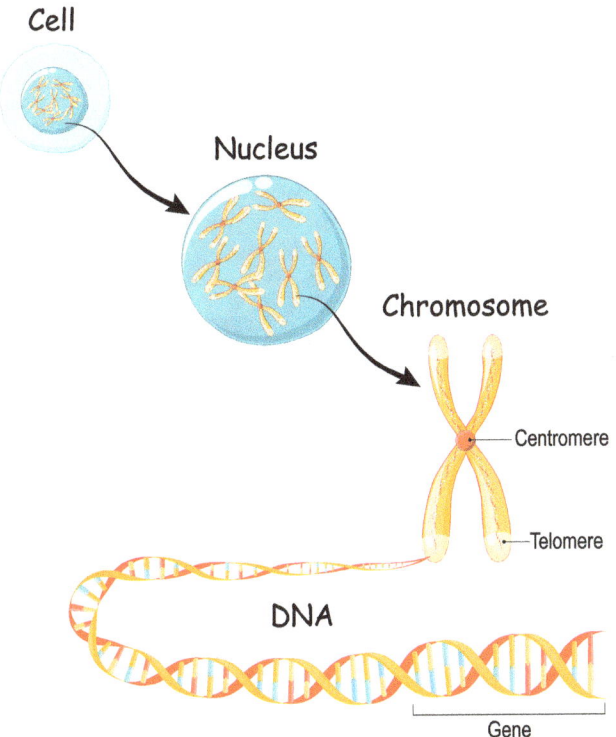

How DNA is organised into chromosomes inside human cells

Genetic code – The genetic code is the code in DNA that provides the instructions for turning a sequence of nucleotides in DNA into the sequence of amino acids in proteins.

Messenger RNA – Messenger RNA (mRNA) is a single-stranded molecule of RNA that carries genetic information from DNA to the ribosome, where it is used to make proteins.

Amino acids – Amino acids are molecules which are the building blocks of proteins.

Enzymes – An enzyme is a biological catalyst that speeds up chemical reactions in living organisms.

ATP – Adenosine triphosphate (ATP) is the energy currency of cells. It provides energy for various cellular processes.

body and have a wide range of functions, e.g. hormones, enzymes, keratin in the nails, collagen in the skin, to name a few.

Mitochondria

Mitochondria are often referred to as the 'powerhouses' of the cell, as they are responsible for releasing energy that can be used by the cell.

- Mitochondria contain *enzymes* that perform the process of cellular respiration. This process breaks down glucose to produce a molecule called *ATP*, the cell's energy currency.

- ATP is vital for various cellular processes, from muscle contraction to protein synthesis.

Recap questions

1. What is meant by a selectively permeable barrier?
2. Name two substances that enter the cell through the membrane.
3. How many chromosomes are found in a normal human body cell?
4. Explain what a gene is.
5. Name two features determined by genes.
6. What is the function of ribosomes?
7. What are the building blocks of proteins called?
8. Why are mitochondria often called the powerhouses of the cell?
9. Name two processes in the body that require ATP energy.

Practice questions

1. Identify the cell structure responsible for protein synthesis

A nucleus   B mitochondria
C ribosomes   D cell membrane

2. Select the correct number of chromosomes found in a human cell.

A 48   B 23   C 92   D 46

3. Cell membranes are described as being selectively permeable. State what is meant by selectively permeable and explain how this benefits the cell.

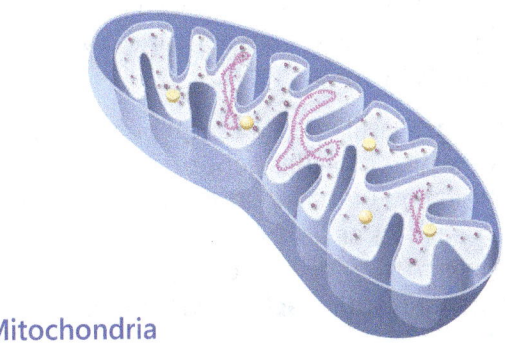

Mitochondria

A2 Tissues

A2.1 The structure, location in organs and organ systems, and function of the main tissue types

A **tissue** is a group of similar cells working together to perform a function. There are four basic types of tissue found within the body: **epithelial, connective, muscular and nervous**. These four tissues make up all the different organs in your body.

Epithelial tissue (also known as **epithelium**) is made up of epithelial cells. It is made up of cells that are tightly packed together to form a continuous sheet. Your skin is an epithelial tissue, but epithelial tissue is also found lining your intestines, your respiratory system, and your sweat glands.

There are two main types: simple and compound.

- **Simple epithelial tissue** is made up of a single layer of cells. It is found in places where substances need to pass through quickly, like the lungs or the blood capillaries. For example, the **alveoli** (tiny air sacs in your lungs) are made of simple epithelium, which is very thin to allow oxygen to pass into the blood.

- **Compound epithelial tissue** is made up of multiple layers of cells. This type is tougher and provides more protection. It is found in places that experience a lot of wear and tear, like your skin. The outer layer of your skin is made of compound epithelium, which helps protect you from damage and infection.

Epithelial tissue has several important jobs:

- **Protection**: it acts as a barrier, protecting your body from pathogens.
- **Absorption**: it absorbs substances, like nutrients in the intestines, or oxygen in the lungs.
- **Excretion**: the epithelial cells in your sweat glands produce and excrete sweat.
- **Filtration**: in your kidneys, the epithelial tissue filters waste substances out of your blood.
- **Sensory reception**: your sense of taste comes from taste buds found in the epithelial tissue on your tongue.

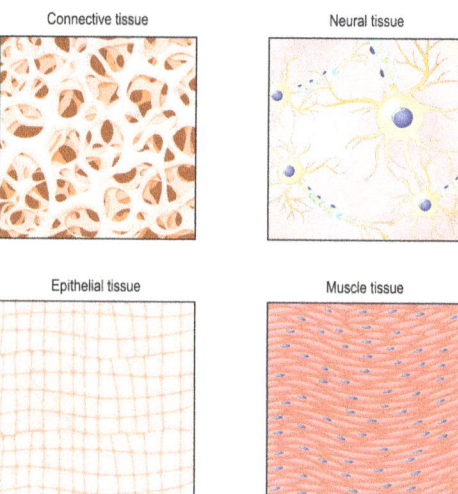

The four types of tissue

Connective tissue (blood, cartilage, bone, areolar and adipose)

Connective tissue is like the scaffolding of your body. It holds everything together, provides support, protection, and insulation and connects the different systems of the body. It is found everywhere, from the bones in your skeleton to the blood flowing through your arteries and veins. There are several different types of connective tissue including **blood, cartilage, bone, areolar and adipose tissue**:

- **Blood**: blood connects all the systems of the body. Through a network of vessels, it transports oxygen and nutrients to body cells and removes waste. Blood is made up of **red blood cells** (which carry oxygen), **white blood cells** (which fight infection), and **platelets** (which help blood clot), and **plasma** which transports dissolved substances (e.g. glucose).

- **Cartilage**: cartilage is a tough but flexible tissue which provides support and cushioning. It is found at the ends of bones (where it acts as a shock absorber and reduces friction on the joints), in your nose, ears, and in your **trachea** (windpipe).

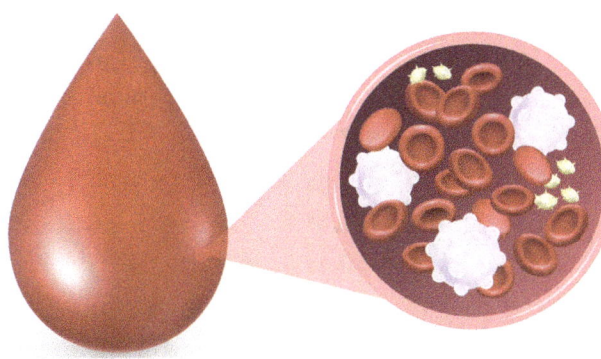

The components of blood

- **Bone**: is a hard connective tissue that makes up your skeleton. It is strong and provides structure and support, which enables movement. It provides protection of organs. For example, your skull protects your brain. Bone also stores minerals like calcium.

- **Areolar tissue**: this is a loose connective tissue found everywhere in the body. It forms a mesh-like structure which is found under the skin, around organs, and in blood vessels. It supports and cushions organs, as well as holding them in place. It contains several types of cells and fibres, including collagen and elastin.

- **Adipose tissue**: Commonly known as fat, it is found beneath the skin, around organs, and in bone marrow. It provides insulation, cushions and protects parts of the body, and is used for energy storage.

Muscle tissue (striated, non-striated, cardiac)

Muscle tissue is made up of muscle cells. These cells are specialised for contraction, allowing movement, posture, and organ function. You have over 600 different muscles in your body which help with breathing, standing, sitting, moving, digestion and many other body functions. There are three main types of muscle tissue: **striated** (also known as **skeletal** muscle), **non-striated** (also called **smooth** muscle) and **cardiac** muscle.

- **Striated muscle**: striated (or skeletal) muscle is what most people think of when they hear the word "muscle". It is attached to bones by tendons and is responsible for voluntary movement. Skeletal muscle cells are long, cylinder shaped, and striated (meaning they have a striped appearance under a

Respiratory system – The organs (like the lungs) and structures used for gas exchange in animals.

Blood capillaries – The smallest blood vessels, forming a vast network that connects arteries to veins and allows the exchange of nutrients, gases, and waste between the blood and body tissues.

Pathogens – A microorganism which causes disease.

Collagen – A protein in the human body. It provides strength, structure, and support to various parts of the body, including skin, bones, muscles, tendons, and ligaments.

Elastin – A protein found in connective tissue throughout the body that gives tissues flexibility and elasticity. It allows tissues to stretch.

Insulation – Fatty tissue keeps us warm by trapping heat and reducing heat loss to the environment.

Posture – The position in which you hold your body when standing, sitting, or lying down.

Tendons – A tough, fibrous connective tissue that connects muscles to bones.

Voluntary movement – Any physical action that is consciously and intentionally initiated and controlled by the individual, such as walking.

Recap questions

1. Name three places where you would find epithelial tissue in the body.
2. What is the difference between simple and compound epithelium?
3. State three functions of epithelial tissue.
4. Name the components of blood.
5. What is the function of areolar tissue?
6. Where is adipose tissue found?

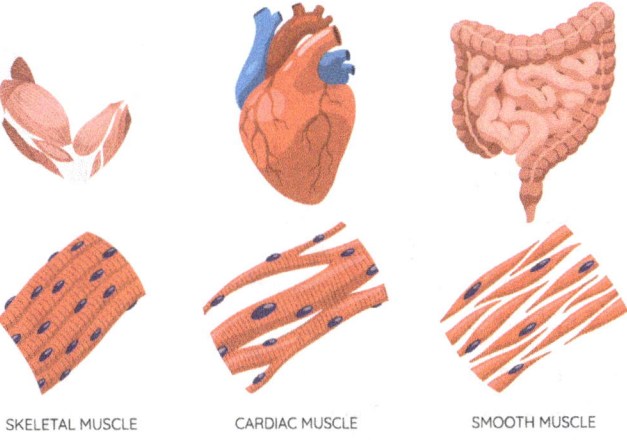

SKELETAL MUSCLE   CARDIAC MUSCLE   SMOOTH MUSCLE

The three types of muscle

microscope). These muscles are controlled by the nervous system. Examples include the biceps, quadriceps, and gluteus maximus.

- **Non-striated muscle**: non-striated (or smooth) muscle is found in the walls of internal organs, such as the stomach, intestines, blood vessels, and bladder. Unlike the other two types, smooth muscle lacks striations. It is **involuntary** (not under conscious control) and contracts slowly and rhythmically to perform functions like digestion, blood flow regulation, and bladder control.

- **Cardiac muscle**: cardiac muscle is only found in the heart. Cardiac muscle is also striated, but has a different appearance to skeletal muscle. Its cells are branched and connected by specialised junctions called intercalated discs. Cardiac muscle is involuntary, meaning it contracts rhythmically without conscious control, ensuring the heart pumps blood continuously.

Nervous tissue (sensory and motor neurones, neuroglia)

Nervous tissue is the specialised tissue that makes up the brain, spinal cord, and nerves. It is responsible for receiving, processing, and transmitting information throughout the body. Nervous tissue is found throughout the body, with the brain and spinal cord forming the **central nervous system (CNS)**, and nerves branching out to every part of the body to form the **peripheral nervous system (PNS)**. This network of nervous tissue enables us to sense our environment, to think, to move, and to respond to a stimulus.

The main cell found in nervous tissue is the **neurone**, or nerve cell. Neurones have a unique structure with a cell body, dendrites, and an **axon**.

- Dendrites receive signals from other neurones or sensory receptors, while the axon carries electrical impulses away from the cell body to transmit information.

- The axon terminals allow the nerve cell to make connections with other nerve cells, or muscles, allowing it to communicate.

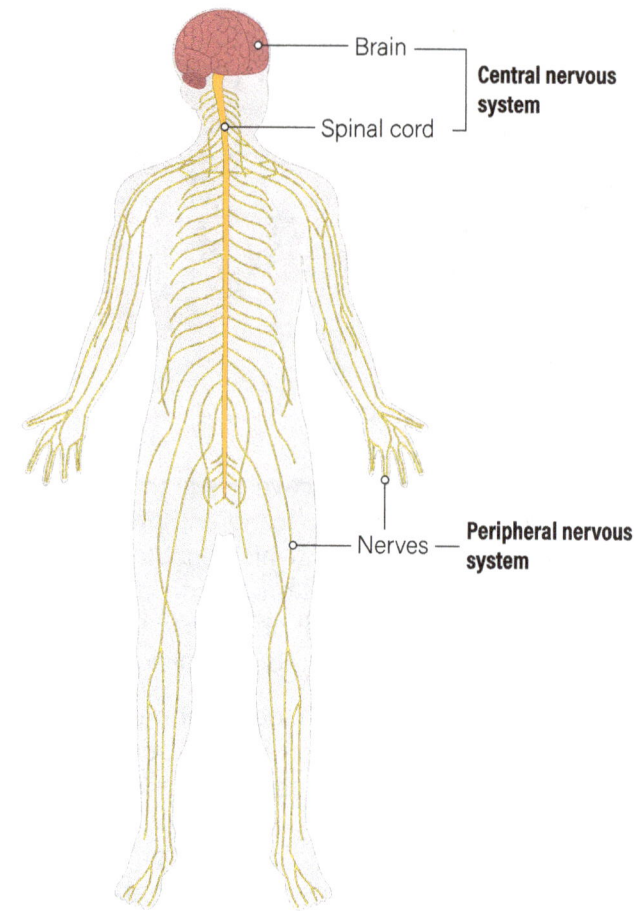

The nervous system

There are several types of neurones, including **sensory neurones** which carry information from the body to the central nervous system, and **motor neurones** which carry signals from the central nervous system to muscles or glands.

- **Sensory neurones** are responsible for transmitting information from the body's sensory receptors to the central nervous system (brain and spinal cord). These receptors can be found in various parts of the body, including the skin, eyes, ears, nose, tongue, and internal organs.

  When a stimulus, such as light, sound,

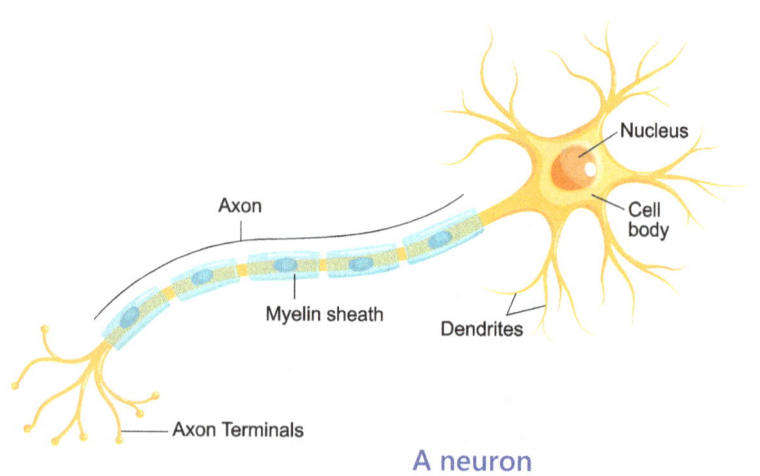

A neuron

touch, taste, or smell, is detected by a sensory receptor, it triggers an electrical signal. This signal travels along the sensory neurone to the brain or spinal cord, where it is processed. This allows us to perceive and respond to our environment. For example, if you touch a hot pan, sensory neurones in your fingertips detect the heat and send a signal to your brain, which interprets it as pain and causes you to withdraw your hand.

- **Motor neurones** are responsible for carrying signals from the central nervous system (brain and spinal cord) to muscles and glands, causing them to contract (muscles) or secrete substances (glands). Motor neurones are the messengers that convert brain signals into actions.

  When you decide to move, the brain sends a signal down the spinal cord and out to the appropriate motor neurones. These neurones then transmit this signal to the target muscle, causing it to contract and produce movement. This process is essential for voluntary actions like walking, talking, and picking up objects.

  Motor neurones also control involuntary actions, such as heart rate, digestion, and respiration. They do this by innervating smooth muscle, cardiac muscle, and glands.

- A third type of cell are called **neuroglia**. They are the supportive cells of the nervous system. The role of neuroglial cells is to maintain the overall health and function of the nervous system. They are often also referred to as **glial cells**.

Their functions include:

- **Support and protection:** Glial cells provide structural support for neurones, anchoring them in place. They also help to protect neurones from injury.
- **Insulation:** Some neuroglial cells produce **myelin**, a fatty substance that insulates axons and speeds up the transmission of nerve impulses.
- **Nutrient and waste management:** Glial cells supply neurones with nutrients and oxygen and remove waste products.
- **Immune defence:** Neuroglia cells help protect the nervous system from pathogens by acting as part of the immune response.
- **Regulation of the cell environment:** Glial cells help to maintain the appropriate chemical balance around neurones, which is essential for them to function properly.

Intercalated discs – Specialised junctions that connect cardiac muscle cells, allowing for rapid and synchronised contraction of the heart.

Conscious control – Refers to the ability to voluntarily initiate and regulate muscle contractions. This is the opposite of involuntary muscle movements which are controlled by the autonomic nervous system.

Stimulus – Any factor that can initiate a nervous response, such as a change in the external or internal environment.

Dendrites – Branched extensions of a neurone. The dendrites receive signals from other neurones and transmit them towards the cell body.

Glands – An organ that produces substances like hormones.

Receptors – Specialised structures or cells within the nervous system that detect and respond to specific stimuli.

Innervating – The process of supplying a particular organ or body part with nerves, allowing for the transmission of nerve impulses to and from that region.

Pathogens – Any microorganism which causes disease.

Recap questions

1. What are the three main types of muscle tissue?
2. What type of movement is striated muscle responsible for?
3. What is the function of non-striated (smooth) muscle?
4. What are intercalated discs?
5. What is the difference between the central nervous system (CNS) and the peripheral nervous system (PNS)?
6. What is the function of sensory neurones?
7. Where are sensory neurones found?
8. What is the role of motor neurones?
9. Which actions do motor neurones control?
10. State three functions of neuroglia.

A3 Energy in the body

Energy **metabolism** is the process by which our bodies convert nutrients into usable energy. At the centre of this process is cellular **respiration**, a series of chemical reactions that occur within the cells to break down glucose and release energy. This energy that gets released is stored in the form of **ATP** (adenosine triphosphate). ATP is the fuel that provides the power for all cell activities, like muscle contractions, nerve impulses, protein synthesis and cell growth.

A3.1 Energy metabolism

Metabolism is made up of two processes: **catabolism** and **anabolism**.

Catabolism

Catabolism is the process of breaking down complex molecules into simpler ones to release energy. This energy is used for all the body's functions, from muscle movement to brain activity. Nutrients like **carbohydrates**, **proteins**, and **fats** get broken down during catabolism.

Anabolism

Anabolism involves using energy to build complex molecules from simpler ones. Anabolism is how our bodies create proteins, carbohydrates, lipids, and **nucleic acids**, which are the building blocks of life.

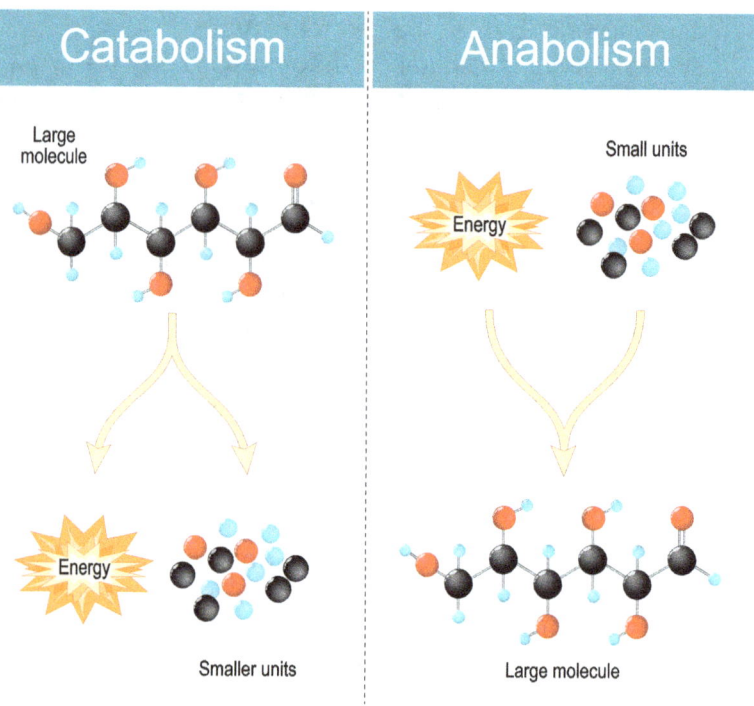

A3.2 Cellular respiration

Aerobic respiration

Aerobic respiration is the process by which cells convert glucose into energy in the presence of oxygen. The process involves a series of chemical reactions which break down glucose step by step. Along the way, energy is released and captured in the form of **ATP**, the **energy currency** of the cell.

This process occurs in several stages.

- The first stage occurs in the **cytoplasm**. Glucose is partially broken down (in a process called **glycolysis**) producing a small amount of ATP. The resulting molecules are transported into the mitochondria.

- Inside the mitochondria, a series of reactions further breaks down the molecules, releasing

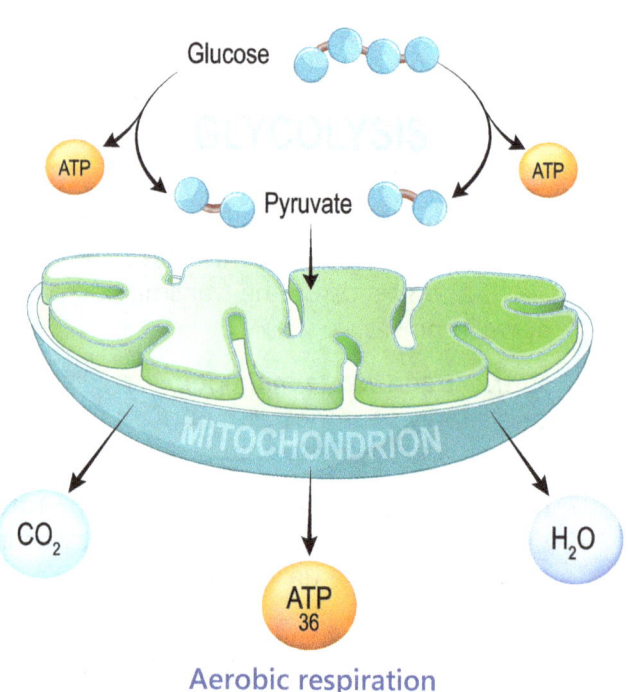

Aerobic respiration

more energy and carbon dioxide. In the final stage, oxygen is used up and water is produced as a byproduct. This process generates a large amount of ATP.

The reaction can be summarised by the equation:

glucose + oxygen ➡ carbon dioxide + water + ATP

Anaerobic respiration

Anaerobic respiration is the process of producing energy without oxygen.

Anaerobic respiration occurs in the **cytoplasm** and is a much less efficient way to produce ATP compared to aerobic respiration.

Anaerobic respiration takes place when oxygen levels are low or absent. Without oxygen, **lactic acid** is created as the end product. This process only produces a small amount of ATP, and quickly leads to a buildup of lactic acid, causing **muscle fatigue**.

> **Recap questions**
>
> 1. What is the difference between anabolism and catabolism?
> 2. What is aerobic respiration?
> 3. What two substances are required for aerobic respiration?
> 4. Where does glycolysis take place?
> 5. How does anaerobic respiration differ from aerobic respiration?
> 6. Which substances get produced in anaerobic respiration?

A3.3 Uses of energy in the body

Our bodies are energy-consuming machines. Energy is needed for every action in our bodies, from breathing to more complex processes like thought and movement. Energy fuels the growth and repair of tissues. It maintains body temperature, it powers our muscles and supports the workings of our organs. Without a constant supply of energy, our bodies would stop working.

Some of the ways our bodies use energy are:

- **Cell division for growth and repair**: Mitosis is the process used for growth and repair in living organisms. During mitosis, a cell divides to create two identical daughter cells. This process is energy intensive, so requires a large amount of ATP.

- **Passage of nerve impulses**: Energy is required for the transmission of nerve impulses. Energy is needed to start the nerve impulse, and to transmit the signal along the neurone. Energy is also required for the production and release of **neurotransmitters** (chemicals which carry signals between neurones).

- **Contraction of muscle tissue**: Energy is needed for muscle contraction. **ATP** powers the muscle fibres, causing them to shorten and contract. This process generates force and movement, allowing us to perform actions like walking and lifting weights.

- **Homeostasis**: Energy is vital for maintaining **homeostasis** (the maintenance of a constant internal environment). It powers processes like temperature regulation, blood sugar control, and hormone production. For example, in heat regulation, shivering to produce heat, or sweating to cool down requires energy. In blood sugar regulation, the liver uses energy to convert glucose into glycogen for storage or break it down when needed.

- **Anabolism**: Energy is essential for anabolism, the process of building complex molecules from simpler ones. Energy is needed to create new tissues, to store nutrients, and to produce hormones and enzymes. Without energy, our bodies couldn't grow or repair damaged cells or store nutrients for future use.

Basal metabolic rate

Basal Metabolic Rate (BMR) is the amount of energy your body burns while at complete rest. It is the amount of energy your body needs to carry out its most basic functions, like:

- breathing
- circulating blood
- respiration

- maintaining body temperature
- keeping your organs functioning.

BMR makes up about 60-70% of the calories we use each day.

Several factors influence BMR, including age, gender, and body composition.

- Younger individuals tend to have higher BMRs.
- Men tend to have higher BMRs than women, due to typically having more muscle mass. Lean muscle tissue burns more calories than fat, so individuals with more muscle will have a higher BMR.
- Other factors, like genetics, hormones, and even climate, can also play a role.

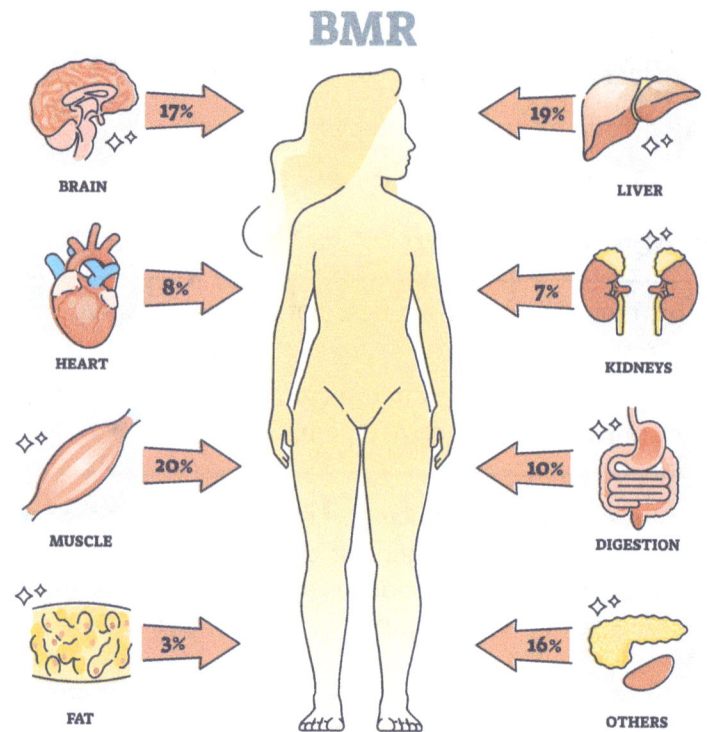

Approximate energy use that makes up the basal metabolic rate

Recap questions

1. State four ways our bodies use energy.
2. What is homeostasis?
3. Give some examples of homeostasis.
4. What is anabolism?
5. What is basal metabolic rate?
6. Why do men typically have a higher BMI than women?
7. Give three examples of basic body functions.

Practice questions

1. Identify the cells that transmit electrical signals away from the spinal cord towards an effector organ.

   A motor neurones   B relay neurones   C neuroglia   D sensory neurones

2. Explain why neuroglial cells are important in maintaining the overall health and function of the nervous system. [3 marks]
3. Discuss the similarities and differences between aerobic and anaerobic respiration. [6 marks]
4. Explain the concept of Basal Metabolic Rate (BMR) and discuss two factors that can influence an individual's BMR. [4 marks]

A4 Homeostatic mechanisms

A4.1 Homeostasis

Homeostasis is defined as "the ability of the body to maintain a stable internal environment despite changes in external conditions". Our bodies constantly monitor and regulate a range of factors, such as temperature, fluid balance, and sugar levels, to ensure optimal conditions for cells and organs to function properly.

A4.2 The role of negative feedback in regulatory mechanisms

Negative feedback is the primary mechanism by which the body maintains homeostasis. It involves a series of steps.

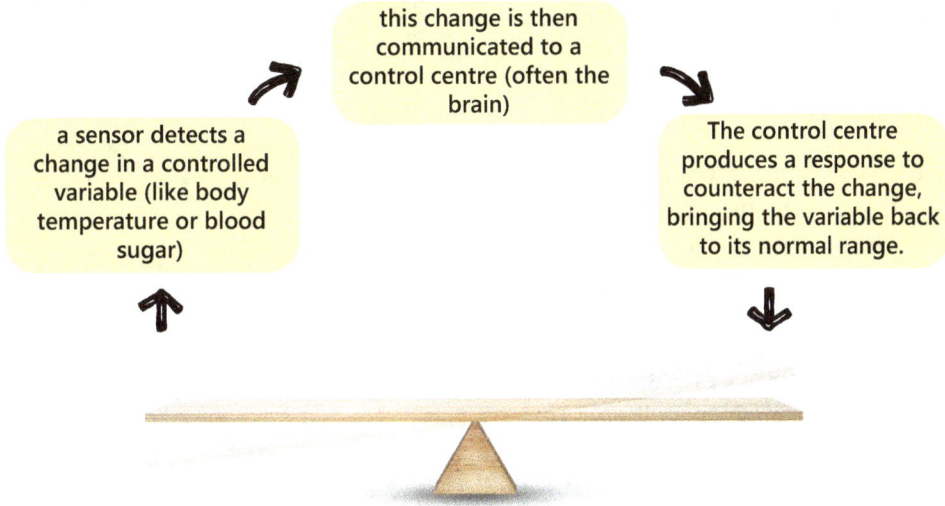

This process is continuous, constantly adjusting to maintain equilibrium within the body.

Thermoregulation

The normal human body temperature lies within the range 36.1°C 37.2°C. **Thermoregulation** uses negative feedback to maintain a stable internal temperature.

- When body temperature rises above the normal range, temperature sensors in the skin and hypothalamus (in the brain) detect the change. The body responds by initiating cooling mechanisms, such as sweating and **vasodilation** (widening of blood vessels).

- When body temperature drops, the body activates warming mechanisms like shivering and **vasoconstriction** (narrowing of blood vessels). These responses work to restore the body's core temperature back to the desired set point.

> Optimal – The ideal or most favourable set point This set point is the target value that the body strives to maintain.
>
> Equilibrium – A balanced state where physiological variables are maintained within a narrow, acceptable range.
>
> Hypothalamus – A small part of the brain, often described as the body's control centre because it plays a crucial role in maintaining homeostasis.

Recap questions

1. State the definition of homeostasis.
2. Give 3 examples of factors our bodies monitor and regulate during homeostasis.
3. Explain what is meant by negative feedback.

Blood glucose regulation

Blood glucose (sugar) regulation is another example of negative feedback. It is important for the body to keep blood sugar levels within a constant range. The brain relies on glucose as a constant source of energy. However, too much glucose in the blood can cause damage to your eyes, kidneys, and other organs.

The **pancreas** plays a vital role in this process.

- When blood sugar levels rise after eating, the pancreas releases **insulin**, a hormone which stimulates glucose uptake by cells and storage as glycogen in the liver and muscles. This reduces blood sugar levels back to normal.

- If blood sugar levels drop too low, the pancreas releases **glucagon**, which breaks down glycogen into glucose and releases it into the bloodstream.

The pancreas constantly monitors blood glucose levels throughout the day to ensure they stay within the correct range.

Osmoregulation

Osmoregulation is the body's process of maintaining a stable water balance. It ensures the correct balance of water and salts in the body, essential for proper cell function. Without it, cells could become dehydrated or swollen, which could lead to organ failure.

Special receptors called **osmoreceptors** detect changes in blood solute concentration.

- If the body is dehydrated, the **hypothalamus** (in the brain) stimulates the release of **antidiuretic hormone** (ADH), which signals the kidneys to reabsorb more water.

- Conversely, if the body is over-hydrated, ADH production decreases, resulting in increased water excretion. This feedback loop ensures that the body's water content remains within a narrow range.

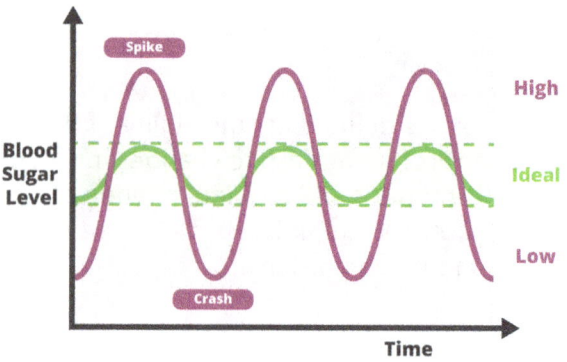

Blood glucose regulation

> Hormone – A chemical messenger produced by glands within the body. They travel through the bloodstream to target organs and tissues, where they regulate a wide range of bodily functions.
>
> Glycogen – Glycogen is the stored form of glucose, the body's primary source of energy. It's a complex carbohydrate made up of many connected glucose molecules.
>
> Solute – A solute is any substance dissolved within blood or within tissue fluid (the fluid that surrounds and bathes the cells of the body's tissues).

Recap questions

1. Why is it important to keep blood sugar levels within a set range?
2. Which hormone is released after eating a meal?
3. Which hormone is released if blood sugar levels decrease?
4. Name the organ in the body responsible for monitoring blood glucose levels?
5. What is osmoregulation?
6. Why is osmoregulation important?
7. Which hormone gets released if you are dehydrated?

Apply your understanding

Sam is 26. They are a running a marathon. It is a very hot and humid day. At mile 20 of the marathon, Sam stops at a drinks station as they feel too hot and slightly dizzy. A paramedic is worried as Sam is very red and covered in sweat.

1. Describe how the body normally regulates its core temperature.
2. Discuss the factors that may be contributing to Sam's current condition, considering the environmental factors and the physiological demands of marathon running.

Learning Aim B: Body systems

Cells are the basic building blocks of life. A group of similar cells working together to perform a particular function is known as a **tissue**. Different tissues, such as muscle, epithelial, connective, and nervous tissue, have distinct roles in the body.

Tissues combine to create **organs**, which are complex structures with specific roles, like the heart, lungs, or liver.

Finally, several organs working together in coordination form organ systems, such as the circulatory, respiratory, or digestive system.

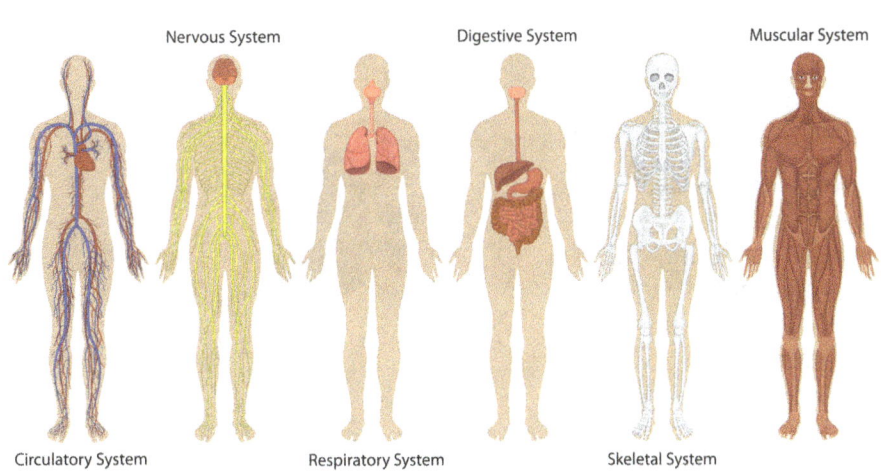

The six major systems in the human body

B1 The cardiovascular system

The **cardiovascular system** is the body's transport network. It is made up of the heart, blood vessels, and blood, and it is responsible for delivering vital substances to all parts of the body.

- The **heart** acts as a powerful pump, pushing blood through a vast network of arteries, veins, and capillaries.
- **Blood** carries **oxygen**, **nutrients**, **hormones**, and **immune cells** to the body's tissues, while also removing **waste products** such as carbon dioxide.

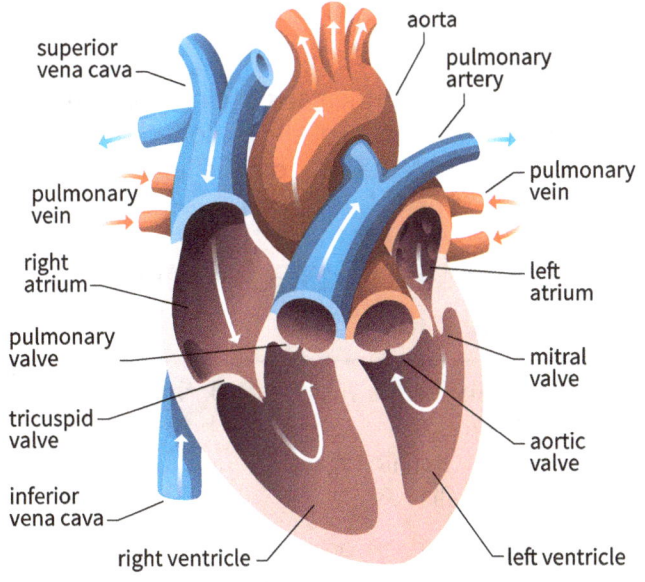

The structure of the heart

The heart and cardiac cycle

The **heart** is a muscular organ roughly the size of a fist. It is divided into four chambers: the **right atrium** and **right ventricle**, and the **left atrium** and **left ventricle**.

- The **atria** are the upper chambers that receive blood being returned from the body, while the ventricles are the lower chambers that pump blood out of the heart.
- The right side of the heart receives deoxygenated blood from the body through the **superior** and **inferior vena cava**. This blood is then pumped to the lungs through the pulmonary artery to pick up oxygen.
- The oxygenated blood then returns to the left side of the heart through the pulmonary veins.
- From the **left atrium**, blood is pumped into the **left ventricle**, which in turn pumps it into the **aorta**, the body's largest artery. This oxygenated blood is then distributed throughout the body through a network of **arteries** and **capillaries**.

Four **valves** control the flow of blood between the chambers and into and out of the heart. The role of the valves is to prevent blood from flowing backward, ensuring a one-way flow of blood.

Specialised muscle cells in the heart, called cardiac muscle cells, generate electrical impulses that cause the heart muscle to contract in a coordinated rhythm.

The cardiac cycle is the sequence of events that occur during one complete heartbeat. This cycle involves the contraction and relaxation of the heart's chambers to pump blood throughout the body.

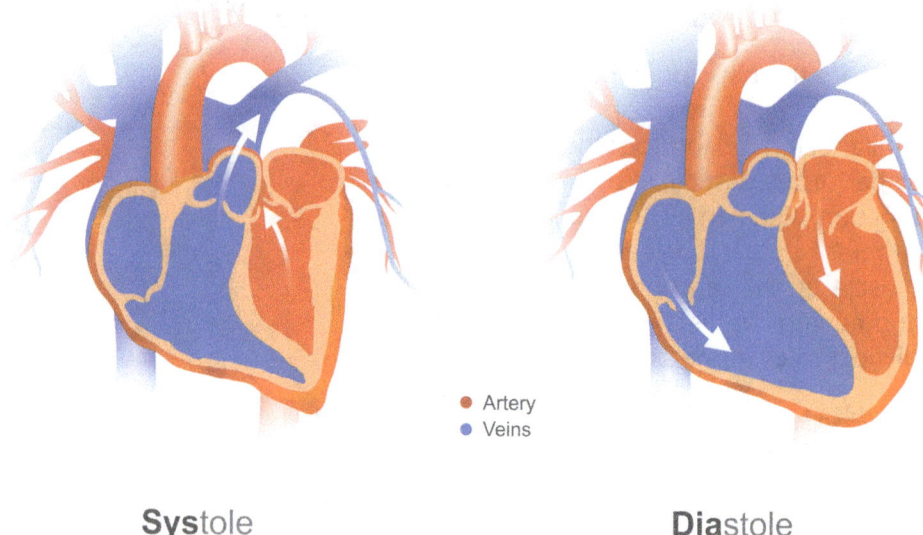

- Artery
- Veins

Systole
(heart pumping)

Diastole
(heart filling)

The cardiac cycle

- The cycle begins with **atrial systole**, where the atria contract, forcing blood into the ventricles. The ventricles are then filled with blood, and the atria relax.

- Next comes **ventricular systole**, where the ventricles contract, pushing blood out of the heart into the arteries. The left ventricle pumps blood into the aorta, which carries oxygenated blood to the body. The right ventricle pumps blood into the pulmonary artery, which carries deoxygenated blood to the lungs.

As the ventricles contract, the atria relax and begin to fill with blood.

Blood vessels: arteries, veins and capillaries

Blood vessels form a vast network that transports blood throughout the body. There are three main types: arteries, veins, and capillaries.

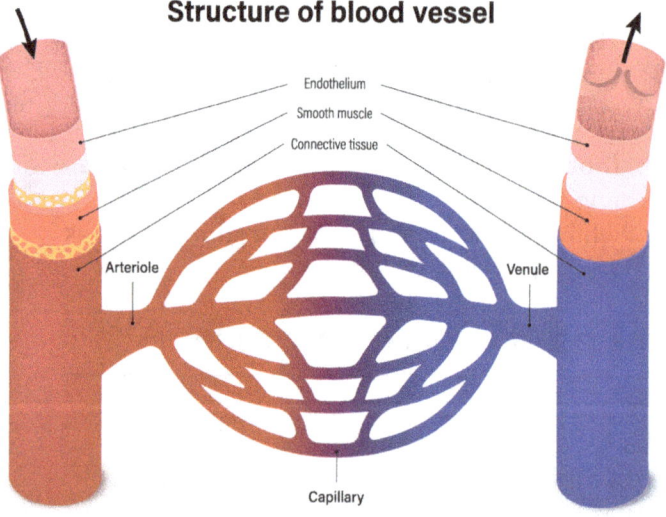

Artery (left), capillaries (middle) and vein (right)

- **Arteries:** carry blood away from the heart. They have thick, muscular walls that can withstand the high pressure of blood pumped by the heart. The largest artery is the aorta, which carries **oxygenated** blood (blood rich in oxygen) from the left ventricle to the rest of the body. As arteries branch into smaller vessels, they become arterioles, which eventually narrow into capillaries.

- **Capillaries:** the smallest blood vessels that form a network that reaches every cell in the body. They have thin walls, which allow for the exchange of oxygen, nutrients, and waste products between the blood and the surrounding tissues.

- **Veins:** carry blood back to the heart. They have thinner walls than arteries and contain valves to prevent blood from flowing backwards. Veins collect **deoxygenated** blood (blood that has low oxygen levels) from the body's tissues and return it to the right atrium of the heart.

Blood: plasma, red blood cells, white blood cells, platelets

Blood is a tissue made up of several components, each with a specific function. These components include plasma, red blood cells, white blood cells, and platelets:

- **Plasma** is the liquid part of the blood, making up about 55% of its total volume. It is a mixture of water, proteins, ions, and other substances. Plasma plays a vital role in maintaining blood pressure, regulating body temperature, and transporting substances around the body.

- **Red blood cells (erythrocytes)** contain **haemoglobin**, a protein that binds to oxygen. Haemoglobin allows red blood cells to transport oxygen from the lungs to the body's tissues. They have a biconcave shape which increases their surface area for the uptake of oxygen. They also have no nucleus which allows them to carry more haemoglobin, and therefore more oxygen.

- **White blood cells**, also known as **leukocytes**, are part of the immune system and help fight infection. There are fewer of them than red blood cells and there are different types each with a specific function. Some white blood cells engulf and destroy bacteria and other pathogens. Others produce antibodies to help neutralise pathogens.

- **Platelets a**re small cell fragments that play a crucial role in blood clotting. When a blood vessel is damaged, platelets clump together and release clotting factors, which help to form a clot and stop bleeding.

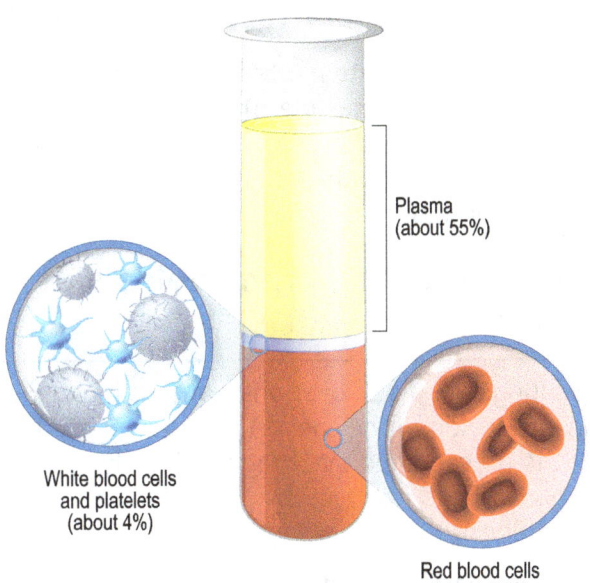

The composition of blood

Antibodies – Antibodies are Y-shaped proteins produced by your immune system to fight off unwanted substances that enter your body.

Pathogens – Any microorganisms which cause disease.

Clotting factors – Clotting factors are proteins in your blood that work together to stop bleeding and form clots following an injury. This process is called coagulation.

Recap questions

2. What is the function of the cardiovascular system?
3. Label the parts of the heart labelled A-D.
4. What is the function of the valves in the heart?
5. What is ventricular systole?
6. Name the three main types of blood vessel.
7. What features do arteries have that allow them to carry out their function?
8. In which vessels does exchange of nutrients occur?
9. What is the purpose of valves?
10. Name two substances carried in blood plasma.

Practice questions

1. State two functions of the cardiovascular system. [2 marks]
2. Describe the systole phase of the cardiac cycle. [5 marks]

B2 The respiratory system

The **respiratory system** takes in oxygen and gets rid of carbon dioxide. This system includes various structures that are specialised for their function: nose, mouth, pharynx, larynx, trachea, bronchi, and lungs.

> Diffuse – The movement of molecules down a concentration gradient i.e. from an area of high concentration to an area of low concentration.

Lungs, bronchi, bronchioles and alveoli

The lungs are a pair of spongy organs located on either side of the chest. They are enclosed by the rib cage and diaphragm, which help to expand and contract the lungs during breathing.

The trachea divides into two **bronchi**, one leading to each lung. The bronchi further divide into smaller and smaller tubes called **bronchioles**. These bronchioles end in tiny air sacs called **alveoli**. The alveoli are where **gas exchange** occurs - where oxygen diffuses into the blood and carbon dioxide diffuses out of the blood.

The walls of the alveoli are very thin, allowing for efficient gas exchange. Surrounding the alveoli are capillaries, which carry blood to and from the lungs. Oxygen from the alveoli diffuses into the blood, while carbon dioxide from the blood diffuses into the alveoli to be exhaled.

Trachea

The **trachea** (or windpipe) is a tube that connects the larynx (voice box) to the bronchi, the passageways leading to the lungs.

The trachea is surrounded by rings of **cartilage**, which provide structural support and prevent it from collapsing. The inner lining of the trachea is lined with a mucous membrane that produces mucus. This mucus traps dust, dirt, and other particles, preventing them from entering the lungs. Tiny hair-like structures called **cilia** move the mucus upwards to the back of the throat, where it can be swallowed or coughed out.

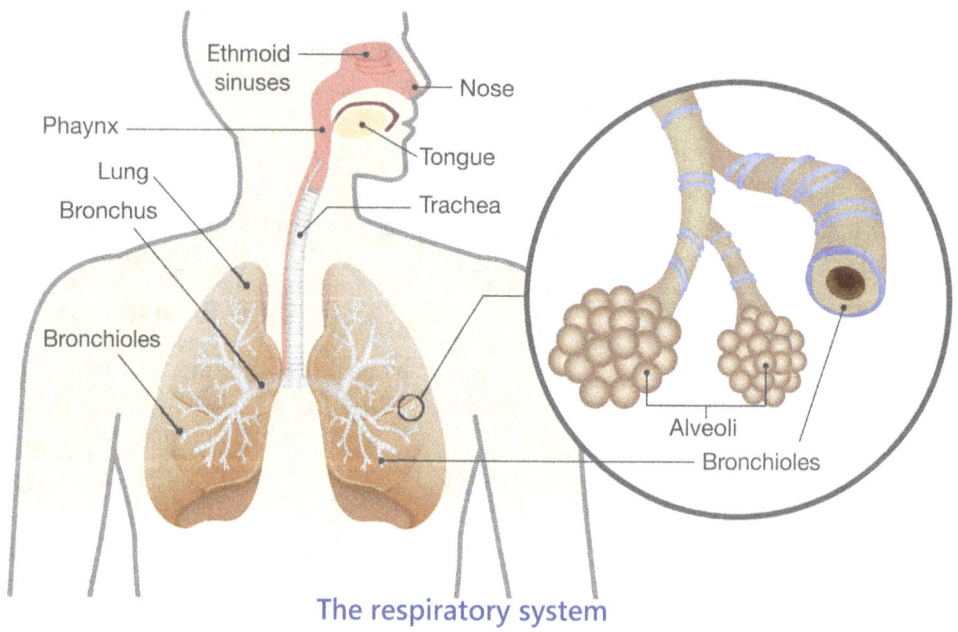

The respiratory system

B2.2 Ventilation

Gaseous exchange

Gaseous exchange is the process by which oxygen is taken into the body and carbon dioxide is expelled. This occurs in the alveoli of the lungs.

The alveoli are tiny, balloon-like structures that are surrounded by a network of capillaries. When you inhale, air travels through the trachea, bronchi, and bronchioles, eventually reaching the alveoli. As oxygen-rich air enters the alveoli, the oxygen molecules diffuse across the thin walls of the alveoli and into the blood capillaries. The oxygen molecules then bind to haemoglobin in red blood cells, which transport the oxygen to the body's tissues.

At the same time, carbon dioxide, a waste product of cellular respiration, diffuses from the blood capillaries into the alveoli. This carbon dioxide is then exhaled when you breathe out.

Action of the diaphragm, ribs and intercostal muscles

The diaphragm and intercostal muscles are responsible for bringing about the process of breathing.

The **diaphragm** is a dome-shaped muscle that separates the **thorax** (chest cavity) from the **abdominal cavity** (the abdominal cavity is the space within the abdomen that contains the liver, pancreas, stomach and intestines). When you inhale, the diaphragm contracts and flattens downward. This increases the volume of the thorax, creating a lower pressure inside the chest cavity. This lower pressure pulls air into the lungs.

The **intercostal muscles** are located between the ribs. When you inhale, these muscles contract, lifting the rib cage upward and outward. This also increases the volume of the chest cavity, helping to draw air into the lungs.

When you exhale, the diaphragm relaxes and moves upward, and the intercostal muscles relax. This decreases the volume of the chest cavity, increasing the pressure inside the thorax and forcing air out.

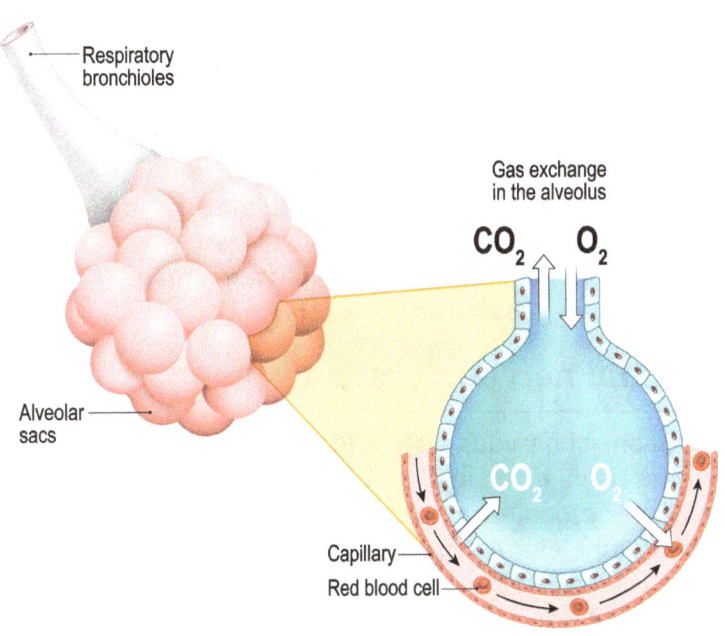

Gas exchange between alveoli and blood capillaries

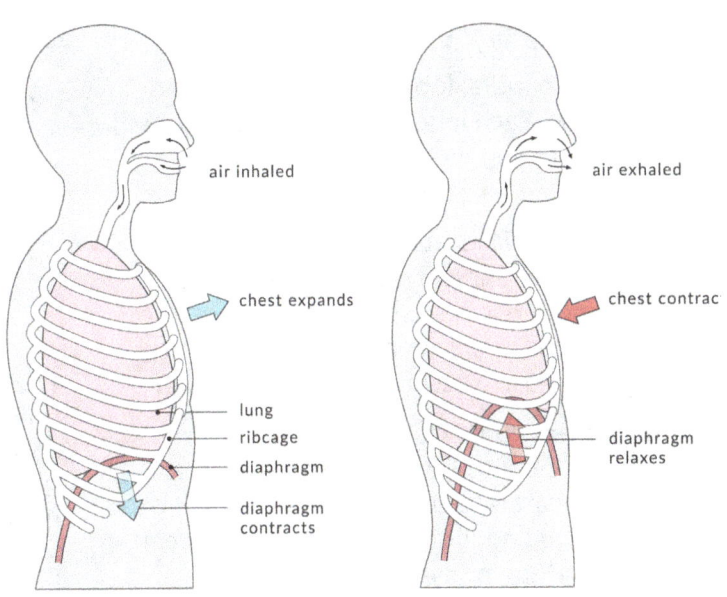

The action of breathing

Practice questions

1. Explain the process of gaseous exchange in the alveoli, including the role of diffusion and the transport of oxygen and carbon dioxide.
2. Describe the structure and function of the trachea, including the role of cartilage rings and the mucous membrane.
3. Explain how the diaphragm and intercostal muscles work together to bring about inhalation and exhalation.

Recap questions

1. What is the function of the cartilage rings in the trachea?
2. What is the role of the mucous membrane in the trachea?
3. How does the trachea divide to reach the lungs?
4. What are the tiny air sacs in the lungs called?
5. Where does the gas exchange between oxygen and carbon dioxide occur?
6. What structures surround the alveoli and facilitate the exchange of gases?

B3 The nervous system

The **nervous system** controls and coordinates all body functions, from simple reflexes to complex thoughts and emotions. It is made up of billions of specialised cells called neurones, which receive, process, and transmit information throughout the body. The nervous system is responsible for everything from movement and sensation to learning and memory.

Central nervous system

The **central nervous system (CNS)** consists of the brain and spinal cord. The brain is a complex organ responsible for functions such as thought, emotion, memory, and movement. It is divided into three main parts: the cerebrum, cerebellum, and brainstem.

The **cerebrum** is the largest part of the brain and is responsible for most conscious activities like thought, perception, and voluntary movement. It is divided into four lobes: the frontal lobe, parietal lobe, temporal lobe, and occipital lobe. Each lobe has specific functions, such as controlling movement, processing sensory information, and regulating emotions.

The **cerebellum** is located at the back of the brain and is primarily responsible for coordinating movement, balance, and posture. It receives sensory information from the body and adjusts muscle activity to maintain balance.

The **brainstem** connects the brain to the spinal cord. It controls vital functions such as breathing, heart rate, and blood pressure. It also relays sensory and motor information between the brain and the body.

The **spinal cord** is a long, thin bundle of nerves that extends from the base of the brain to the lower back. It is protected by the **vertebrae** (bones) of the spine. The spinal cord transmits sensory information from the body to the brain, and motor signals from the brain to the body. It also plays a role in **reflexes**, which are rapid, involuntary movements that help protect the body from injury, such as withdrawing your hand quickly from a hot object.

Peripheral nervous system

The peripheral nervous system (PNS) is the network of nerves that connect the central nervous system (brain and spinal cord) to the rest of the body.

It has many functions including:

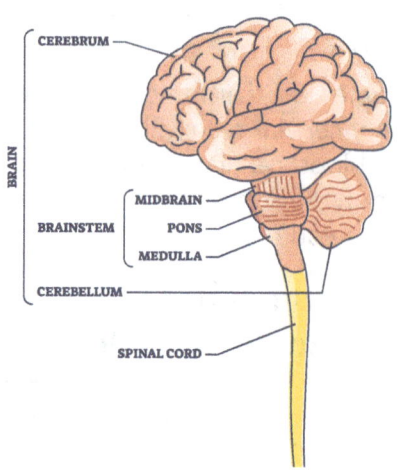

CENTRAL NERVOUS SYSTEM

The central nervous system

- **Sensory functions**: Sending information from the senses (sight, hearing, touch, taste, smell) to the brain.
- **Motor functions**: Carrying instructions from the brain to muscles and organs in order to control movement, breathing, digestion, etc.
- **Autonomic functions**: Regulating involuntary processes like heart rate, blood pressure, and body temperature.

The peripheral nervous system (PNS) is made up of nerves (bundles of nerve fibres) and ganglia (collections of nerve cell bodies outside the central nervous system). Nerves connect the CNS to peripheral organs like muscles and glands, transmitting impulses to and from the brain and spinal cord.

The PNS is divided into the sensory and motor divisions:

Perception – The process of interpreting and organising sensory information to understand and make sense of the world around us.

Voluntary movement – Any action that is consciously and intentionally initiated and controlled by the individual.

Sensory information – Sensory information refers to the data gathered by the body's sensory organs (like eyes, ears, skin, etc.) about the internal and external environment.

Motor signals – Messages sent from the brain or spinal cord to muscles, instructing them to contract or relax, thereby producing movement.

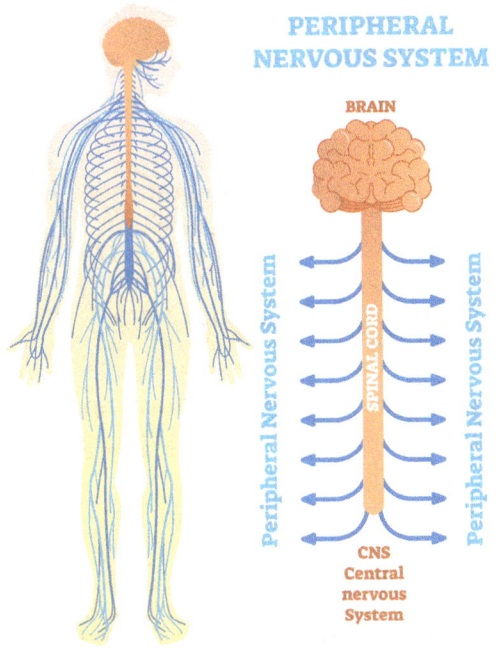
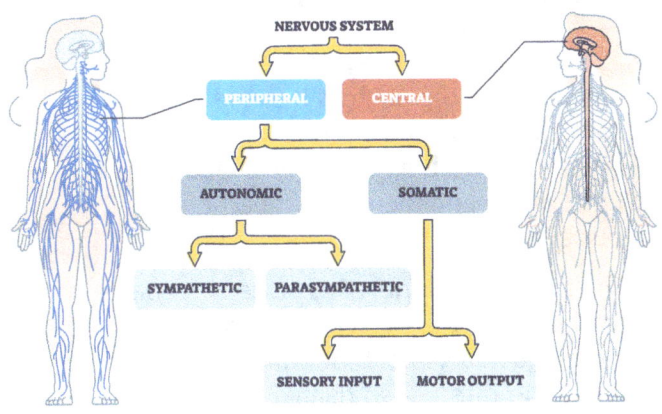

Above: The divisions of the nervous system

Left: the CNS and PNS

- The **sensory division** transmits impulses from peripheral organs to the CNS, providing information about the body's environment.
- The **motor division** transmits impulses from the CNS to peripheral organs, causing actions or effects.

The motor division can be further divided into the somatic nervous system and the autonomic nervous system:

- The **somatic nervous system** controls skeletal muscles, allowing for conscious movement.
- The **autonomic nervous system** regulates involuntary functions like heart rate, digestion, and respiration, controlling cardiac muscle.

Recap questions

1. What are the two main components of the central nervous system?
2. Which part of the brain is responsible for most conscious activities?
3. Name the four lobes of the cerebrum.
4. What is the primary function of the cerebellum?
5. What vital functions does the brainstem control?
6. What is the role of the spinal cord in transmitting information?
7. List three major functions of the PNS.
8. What are the two main components of the PNS?
9. How is the PNS divided based on its function?
10. What is the role of the somatic nervous system?
11. Which part of the nervous system regulates involuntary functions like heart rate?

Autonomic nervous system

The **autonomic nervous system** controls involuntary functions such as heart rate, blood pressure, digestion, and body temperature. It is divided into two branches: the sympathetic nervous system and the parasympathetic nervous system:

- The **sympathetic nervous system** prepares the body for a fight-or-flight response. It increases heart rate, blood pressure, and breathing rate. It also dilates the pupils and diverts blood flow to the muscles. The sympathetic nervous system is activated in response to stress, danger, or excitement.

- The **parasympathetic nervous system** is responsible for the body's "rest and digest" response. It slows heart rate, lowers blood pressure, and stimulates digestion. The parasympathetic nervous system is activated when the body is at rest and does not need to be alert.

Recap questions

1. What are some of the involuntary functions controlled by the autonomic nervous system?
2. What are the two main branches of the autonomic nervous system?
3. How does the sympathetic nervous system prepare the body for a "fight-or-flight" response?
4. What is the role of the parasympathetic nervous system in the "rest and digest" response?

Practice questions

1. Describe the functions of the cerebrum, cerebellum, and brainstem.
2. Explain the difference between the sensory and motor divisions of the peripheral nervous system.
3. Discuss the similarities and the differences between the sympathetic and parasympathetic nervous systems.
4. Explain the relationship between the central nervous system, peripheral nervous system, and autonomic nervous system.

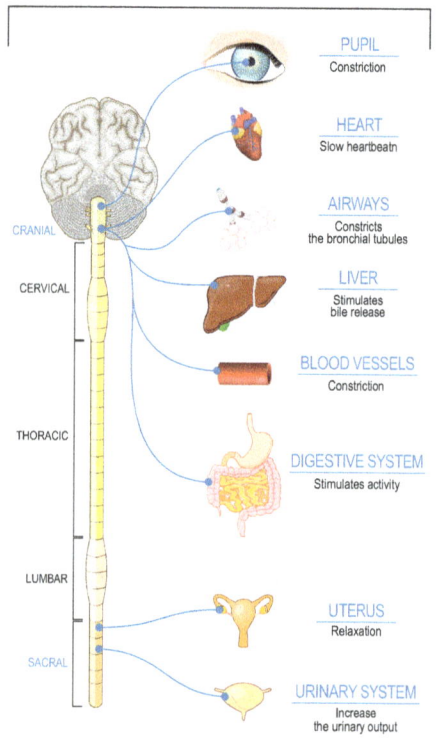
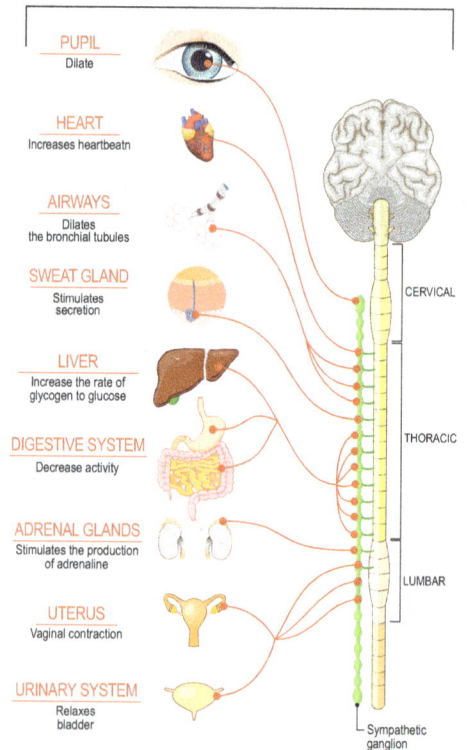

The sympathetic and parasympathetic nervous systems

B4 The endocrine and renal systems

The endocrine and renal systems are two organ systems that work together to maintain the body's internal balance.

The **endocrine system** is made up of glands that secrete hormones. The hormones regulate various bodily functions such as metabolism, growth, and reproduction.

The **renal system** is made up of the kidneys and associated structures (like the ureters) and is responsible for filtering waste products from the blood and maintaining fluid balance in the body.

These two systems interact closely, with hormones produced by the endocrine system influencing kidney function.

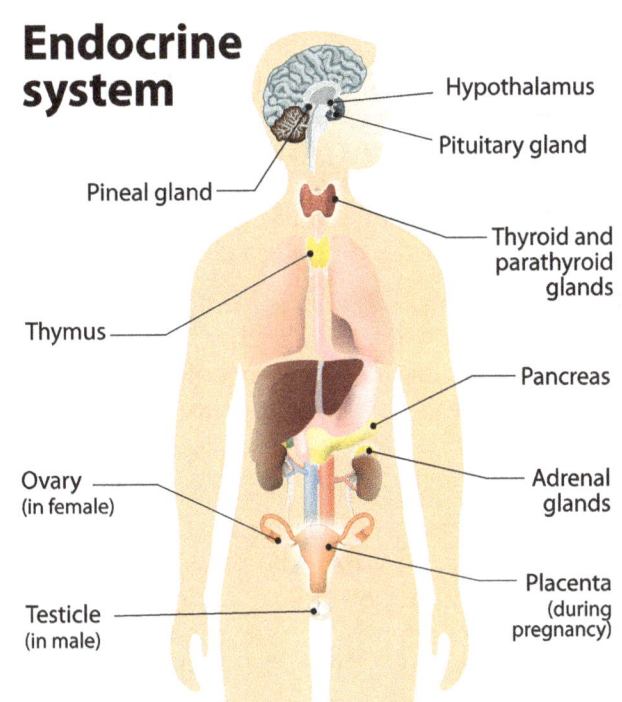

B4.1 The role of the hypothalamus in controlling the endocrine system

The **hypothalamus** is a small region deep within the brain, which plays a role in controlling the endocrine system. It serves as a communication hub, linking the nervous and endocrine systems. The hypothalamus receives information from various parts of the body, including the **brain**, **spinal cord**, and **peripheral nervous system**. It then processes this information and responds by regulating the secretion of hormones from the **pituitary gland**.

The pituitary gland is located just below the hypothalamus. The hypothalamus produces hormones that stimulate or inhibit the release of hormones from the pituitary. These hormones in turn regulate a wide range of bodily functions, including growth, metabolism, reproduction, and stress response.

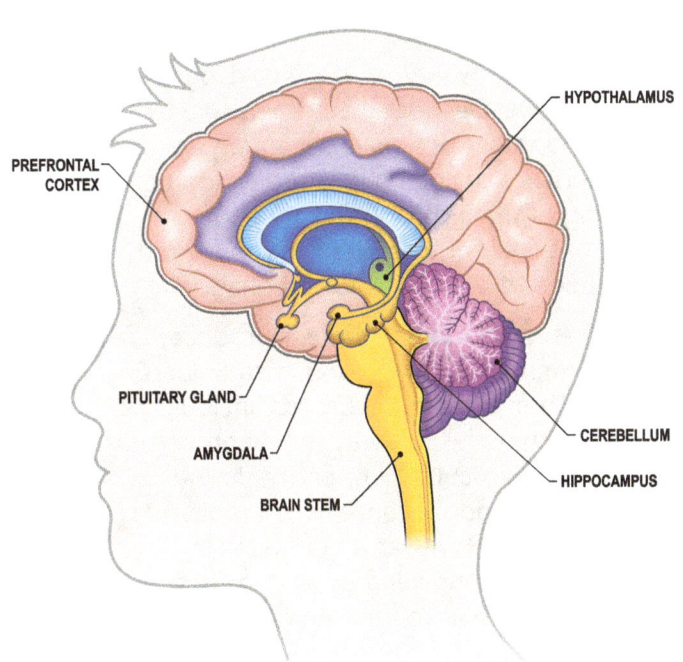

The location of the hypothalamus and pituitary gland

Recap questions

1. What is the hypothalamus?
2. What is the role of the hypothalamus in the endocrine system?
3. How does the hypothalamus communicate with the body?
4. Where is the pituitary gland located in relation to the hypothalamus?
5. How does the hypothalamus control the pituitary gland?
6. What are some of the bodily functions regulated by hormones released from the pituitary gland?

B4.2 The role of the endocrine system in the following processes:

Control and regulation of growth

The endocrine system releases hormones which regulate growth and development. Several hormones produced by various endocrine glands contribute to this process.

The thyroid gland secretes **thyroid hormone**, which is essential for overall growth and development. It influences metabolic rate, protein synthesis, and bone growth. Insufficient thyroid hormone production can lead to stunted growth and other developmental issues.

In males, the testes produce **testosterone**, a hormone that controls male sexual development and growth. Testosterone stimulates muscle growth, bone development, and the deepening of the voice. It also stimulates the development of **secondary sexual characteristics**, such as facial hair, pubic hair, and increased body mass.

In females, the ovaries produce **oestrogen** and **progesterone**. Oestrogen is responsible for the development of female secondary sexual characteristics, including breast development, widening of the hips, and the onset of menstruation. Progesterone is involved in the preparation of the uterus for pregnancy.

Growth stimulating hormone is produced by the anterior pituitary gland. It stimulates the growth of tissues and organs, including bones and muscles. Growth stimulating hormone is particularly important during childhood and adolescence, when rapid growth occurs. However, it continues to play a role in maintaining bone density and muscle mass throughout life.

Osmoregulation

The endocrine system is responsible for maintaining the body's water balance, a process known as **osmoregulation**. Osmoregulation is essential for various physiological functions, including cell volume, blood pressure, and ion concentration. One of the most important hormones involved in osmoregulation is **antidiuretic hormone (ADH)**.

ADH is produced by the hypothalamus. The hypothalamus monitors blood volume and solute concentration (the concentration of dissolvable substances in the blood). When blood volume decreases or solute concentration increases (indicating dehydration), the hypothalamus releases ADH into the bloodstream. ADH travels to the kidneys, where it acts on the collecting ducts to increase water reabsorption. This means that more water is returned to the bloodstream, reducing urine output and helping to conserve water.

Conversely, when blood volume increases or solute concentration decreases (indicating excess fluid), ADH secretion is reduced. This allows more water to be excreted in the urine.

Regulation of blood sugar

The endocrine system is responsible for maintaining a stable blood glucose level, a process known as **glucoregulation**. Two hormones, **insulin** and **glucagon**, produced by the **pancreas**, play key roles in regulating blood glucose levels.

Insulin is secreted by the **beta cells** of the pancreas when blood glucose levels increase, typically after a meal. Insulin acts on target tissues, such as muscle, liver, and adipose (fatty) tissue, promoting them to take up glucose and store it. In the liver, insulin is responsible for the conversion of excess glucose into **glycogen**, a storage form of glucose.

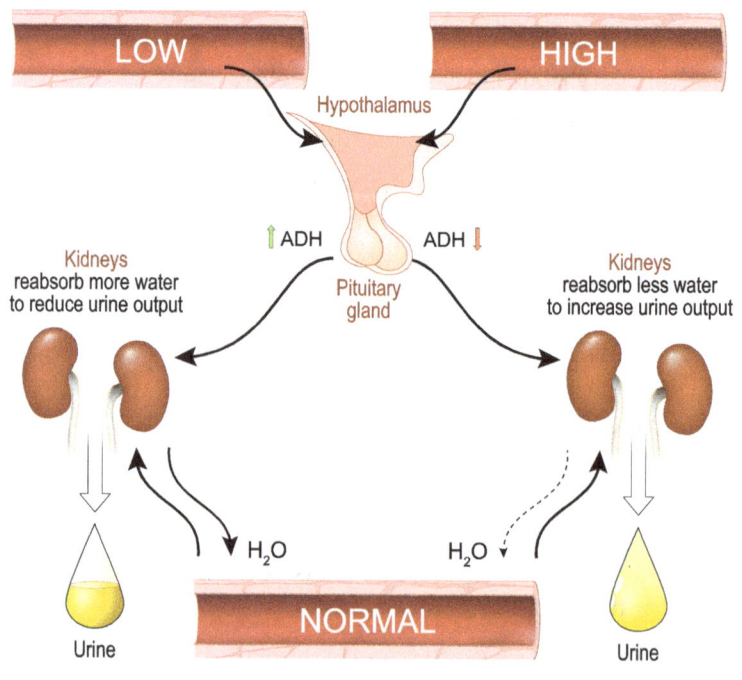

Osmotic homeostasis

Glucagon is secreted by the **alpha cells** of the pancreas and has the opposite effect of insulin. It is released in response to low blood glucose levels, such as during fasting or exercise. Glucagon primarily acts on the liver, stimulating the breakdown of glycogen into glucose and the synthesis of new glucose molecules from non-carbohydrate sources (amino acids or fatty acids).

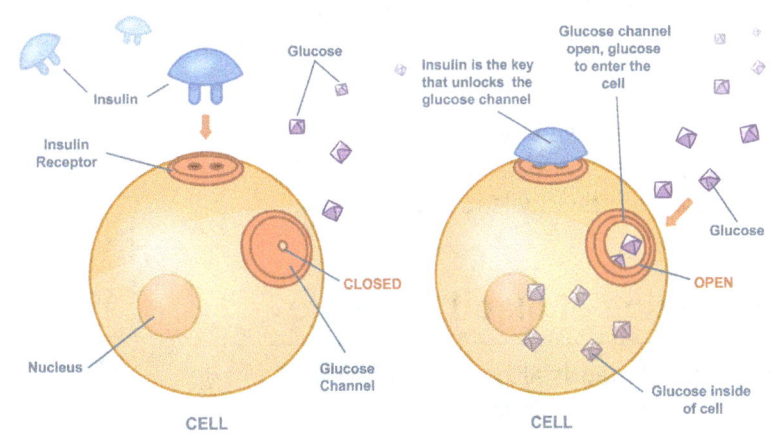

How insulin works

Recap questions

1. What hormone does the thyroid gland secrete, and what are its functions?
2. What hormones are produced by the ovaries, and what are their roles in female development?
3. Where is growth stimulating hormone produced, and what is its main function?
4. What is the endocrine system's role in maintaining body water balance?
5. What hormone plays a crucial role in osmoregulation?
6. What factors stimulate the release of ADH from the hypothalamus?

'Fight or flight' response

The endocrine system plays a crucial role in preparing the body for a stress response, often referred to as the **fight-or-flight** response. This physiological reaction is triggered by perceived threats or danger and results in hormonal and physiological changes designed to enhance the body's ability to respond to danger.

The **adrenal glands**, found on top of the kidneys, are responsible for releasing **adrenaline** – the main hormone in the flight or fight response.

When faced with a threat, the hypothalamus sends signals to the adrenal glands. This stimulation triggers the release of adrenaline into the bloodstream. Adrenaline has a wide range of effects on the body, including:

- Increased heart rate and blood pressure: Adrenaline stimulates the heart to beat faster and stronger, increasing blood flow to vital organs.
- Dilated airways: Adrenaline relaxes the muscles in the airways to increase airflow. This brings more air into the lungs and allows for more oxygen to diffuse into the blood stream.

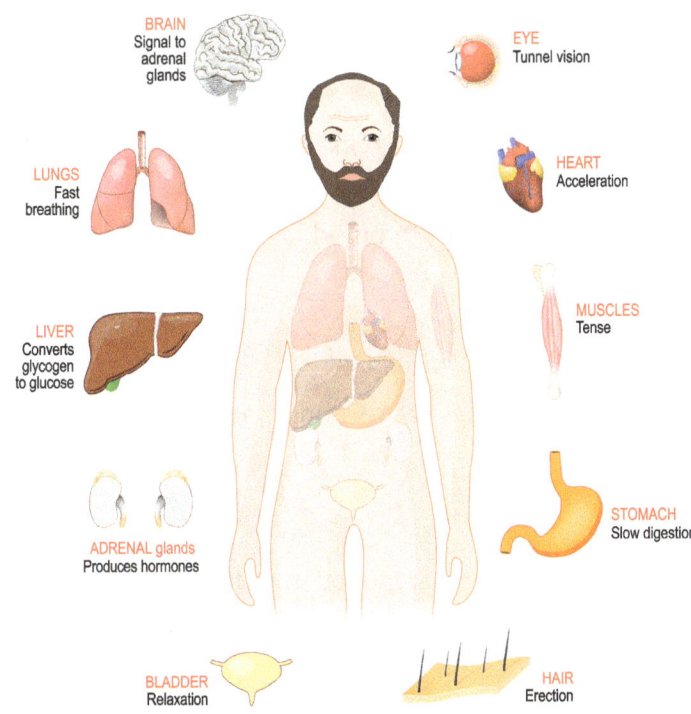

What happens in the body during the fight or flight response

- Breakdown of energy stores: Adrenaline promotes the breakdown of glycogen in the liver and muscles, releasing glucose into the bloodstream to be used in respiration to release energy.

- Increased blood clotting: Adrenaline helps to prepare the body for potential injuries by promoting blood clotting.
- Reduced sensitivity to pain: Adrenaline can temporarily reduce the sensation of pain, allowing individuals to focus on the task at hand.

Regulation of blood pressure

The adrenal glands also play a role in maintaining blood pressure.

The **adrenal cortex**, the outer layer of the adrenal gland, produces a hormone called **aldosterone**. Aldosterone is a key hormone in regulating blood pressure by influencing the body's sodium levels and water balance.

When blood pressure decreases, specialised cells in the kidneys detect the change and signal the adrenal glands to increase aldosterone production. Aldosterone acts on the kidneys, mainly in the distal convoluted tubules and collecting ducts, where it promotes the reabsorption of sodium ions from the filtrate back into the bloodstream. As sodium is reabsorbed, water is also taken up, leading to an increase in blood volume and ultimately, blood pressure.

When blood pressure increases, aldosterone secretion is reduced, allowing more sodium and water to remain in the kidney filtrate, leading to a decrease in blood volume and blood pressure.

> Metabolic rate – The rate at which the body uses energy to carry out its vital functions, such as breathing, circulating blood, and maintaining body temperature.
>
> Protein synthesis – The process by which cells build proteins from individual amino acids, following instructions encoded in DNA.
>
> Physiological – The normal functions and processes of living organisms, including physical and chemical changes within the body.

Recap questions

1. Which two hormones are primarily responsible for regulating blood glucose levels?
2. Which cells in the pancreas produce insulin?
3. What happens to blood glucose levels after a meal?
4. What is the primary role of glucagon in blood glucose regulation?
5. Which glands are responsible for releasing adrenaline?
6. What is one way adrenaline helps the body prepare for potential injuries?
7. Which hormone produced by the adrenal cortex regulates blood pressure?
8. How does aldosterone influence blood pressure?
9. What happens to aldosterone secretion when blood pressure increases?

Practice questions

1. State the primary function of the hypothalamus in the endocrine system. [1 mark]
2. Name the hormone produced by the testes which is responsible for male sexual development. [1 mark]
3. Describe the role of insulin in regulating blood glucose levels. [3 marks]
4. Explain how the endocrine system contributes to the fight-or-flight response. [4 marks]
5. Discuss the role of the endocrine system in osmoregulation. [6 marks]
6. Explain how the endocrine system contributes to growth and development.

B5 The musculoskeletal system

The musculoskeletal system is made up of bones, muscles, tendons, ligaments, and cartilage that provides structure, support, and movement to the human body. It acts as a framework, allowing us to stand upright, walk, run, and perform countless other activities. The musculoskeletal system works with the nervous system to coordinate movement and maintain posture.

B5.1 How the musculoskeletal system enables movement and provides support and structure

Ligaments

Ligaments are tough, fibrous bands of connective tissue that provide stability, support, and structure to the musculoskeletal system. They connect bones to bones to hold the skeleton together.

While ligaments provide stability, they also allow for flexibility, enabling a wide range of movements. For example, the ligaments in the knee joint allow for bending, straightening, and twisting, while also preventing excessive movement that could lead to injury. The ligaments in the shoulder joint provide stability for the shoulder joint, but also allow for a wide range of arm movements, including abduction, adduction, rotation, and flexion.

Tendons

Tendons connect muscles to bones, allowing muscles to exert force and produce movement. Tendons are typically composed of dense, fibrous tissue that is highly resistant to tension.

Tendons allow muscles to transmit their force to the skeleton. This allows us to perform a wide range of movements, from walking and running to lifting heavy objects and playing sports. Tendons also help to stabilise joints and prevent excessive movement that could lead to injury.

Cartilage

Cartilage provides support, structure, and flexibility to the musculoskeletal system. Cartilage is a tough yet flexible tissue that can withstand significant forces without breaking.

Cartilage is found in various parts of the body, including joints, the nose, the ears, the trachea, and the **intervertebral discs** (between the vertebrae). In joints, cartilage acts as a cushion, reducing friction between bones and preventing wear and tear. It also provides stability and flexibility, allowing for smooth and efficient movement.

Bone

Bones form the rigid framework of the human body, providing structural support, protection for vital organs, and a surface for muscle attachment. They are composed of a hard, mineralised **matrix** (scaffolding) that gives them strength and rigidity. Bones act as anchors for muscles, allowing them to exert force and produce movement.

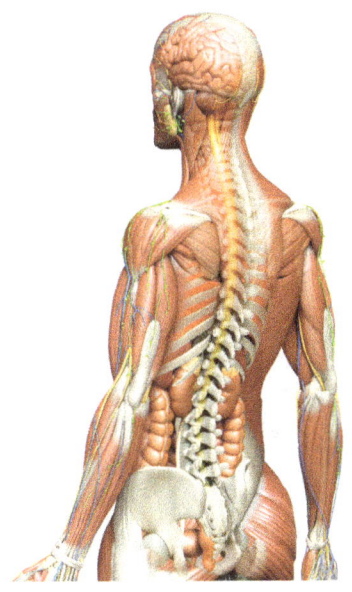

Bones are classified into two main types: long bones, such as the femur and tibia, which are longer than they are wide; and short bones, such as the carpals and tarsals, which are roughly cube shaped. Long bones provide support and leverage for movement, while short bones provide stability and support in areas like the hands and feet.

Recap questions

1. What are ligaments made of?
2. What is the primary function of ligaments?
3. What is the difference between ligaments and tendons?
4. What is cartilage?
5. Where in the body can cartilage be found?
6. What are the two main types of bones?

Types of muscle interactions

The human body relies on muscles to produce movement. Muscles often work in groups which allows them to achieve coordinated and controlled motion.

Three main types of muscle interactions are essential for movement: **antagonistic pairs**, **synergistic muscles**, and **fixator muscles**.

- **Antagonistic pairs:** These are muscles that work in opposition to each other. When one muscle contracts, its antagonist relaxes, allowing for controlled movement. For example, the biceps brachii and triceps brachii are antagonistic pairs in the arm. Contraction of the biceps brachii flexes the elbow, while contraction of the triceps brachii extends the elbow.

- **Synergistic muscles:** These are muscles that work together to produce a specific movement. Synergists can assist the primary mover, or agonist, in a movement, or they can help to stabilise a joint. For example, several muscles work together to flex the wrist, including the flexor carpi radialis, flexor carpi ulnaris, and palmaris longus.

- **Fixator muscles:** these are muscles that stabilise a joint or body part while other muscles produce movement. For example, when lifting a heavy object, the muscles of the shoulder girdle act as fixators, stabilising the shoulder joint and preventing unwanted movement. This allows the muscles of the arm to focus on lifting the object.

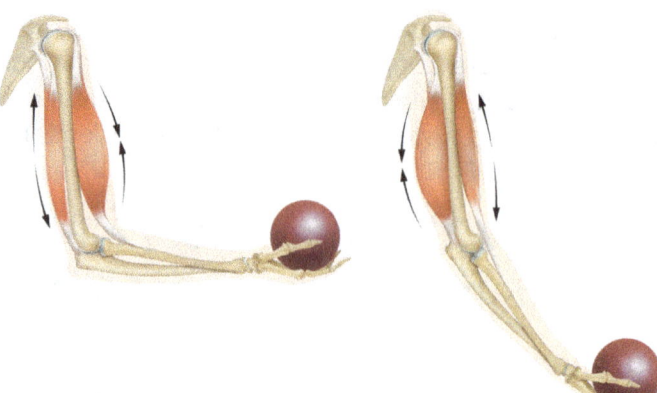

The biceps and triceps are an antagonistic pair

Fibrous joints

Fibrous joints are those that are held together by collagen fibres. These joints are characterised by their lack of movement or very limited mobility. They provide stability and support to the body by firmly connecting bones together.

While fibrous joints do not allow for much movement, they play an essential role in providing structural support and protecting vital organs. For example, the sutures of the skull protect the brain, while the fibrous joint between the tibia and fibula provides stability to the ankle.

Cartilaginous joints

Cartilaginous joints are joints that are held together by cartilage. These joints allow for a limited amount of movement, making them more flexible than **fibrous joints** but less mobile than **synovial joints**.

They are found in areas of the body that require both stability and flexibility, such as the intervertebral discs and the pubic symphysis (the joint which connects the two pubic bones in the pelvis). The fibrocartilage in these joints provides cushioning and allows for a limited amount of movement, such as bending and twisting.

Synovial joints

Synovial joints are the most movable type of joint in the human body. They are characterised by a fluid-filled joint cavity, cartilage, a synovial membrane, and ligaments. Synovial joints are surrounded by a fibrous capsule that provides stability and support.

Within the joint cavity, cartilage covers the ends of the bones, providing a smooth, low-friction surface for movement. **Synovial fluid**, produced by the synovial membrane, nourishes the cartilage and removes waste products. Ligaments and tendons also play a role in stabilising synovial joints and limiting excessive movement.

Synovial joints are responsible for a wide range of movements, including flexion, extension, abduction, adduction, rotation, and circumduction. They are found in most of the major joints in the body, such as the shoulder, elbow, wrist, hip, knee, and ankle.

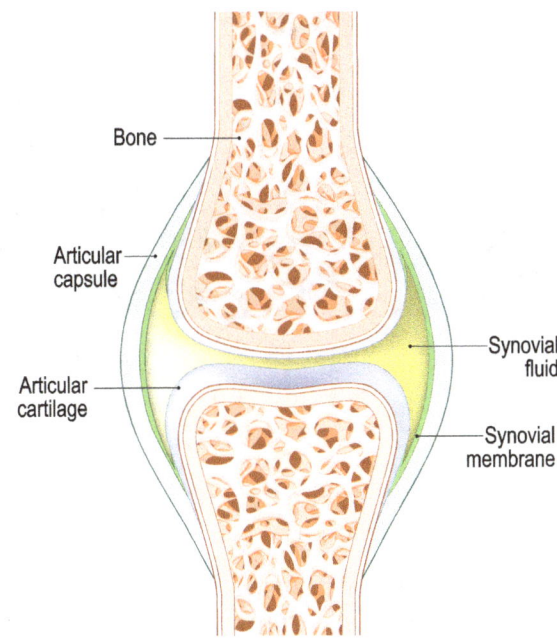

The structure of synovial joints

Recap questions

1. What are two functions of bones?
2. What type of tissue connects bones in fibrous joints?
3. What is the primary characteristic of fibrous joints in terms of movement?
4. How are cartilaginous joints held together?
5. What is the most movable type of joint in the human body?
6. What are the key features of a synovial joint?
7. What type of movement do synovial joints allow?

Practice questions

1. Identify the type of joint which provides the least amount of movement. [1 mark]

   A cartilaginous
   B fibrous
   C synovial
   D rotator

2. Identify the function of tendons. [1 mark]

   A to connect bone to bone
   B to connect muscle to bone
   C to cushion the joint
   D to prevent movement

3. Describe the role of antagonistic muscle pairs in producing movement. Give an example of an antagonistic muscle pair. [4 marks]

4. Explain the importance of cartilage in the musculoskeletal system. [4 marks]

5. Discuss the different types of joints found in the human body, highlighting their key characteristics and functions. [6 marks]

6. Explain how muscles work together to produce coordinated movement. [6 marks]

B6 The function of further body systems

B6.1 Additional body systems and how they link to other systems

Beyond the musculoskeletal, nervous, endocrine, and circulatory systems, there are several other essential systems that work together to maintain life and health. The immune system defends against pathogens, the lymphatic system circulates fluid and aids in immunity, the reproductive system ensures the continuation of the species, and the digestive system processes food for energy and nutrients.

B6.1.1 Immune system

The immune system is the body's defence mechanism, responsible for protecting against **pathogens** (disease-causing microorganisms) such as bacteria, viruses, fungi, and parasites. Its various components work together to identify and eliminate pathogens.

The immune system consists of two main components: the **innate immune system** and the **adaptive immune system**.

- The **innate immune system** is the body's first line of defence, providing a rapid but non-specific response to pathogens. It includes **physical barriers** like the skin and mucous membranes, as well as cells such as neutrophils, macrophages, and natural killer cells.
- The **adaptive immune system** is a slower but more **specific** response that develops over time. It involves the production of antibodies and T cells, which can recognise and target specific pathogens.

White blood cells (**leukocytes**) are a major part of the immune response. There are different types, each with its own specific functions.

- **Neutrophils** are the most common type of white blood cell and are crucial for fighting bacterial infections. **Macrophages** are large white blood cells that engulf and destroy pathogens. **Natural killer cells** are specialised white blood cells that can kill virus-infected cells and cancer cells.
- **Antibodies** are proteins produced by B cells, a type of white blood cell. They bind to **antigens**, which are foreign proteins on the surface of pathogens. This binding helps to neutralise pathogens and mark them for destruction by other immune cells.

The immune system works alongside other body systems. For example, the **lymphatic system**, which is responsible for draining fluid from tissues and transporting immune cells, plays a role in the immune response. The **circulatory system** is involved as it transports immune cells and antibodies throughout the body, allowing them to reach sites of infection or inflammation. The digestive system also interacts with the immune system, as it is a potential entry point for pathogens and therefore produces **hydrochloric acid** in the stomach to kill them.

While the musculoskeletal system is primarily associated with movement and support, it also plays a role in the immune response. The **bone marrow**, a soft tissue found within bones, is the primary site of blood cell production, including immune cells such as lymphocytes and neutrophils. These cells are essential for fighting infections and other immune responses.

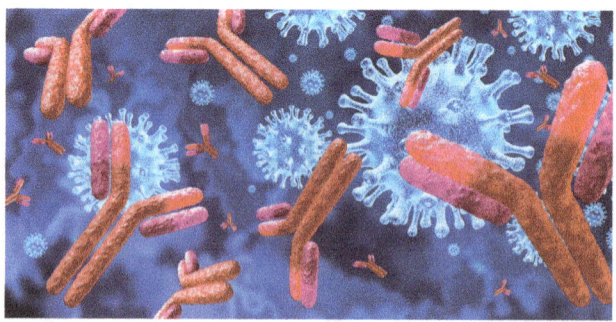

Antibodies

Recap questions

1. What is the primary function of the immune system?
2. What are the two main components of the immune system?
3. What are white blood cells, and what is their role in the immune response?
4. What are antibodies, and how do they help fight infections?
5. How does the lymphatic system interact with the immune system?
6. What is the role of the musculoskeletal system in the immune response?

Lymphatic system

The **lymphatic system** is a network of vessels, nodes, and organs that play a role in the body's immune function and fluid balance. It serves as a drainage system, collecting excess fluid (lymph) from tissues and returning it to the bloodstream. This helps to prevent swelling.

The lymphatic system works closely with the circulatory system.

- **Lymphatic vessels** are similar to blood vessels and transport **lymphatic fluid** throughout the body.
- **Lymphatic nodes**, located along the lymphatic vessels, act as filters, trapping and destroying pathogens and debris (cellular waste).

The lymphatic system also plays a crucial role in the immune response by transporting immune cells and antibodies to areas of infection or **inflammation**.

The lymphatic system interacts with the immune system, as lymph nodes are important sites for immune cell activity.

Additionally, the lymphatic system works with the digestive system, as it plays a role in the absorption of fats in the small intestine. Fatty acids and glycerol are first absorbed into lymphatic vessels before being transported to the bloodstream.

Reproductive system

While the male and female reproductive systems have distinct structures and functions, they share the common goal of producing **gametes** (sperm and eggs) and facilitating fertilisation.

Male reproductive system

The male reproductive system is designed to produce sperm and deliver them to the female reproductive system during sexual intercourse. It consists of several key organs, including the **penis** and **testes**.

The testes are two oval-shaped organs located in the **scrotum**, a sac of skin that hangs outside the body. They are responsible for producing **sperm**, which are the male reproductive cells. The testes also produce **testosterone**, a hormone that controls male sexual development and function.

The **penis** is the male organ of sexual intercourse. It contains the urethra, a tube that carries sperm and urine out of the body. During sexual arousal, the penis becomes erect, allowing for the delivery of sperm into the vagina.

Female reproductive system

The female reproductive system is designed to produce eggs, receive sperm, and grow the developing foetus. It consists of several key components, including the **breasts, uterus, ovaries,** and **vagina**.

The breasts are **mammary glands** that produce milk to nourish a newborn baby. They are made up of glandular tissue and fatty tissue.

The uterus, also known as the womb, is the organ where the developing **foetus** grows. It is lined with a tissue called the **endometrium**, which thickens and prepares for implantation of a **fertilised egg** during the menstrual cycle.

The ovaries are two small organs located on either side of the uterus. They produce eggs and hormones, including **oestrogen** and **progesterone**, which regulate the menstrual cycle and pregnancy.

The vagina is a muscular tube that connects the uterus to the outside of the body. It serves as the passageway for sperm during sexual intercourse and for the delivery of a baby.

The reproductive systems work alongside other body systems. For example, the pituitary gland in the endocrine system produces some of the reproductive hormones. **FSH** and **LH** are hormones produced by the pituitary gland which control oestrogen secretion and ovulation. The circulatory system transports hormones throughout the body. The nervous

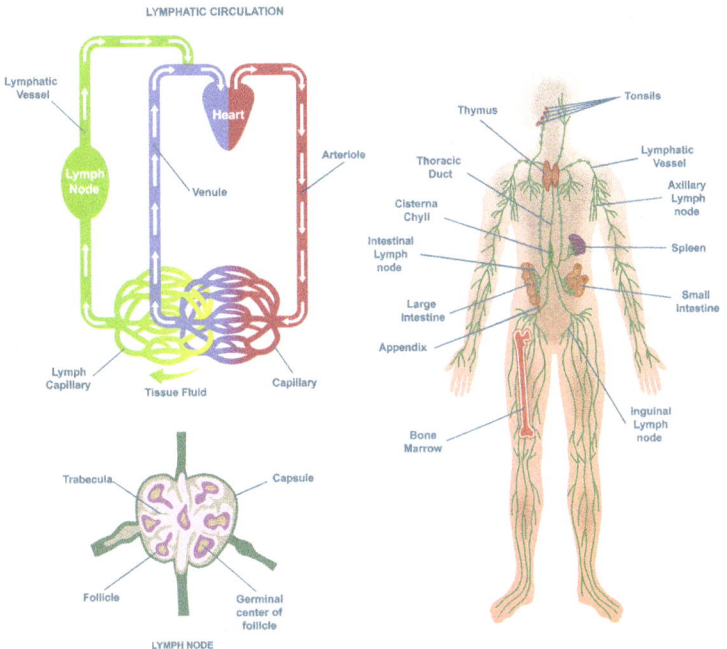

The lymphatic system

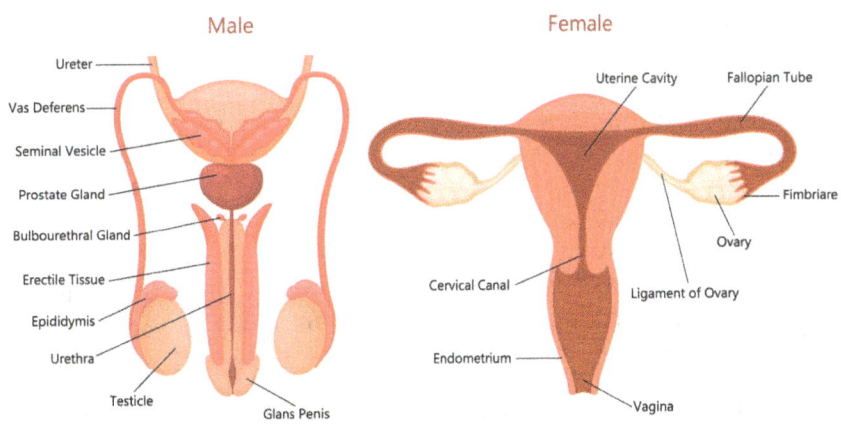

The reproductive system

system controls the physiological processes involved in reproduction, such as sexual arousal and childbirth. Additionally, the immune system plays a role in protecting the reproductive organs and preventing infections.

Digestive system

The digestive system is responsible for breaking down food into smaller soluble molecules that the body can absorb and use for energy and growth. This process, known as digestion, involves a series of mechanical and chemical processes that occur along the alimentary canal.

The alimentary canal is a long, muscular tube that extends from the mouth to the anus. It includes:

- The **oesophagus** is a muscular tube that transports food from the mouth to the stomach.
- The **stomach** is a muscular sac that stores and breaks down food using gastric juices (hydrochloric acid and a protease enzyme called pepsin).
- The **duodenum** is the first part of the small intestine, where most of the digestion and absorption of nutrients occurs.
- The **ileum** is the final part of the small intestine, where the remaining nutrients are absorbed.
- The **colon**, or **large intestine**, absorbs water and electrolytes before the waste material is eliminated from the body.

Accessory organs, like the liver, pancreas, gallbladder, and salivary glands, also play important roles in digestion:

- The **liver** produces **bile**, which emulsifies fats (breaks them up into smaller droplets to increase the surface area). The increased surface area then allows lipase enzyme to break the fats down faster.
- The **pancreas** produces digestive **enzymes** (lipase, proteases and carbohydrates) that aid in the breakdown of fats, proteins, and carbohydrates.
- The **gallbladder** stores bile and releases it into the small intestine when needed.

Recap questions

1. What is the primary function of the lymphatic system?
2. How does the lymphatic system help prevent swelling?
3. What are lymphatic nodes, and what is their role in the immune system?
4. How does the lymphatic system interact with the circulatory system?
5. How does the lymphatic system interact with the digestive system?
6. What role do lymphatic vessels play in the transport of fats?
7. What is the primary function of both the male and female reproductive systems?
8. What are the male sex organs responsible for producing sperm?
9. What hormone is responsible for controlling male sexual development?

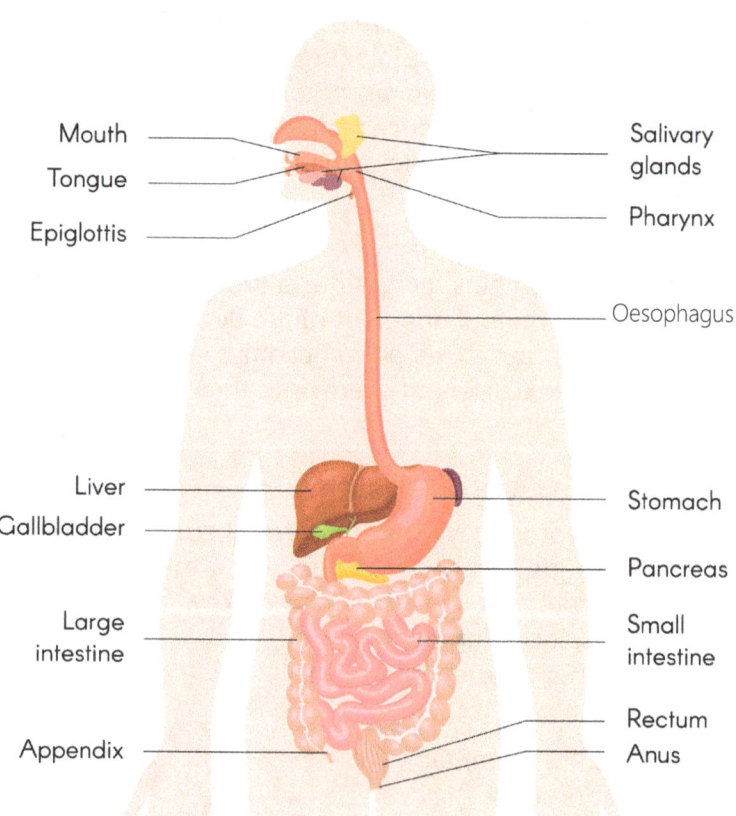

The human digestive system

- The salivary glands produce saliva, which contains an enzyme (amylase) that begins the breakdown of carbohydrates.

The digestive system is closely linked to other body systems. For example, the nervous system controls the movement of food through the digestive tract and regulates the secretion of digestive enzymes. The circulatory system transports nutrients absorbed from the digestive system to other parts of the body. The endocrine system produces hormones that regulate appetite, digestion, and metabolism. And the immune system plays a role in protecting the digestive tract from pathogens.

Recap questions

1. What is the primary function of the uterus?
2. Which organs produce female sex hormones?
3. What is the role of the vagina in the female reproductive system?
4. What is the function of the digestive system?
5. What is the alimentary canal?
6. Which organ is responsible for the production of bile?
7. What is the role of the pancreas in digestion?
8. What is the function of saliva in digestion?
9. How does the nervous system interact with the digestive system?

Apply your understanding

Mr Jones is a 55-year-old man. He recently underwent a cholecystectomy, a surgical procedure to remove his gallbladder. Without the gallbladder, bile is released directly into the small intestine, which can sometimes lead to digestive issues.

He has been experiencing some digestive discomfort since the surgery, including occasional bouts of diarrhoea and mild abdominal cramps, particularly after consuming fatty foods.

2. State the function of the gallbladder in digestion. (1 mark)
3. Describe the role of bile in fat digestion. (2 marks)
4. Describe how the removal of the gallbladder affects the flow of bile. (2 marks)
5. Explain why Mr Jones might be experiencing diarrhoea after his gallbladder removal. (3 marks)
6. Discuss what dietary changes Mr Jones could consider to alleviate his digestive symptoms. (3 marks)

Practice questions

1. Identify the organ in the picture on the right which produces bile. [1 mark]
2. Describe the role of the lymphatic system in the immune response. [3 marks]
3. Describe the key functions of the male reproductive system. [3 marks]
4. Discuss the interactions between the digestive system and other body systems. [6 marks]
5. Describe the process of digestion, including the key organs and enzymes involved. [6 marks]

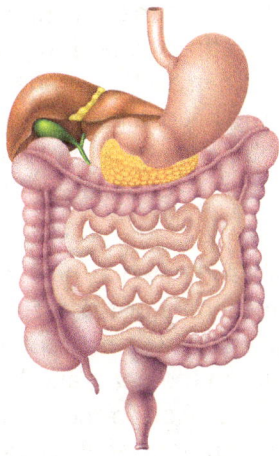

Learning Aim C: Disorders of the body and the effect on body systems

C1 The main disorders of the body systems

In this topic you will learn about the main disorders of the body systems. You will also learn about the primary and secondary effects the disorders have on the body systems.

- coronary heart disease
- stroke
- chronic obstructive pulmonary disorder – emphysema and chronic bronchitis
- asthma
- diabetes – type 1 and type 2
- dementia
- acquired brain injury: traumatic and non-traumatic
- cancer: breast, bowel, and lung

C1.1 Coronary heart disease

Coronary heart disease (CHD) is a leading cause of death worldwide. It occurs when the arteries that supply blood to the heart become narrowed or blocked by a buildup of **plaque**. This buildup, known as **atherosclerosis**, can lead to a heart attack or stroke if the blood flow to the heart is significantly reduced or cut off entirely.

Causes of CHD

Two of the most significant causes of coronary heart disease (CHD) are atherosclerosis and hypertension.

Atherosclerosis occurs when plaque, a substance composed of cholesterol, fatty substances, cellular waste products, calcium, and fibrin, builds up in the **coronary arteries** (the arteries that supply blood to the heart). This buildup can narrow the arteries, reducing blood flow to the heart muscle. Over time, the plaque can rupture, leading to blood clots that can block the arteries completely, causing a heart attack.

Hypertension, also known as high blood pressure, is another major risk factor for CHD. When blood pressure is consistently raised, it puts extra strain on the heart and blood vessels. This can lead to damage to the artery walls and lead to the development of atherosclerosis. Additionally, high blood pressure can increase the risk of blood clots forming in the coronary arteries.

Primary effects of CHD

Coronary heart disease (CHD) can have a variety of serious consequences:

Heart Attack: A heart attack occurs when a coronary artery becomes completely blocked, cutting off blood flow to a portion of the heart muscle. This can cause chest pain, shortness of breath, sweating, nausea, and vomiting. If the blockage is not treated promptly, it can lead to heart muscle damage or death.

Angina: Angina is a condition characterised by chest pain or discomfort that occurs when the heart muscle does not receive enough oxygen. This can happen when the coronary arteries become narrowed, reducing blood flow to the heart. Angina can be a warning sign of a heart attack.

Heart Failure: Heart failure occurs when the heart muscle is unable to pump enough blood to meet the body's needs. This can be caused by damage to the heart muscle due to a heart attack or other conditions. Heart failure can lead to shortness of breath, fatigue, and swelling in the legs and ankles.

Secondary effects of CHD

In addition to the primary effects of coronary heart disease (CHD), there are also several secondary effects that can occur. These secondary effects can significantly impact a person's quality of life and daily activities.

- **Shortness of Breath:** Shortness of breath is a common symptom of CHD, especially when the heart muscle is weakened or unable to pump blood efficiently. It can be caused by a variety of factors, such as fluid buildup in the lungs or decreased blood flow to the heart.

- **Dizziness:** Dizziness can be another symptom of CHD, particularly if the heart is unable to pump enough blood to the brain. This can lead to a decrease in blood pressure and reduced oxygen supply to the brain.

- **Nausea and Vomiting:** Nausea and vomiting can occur in some individuals with CHD, especially during or after a heart attack. When the heart doesn't work properly, fluid can build up in the liver and stomach, which can cause nausea and loss of appetite. This is because blood is being diverted away from the digestive system.

NORMAL FUNCTIONS

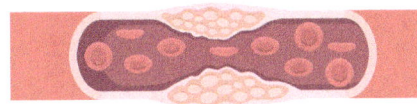

CHOLESTEROL PLAQUE FORMATION

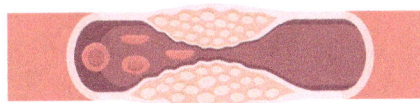

COMPLETE BLOCKAGE

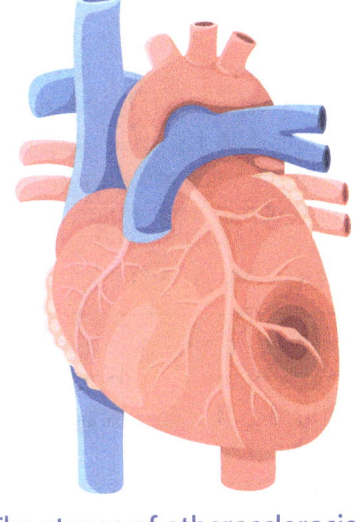

The stages of atherosclerosis

Body systems affected

Coronary heart disease (CHD) can have far-reaching effects on the body, impacting not only the cardiovascular system but also other vital organs and systems.

Cardiovascular System: The primary impact of CHD is on the cardiovascular system itself. Reduced blood flow to the heart muscle can lead to heart failure, **arrhythmias** (irregular heart rhythms), and sudden cardiac death. CHD can increase the risk of stroke, as blood clots can break off from the heart and travel to the brain.

Respiratory System: CHD can also affect the respiratory system. When the heart is unable to pump blood efficiently, it can lead to fluid buildup in the lungs, a condition known as **pulmonary oedema**. This can cause shortness of breath, difficulty breathing, and even respiratory failure.

Digestive System: CHD can impact the digestive system in several ways. Reduced blood flow to the digestive organs can lead to decreased digestive function and symptoms such as nausea, vomiting, and loss of appetite.

Recap questions

1. What are the two main causes of coronary heart disease (CHD)?
2. What is plaque made up of?
3. What are the common symptoms of a heart attack?
4. What is angina, and what causes it?
5. What are some common symptoms of heart failure?
6. Which other body systems can be impacted by CHD?
7. What is pulmonary oedema, and how is it related to CHD?
8. How can CHD affect the digestive system?
9. How can CHD increase the risk of stroke?

C1.2 Stroke

Strokes are a serious neurological condition that occur when blood flow to the brain is interrupted or reduced. This can lead to damage to brain cells and a range of symptoms, from mild to severe.

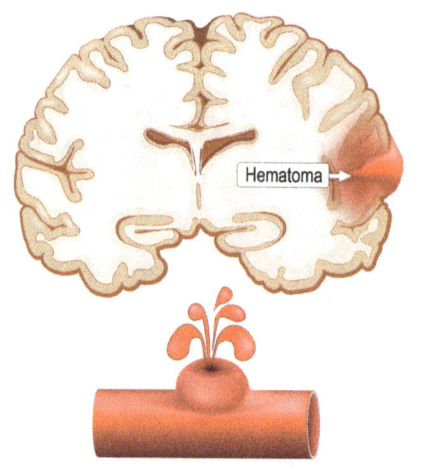
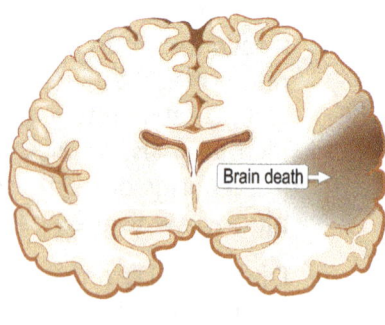

Causes of strokes

Strokes occur when blood flow to the brain is interrupted or reduced. This can happen in two main ways:

Ischaemic stroke: This is the most common type of stroke and occurs when a blood vessel that supplies blood to the brain becomes blocked. This blockage can be caused by a blood clot (**thrombosis**) or an **embolus** (a clot that travels from another part of the body to the brain). When a blood vessel is blocked, the brain tissue beyond the blockage becomes deprived of oxygen and nutrients, leading to cell death.

Haemorrhagic stroke: This type of stroke occurs when a blood vessel in the brain bursts and bleeds. This can be caused by a variety of factors, including high blood pressure, aneurysms, and blood clotting disorders. When a blood vessel ruptures, the blood leaks into the brain tissue which can put pressure on brain tissue and cause damage to brain cells.

The two main types of strokes: haemorrhagic stroke (left) and ischaemic stroke (right)

Aneurysm – A bulging, weakened area in the wall of a blood vessel, like a balloon.

Primary effects of strokes

Strokes can have a wide range of effects on the brain, depending on the location and severity of the damage. Some of the primary effects of strokes include:

- **Brain damage**: When blood flow to the brain is interrupted, brain cells can become damaged or die. This damage can lead to neurological problems, including weakness or paralysis, difficulty speaking or understanding language, and changes in vision.

- **Bleeding**: In haemorrhagic strokes, bleeding into the brain can cause significant damage to brain tissue. The pressure from the blood can compress brain cells and disrupt their function.

- **Clotting**: In ischaemic strokes, blood clots can block blood flow to the brain, leading to tissue damage. The clots can also break off and travel to other parts of the brain, causing multiple strokes.

The specific effects of a stroke that a patient will experience will depend on the location of the brain damage. For example, a stroke in the left hemisphere of the brain may affect language and speech, while a stroke in the right hemisphere may affect spatial awareness and problem-solving.

Secondary effects of strokes

Strokes can have a wide range of effects on the body, both physically and mentally. In addition to the primary effects of brain damage, bleeding, and clotting, strokes can also cause a number of secondary effects. These secondary effects can significantly impact a person's quality of life and daily activities:

- **Muscle weakness**: strokes can cause muscle weakness or paralysis, particularly on one side of the body. This can make it difficult to perform daily activities such as walking, dressing, or eating and can lead to a loss of independence.

- **Lack of coordination**: Strokes can also affect coordination, making it difficult to perform tasks that require fine motor skills, such as writing or buttoning clothes.

- **Dysphasia**: Dysphasia is a language disorder that can occur after a stroke. It can affect a person's ability to understand or express language, making communication difficult.

- **Increased risk of respiratory infections**: Strokes can increase the risk of respiratory infections, such as pneumonia, due to weakened muscles involved in breathing and swallowing. This can lead to pneumonia and other complications.

These secondary effects can vary widely depending on the severity and location of the stroke. Over time, with appropriate rehabilitation, many individuals who have experienced a stroke can regain some or all of their lost functions. However, some individuals may continue to experience long-term effects that can impact their daily lives.

Body systems affected by strokes

Strokes can also have consequences on other body systems:

- **Cardiovascular System:** Strokes can increase the risk of future cardiovascular events, such as heart attacks and strokes. This is because the underlying conditions that contribute to stroke, such as high blood pressure and atherosclerosis, can also increase the risk of heart disease. Additionally, strokes can damage the heart muscle, leading to heart failure or arrhythmias.

- **Nervous System:** Beyond the initial brain damage caused by the stroke, the nervous system can experience other effects. Strokes can disrupt the communication pathways between the brain and other parts of the body, leading to problems with sensation, movement, and coordination. This can lead to long-term neurological consequences, such as changes in mood, personality, and cognitive function. The nervous system also controls other bodily functions, so damage to the brain can impact everything from bladder control to swallowing.

- **Musculoskeletal System:** Strokes can cause muscle weakness or paralysis, particularly on one side of the body. This can lead to difficulties with movement, balance, and coordination. Over time, the affected muscles may atrophy due to lack of use, further impacting mobility. Additionally, the nervous system controls the muscles, so damage to the brain can disrupt muscle function and coordination.

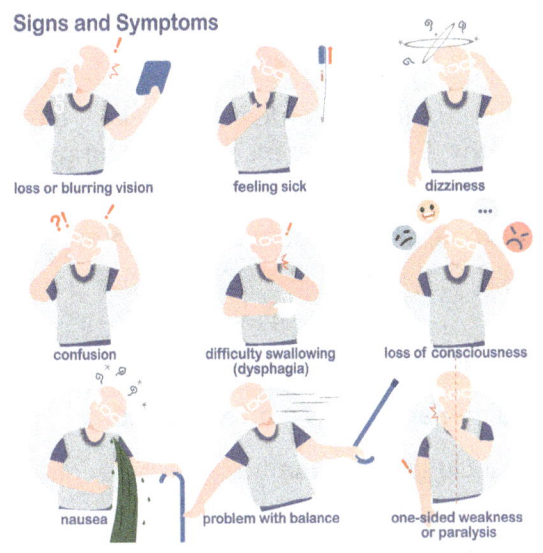

Signs and symptoms of a stroke

Recap questions

1. What is the primary cause of a stroke?
2. What are the two main types of stroke?
3. What are the primary effects of a stroke on the brain?
4. How does clotting affect the brain in an ischaemic stroke?
5. What are some neurological consequences of a stroke beyond the initial brain damage?
6. How can a stroke impact the musculoskeletal system?
7. How can a stroke increase the risk of future cardiovascular events?

C1.3 Chronic obstructive pulmonary disorder

Chronic obstructive pulmonary disorder (COPD) is a group of lung disorders that make it hard to breathe. COPD happens when the lungs become damaged.

- Chronic means that it is a long-term disorder which gets worse over time.
- Obstructive means that it is restricting the movement of air in and out of the lungs.
- Pulmonary means it affects the lungs.

COPD includes the conditions emphysema and chronic bronchitis.

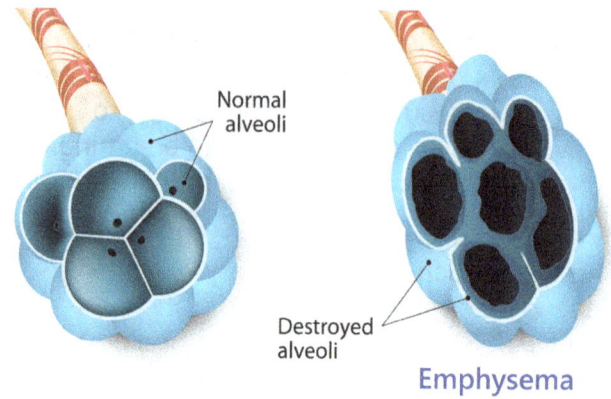

Emphysema

Causes of COPD

COPD is caused by long-term exposure to breathing in harmful substances. The main causes are:

- smoking cigarettes, and
- breathing in harmful substances, like pollution or chemicals.

Over time, these substances irritate the lungs, causing damage. COPD is a serious condition which gets worse over time.

- **Emphysema** develops when cigarette smoke damages the walls of tiny air sacs in the lungs called **alveoli**. The alveoli normally fill with air when we breathe in and deflate when we breathe out. Because of the damage, the walls of the alveoli break down, enlarging the alveoli and making them an uneven shape. This makes the alveoli less effective in exchanging gases. As a result, less oxygen is transferred into the blood, which means cells and organs do not get enough oxygen to work well.

- **Chronic bronchitis** develops when your airways (**trachea**, **bronchi**, and **bronchioles**) become permanently inflamed. The airways become swollen which make them narrower. In addition, the airways start to produce large amounts of **mucus**. This makes it harder to get air into and out of the lungs and leaves the person feeling out of breath.

People with COPD often have damage to both their alveoli and airways, so will show symptoms of both emphysema and chronic bronchitis.

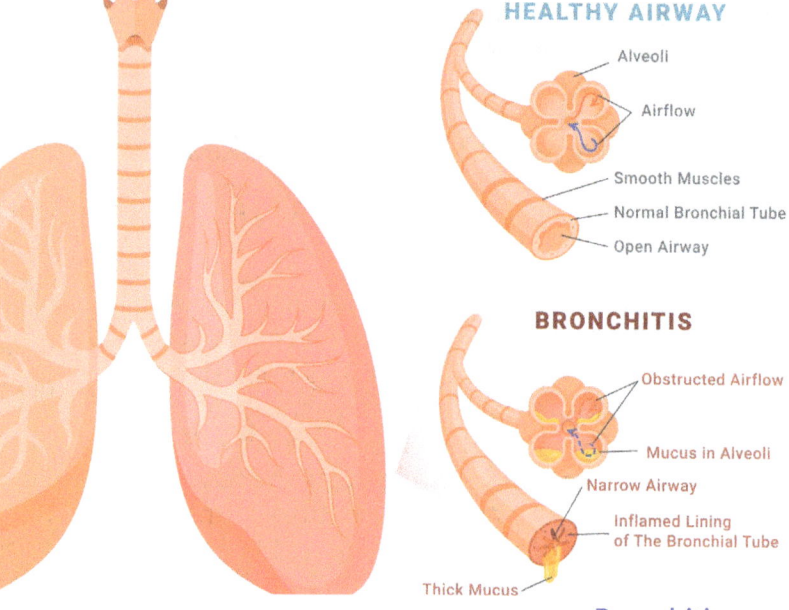

Bronchitis

C1.2.2 Primary effects of COPD

The most common symptoms of COPD are:

- a persistent cough
- large amounts of mucus
- being out of breath
- feeling tired
- wheezing
- frequent chest infections
- increased heart rate.

A persistent cough is one of the first symptoms of COPD. 'Persistent' means that the cough lasts for a long period of time. Coughing is the way in which our airways try to clear out mucus. People with COPD cough a lot because their airways continually make too much mucus.

The large amount of mucus clogs the airways,

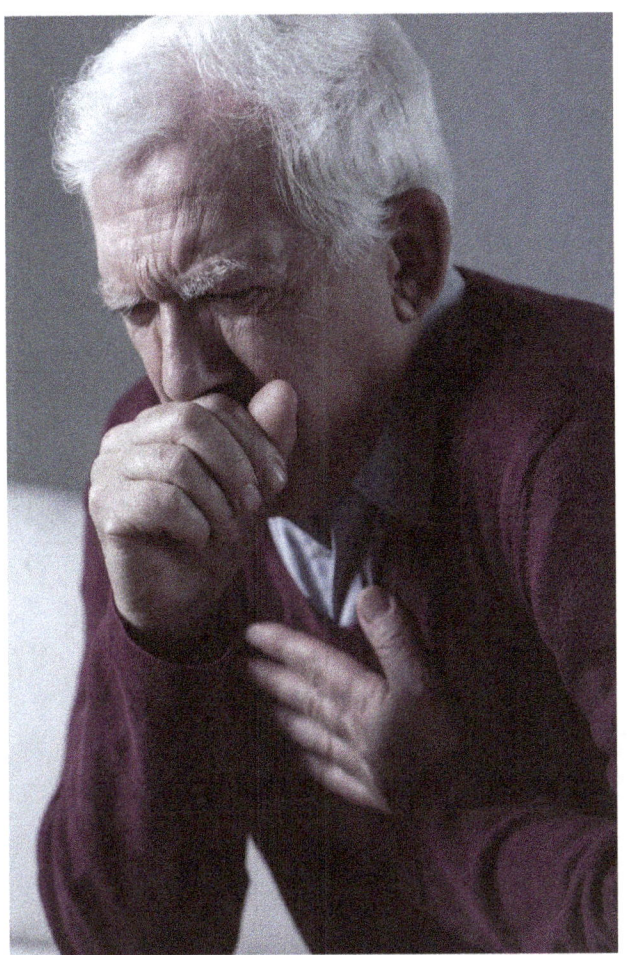

making it harder for air to move in or out. Inflammation in the airways also makes them narrower. The narrowing of the airways makes it much harder to move air in and out of the lungs. People with COPD have trouble breathing, especially when they are active. This can also make them feel tired as they are not delivering enough oxygen to their muscles.

Wheezing is a whistling sound that happens when breathing. It happens when the airways are inflamed or blocked with mucus. The air that is being inhaled (or exhaled) is being forced through a narrower space. This creates the whistling, or wheezing, sound.

The mucus in the airways also traps **pathogens** (microorganisms that cause disease). The mucus is an ideal breeding ground for bacteria and viruses, which can cause infections in the lungs and chest. People with COPD will often have frequent chest infections like **pneumonia**.

Because people with COPD have difficulty breathing, the lungs have trouble getting enough oxygen into the blood. This means less oxygen reaches the body's tissues and organs. When the body detects low oxygen levels, it

Recap questions

1. What does the term 'chronic' mean in the context of COPD?
2. What are the two main conditions that are associated with COPD?
3. What is the primary cause of COPD?
4. What is the name of the tiny air sacs in the lungs that are damaged in emphysema?
5. What is the main symptom of chronic bronchitis?
6. What is one of the first symptoms of COPD?
7. What causes a persistent cough in people with COPD?
8. What is wheezing and how does it occur in COPD?
9. Why are people with COPD more prone to chest infections?
10. How does COPD affect heart rate?
11. What is the main consequence of reduced oxygen levels in the body for people with COPD?
12. What is the main symptom of chronic bronchitis?

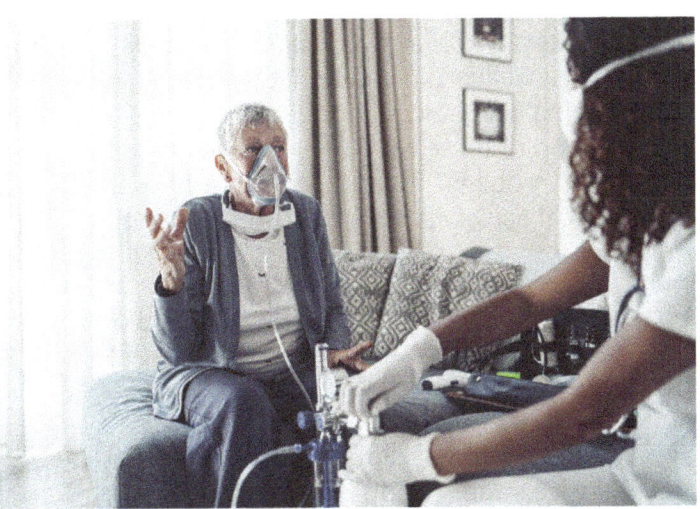

People with severe COPD may require oxygen to help them breathe

signals to the heart to beat faster. The **faster heart rate** pumps more oxygen-rich blood around the body. This is a natural response to try to deliver more oxygen to the tissues and organs.

Secondary effects of COPD

While COPD is a lung disorder, it also impacts on overall health and wellbeing. The secondary effects of COPD include:

- weight loss
- muscle weakness
- reduced mobility

All of these can affect daily functioning and lead to a poorer quality of life for individuals living with COPD.

Weight loss is common in people with COPD. Breathing with COPD uses a lot of energy, so your body burns more calories just to breathe. COPD can also make you feel less hungry because of inflammation in your body. This means you might not eat as much as you need to. Over time, if the calories you are eating are less than the calories you are burning, you can start losing weight.

As COPD makes it hard to breathe, especially after physical activity, people with COPD often become physically inactive. As there is less oxygen reaching the muscles, people with COPD will tire easily when trying to do physical activities. This often means that they will stop doing simple daily activities like walking. Over time, this makes their muscles weaker.

As the disorder progresses, people with COPD will often lose some of their mobility. This is due to a combination of factors. Shortness of breath means they are less likely to do physical activity. Less physical activity means that their muscles will weaken. In addition, they are experiencing weight loss and tiredness. The combination of these will make the person less likely to be mobile. This leads to a cycle of even less physical activity and further reduction in mobility.

Body systems affected by COPD

COPD is an inflammatory disease. As described above, COPD not only impacts the respiratory system but also the cardiovascular system, the digestive system, and the musculoskeletal system.

- **Respiratory system**: Long term exposure to harmful chemicals causes the airways to produce excess mucus. The airways (trachea, bronchi, and bronchioles) become inflamed and constrict. The alveoli become damaged and breakdown, reducing the

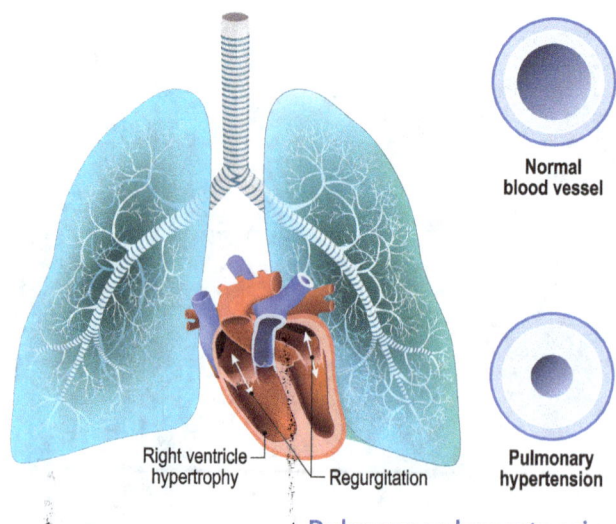

Pulmonary hypertension

surface area for gas exchange. Breathing becomes difficult and, as a result, less oxygen enters the blood stream.

- **Cardiovascular system**: COPD causes lower levels of oxygen in the blood, which causes the heart rate to increase. Over time, this can lead to a condition called **pulmonary hypertension**. Pulmonary hypertension is where the blood pressure in the **pulmonary artery** (the artery which carries blood from the heart to the lungs) becomes dangerously high. The extra strain on the heart can also cause the **right ventricle** to weaken, leading to heart failure.

The long-term inflammation caused by COPD can also cause the development of **atherosclerosis**, a condition where plaque builds up inside the **arteries**, restricting blood flow to the heart and to the brain. This increases the risk of cardiovascular disease like coronary artery disease, heart attack and strokes.

- **Digestive system**: The main impact of COPD on the digestive system is weight loss and malnutrition. The increased effort required to breathe can result in the individual burning more energy than they consume. People with COPD will often have a reduced appetite due to the impact of the inflammation and the medications they take for COPD. This will also contribute to their weight loss and malnutrition.

The chronic coughing due to COPD can also weaken the muscles that control the opening between the oesophagus and the stomach. If this opening becomes damaged, it can lead to a condition known as **gastroesophageal reflux disease (GERD)**. In people with GERD the

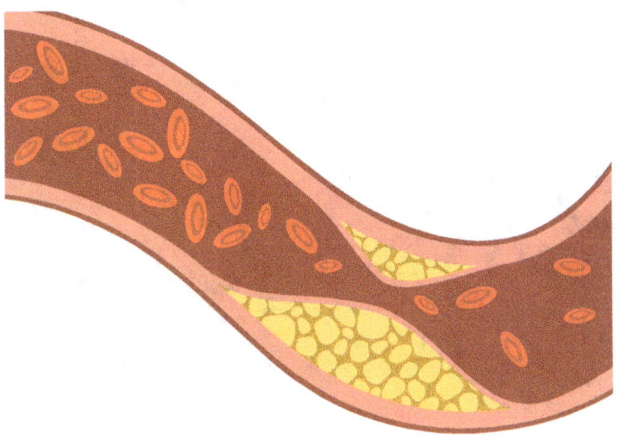

Atherosclerosis

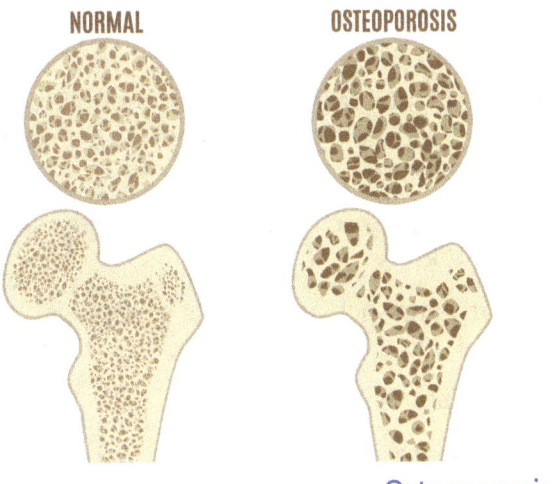

GERD is when stomach acid enters the oesopahgus

stomach acid can move into the oesophagus causing heartburn and damage to the oesophagus.

- **Musculoskeletal system**: The reduced lung function in COPD often leads to reduced physical activity. This can result in muscle weakness and over time the muscles start to **atrophy** (waste away). This will lead to even less physical activity and reduced mobility.

Reduced physical activity, poor nutrition and the use of steroid medication can lead to a decrease in bone density. This puts the individual at greater risk of developing osteoporosis and bone fractures.

Osteoporosis

Recap questions

1. What is one of the secondary effects of COPD on overall health?
2. How does COPD contribute to muscle weakness?
3. What is pulmonary hypertension and how is it related to COPD?
4. How does COPD increase the risk of cardiovascular disease?
5. What are the main digestive system issues associated with COPD?
6. What factors contribute to decreased bone density in individuals with COPD?

Practice questions

1. Explain how atherosclerosis contributes to the development of coronary heart disease. [3 marks]
2. Describe two secondary effects of CHD on the body. [2 marks]
3. Describe the primary effects of a stroke on the brain. [3 marks]
4. Explain how a stroke can affect the musculoskeletal system. [6 marks]
5. Describe the impact of COPD on the cardiovascular system. [3 marks]
6. Discuss the secondary effects of COPD on overall health and well-being. [5 marks]

C1.4 Asthma

Asthma is a chronic lung condition that is characterised by inflammation and narrowing of the airways, leading to wheezing, coughing, shortness of breath, and chest tightness. These symptoms can be triggered by various factors, including allergens, irritants, respiratory infections, and exercise.

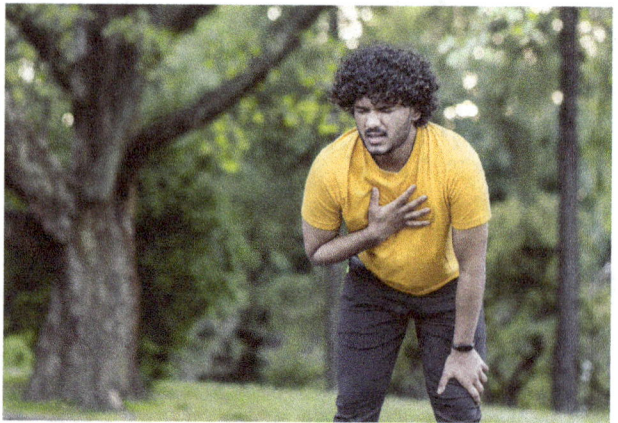

Causes of asthma

Asthma is caused by a combination of genetic and environmental factors. The genetic factors may make an individual more likely to have an exaggerated immune response to certain triggers, leading to inflammation and narrowing of the airways.

Environmental factors also play a significant role in the development of asthma. Common triggers include:

- **allergens** such as pollen, dust mites, and mould
- **irritants** such as cigarette smoke, air pollution, and strong odours (e.g. perfumes)
- respiratory **infections**
- **exercise**.

These triggers can cause inflammation and muscle spasms in the airways, leading to the symptoms of asthma. Being exposed to certain environmental pollutants (e.g. traffic fumes) during early childhood may also increase the risk of developing asthma.

Primary effects of asthma

The primary effects of asthma include:

- **Shortness of breath**: this is a common symptom of asthma, and it occurs when the airways become narrowed, making it difficult to breathe.
- **Wheezing**: a high-pitched whistling sound that occurs when air is forced through the narrowed airways.
- **Tight chest**.
- **Coughing**.

During an asthma attack, these symptoms can become severe and constant, leading to:

- **Breathlessness**.
- **Faster breathing and heartbeat**: the body's natural response to an asthma attack is to increase breathing and heart rate in an attempt to get more oxygen into the lungs.
- **Confusion, drowsiness, and dizziness**: these symptoms can occur if the brain is not receiving enough oxygen due to the difficulty breathing.
- **Fainting**: in severe cases of asthma, a person may faint due to a lack of oxygen.
- **Blue lips and fingers**: this is a sign of severe oxygen deprivation and is a medical emergency.

Secondary effects of asthma

Some of the secondary effects of asthma include:

Anxiety and depression: Chronic asthma can lead to anxiety and depression, as individuals may worry about having an asthma attack or feel limited by their condition.

Pneumonia: People with asthma are at a higher risk of developing pneumonia, a lung infection. This is because the inflammation and narrowing of the airways can make it more difficult to clear mucus and pathogens from the lungs.

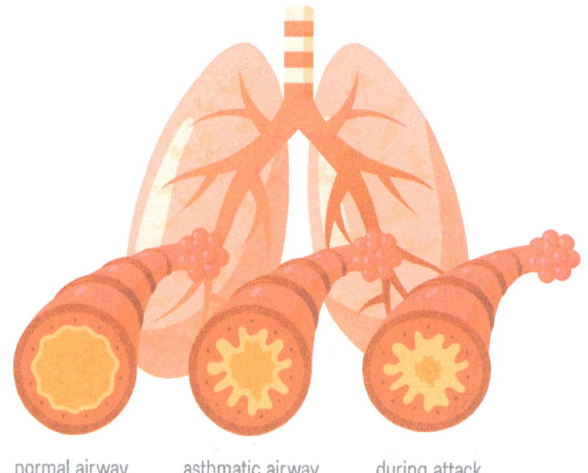

The effect of asthma on the airways

Delays in growth: Children with asthma may experience delays in growth and development. This can be due to issues including poor sleep, difficulty eating, and reduced physical activity.

Body systems affected by asthma

Asthma can also have an impact on other vital organs and systems.

Respiratory System: Chronic inflammation and narrowing of the airways can lead to a variety of respiratory complications, including:

Pneumonia: People with asthma are at a higher risk of developing pneumonia due to the difficulty in clearing mucus and pathogens from the lungs.

Respiratory failure: In severe cases of asthma, the airways can become so narrowed that the lungs are unable to deliver enough oxygen to the body, leading to respiratory failure. In respiratory failure the lungs can't get enough oxygen into the blood, which can be fatal.

Sleep apnoea: Asthma can contribute to sleep apnoea, a condition where breathing is interrupted during sleep. People with sleep apnoea will often wake up several times throughout the night. This can lead to fatigue, daytime sleepiness, and other health problems. People with sleep apnoea will often have to wear a special mask while they sleep. The mask holds their airways open and allows a continuous flow of oxygen into the lungs.

Cardiovascular System: Asthma can also affect the cardiovascular system. When the lungs are struggling to get enough oxygen,

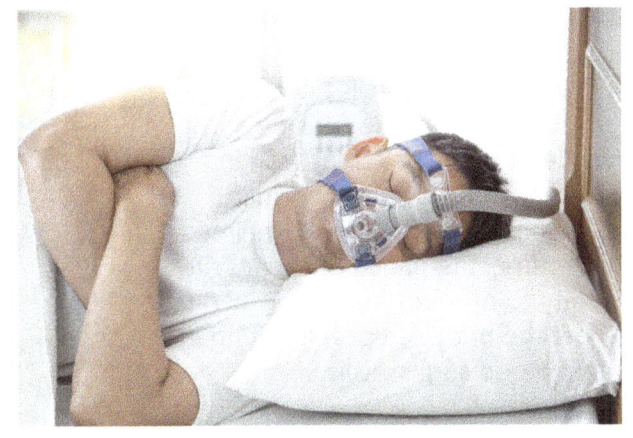

the heart must work harder to pump blood. This increased workload can put strain on the heart and lead to conditions such as high blood pressure, heart rate irregularities, and even heart failure. The chronic inflammation associated with asthma can also contribute to the development of atherosclerosis, a condition where plaque builds up in the arteries, increasing the risk of heart attack and stroke.

> **Recap questions**
>
> 1. What are the four main symptoms of asthma?
> 2. What two main factors contribute to the development of asthma?
> 3. What lung infections are people with asthma at increased risk of?
> 4. How can asthma contribute to sleep apnoea?
> 5. What are two cardiovascular effects of asthma?

C1.5 Diabetes – type 1 and type 2

Diabetes is a chronic condition that occurs when the body cannot produce enough insulin or cannot effectively use the insulin it produces. Insulin is the hormone that helps to regulate blood sugar levels. When blood sugar levels are too high, it can damage the body's organs and tissues. There are two main types of diabetes: Type 1 and Type 2.

Causes of diabetes

Type 1 diabetes is an autoimmune disorder, meaning the body's immune system mistakenly attacks and destroys the cells in the pancreas which produce insulin. There are different factors which can lead to Type 1 diabetes:

- Genetic predisposition - individuals with family members who have type 1 diabetes are at a higher risk.

- Environmental factors - exposure to viruses or toxins, may also trigger the autoimmune response in susceptible individuals.

Type 2 diabetes occurs when the body either doesn't produce enough insulin or doesn't use insulin effectively. Unlike type 1 diabetes, which is an autoimmune disorder, type 2 diabetes is primarily caused by lifestyle factors. Risk factors include obesity, a sedentary lifestyle, and a diet high in unhealthy foods.

A key factor in Type 2 diabetes is insulin resistance, a condition where the body's cells become less responsive to insulin. This resistance can lead to the pancreas working harder to produce more insulin, eventually becoming overwhelmed. Over time, the pancreas can lose its ability to produce enough insulin to meet the body's needs, resulting in high blood sugar levels.

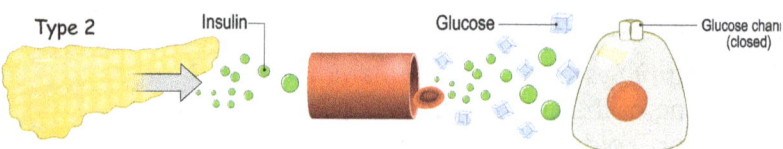

Type 1 and Type 2 diabetes

Primary effects of diabetes

Uncontrolled blood sugar levels can lead to a variety of health problems. One common effect is weight change. When blood sugar levels are high, the body may try to compensate by increasing appetite and reducing energy expenditure, leading to weight gain. Conversely, when blood sugar levels are low, the body may experience **hypoglycaemia**, which can cause symptoms such as sweating, shaking, and confusion. These symptoms can lead to weight loss.

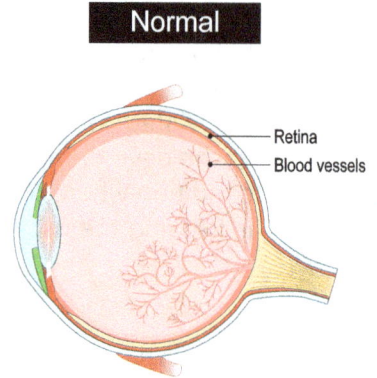
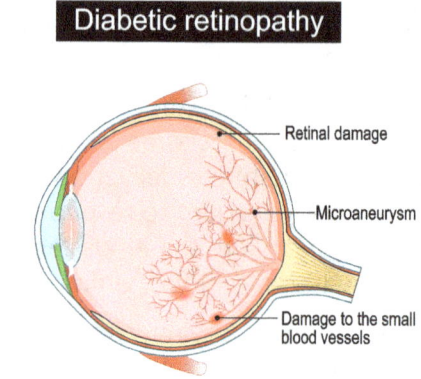

Diabetic retinopathy

High blood sugar levels can also affect vision. High blood sugar levels can cause the lens of the eye to become cloudy, which can cause blurred vision or **cataracts**. High blood sugar levels can also damage the nerves in the **retina**, leading to **diabetic retinopathy**. If left untreated, diabetic retinopathy can cause blindness.

Other common symptoms of diabetes include feeling thirsty, hungry, and experiencing mood changes. When blood sugar levels are high, the body may try to eliminate excess glucose through the urine, which can lead to dehydration and increased thirst. High blood sugar levels can also affect the body's ability to use glucose for energy, leading to increased hunger. Fluctuating blood sugar levels can cause mood changes, such as irritability, depression, and anxiety.

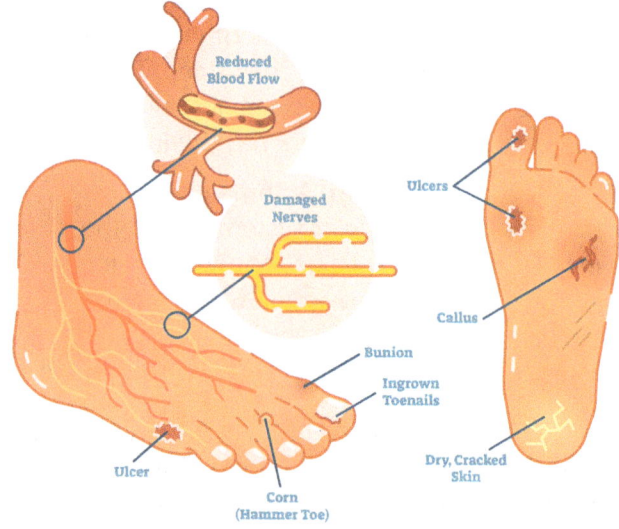

Diabetic foot

Diabetes can also cause:

- **Tiredness** – When blood sugar levels are high, the body's cells may not be able to use glucose for energy efficiently, leading to fatigue.
- **Excessive urination.**
- **Itching** – Can occur due to dry skin, which can be caused by dehydration
- **Thrush infections** – High sugar levels can lead to an overgrowth of yeast-like fungi in the mouth, vagina, or skin folds.
- **Slow-healing cuts and wounds** – High blood sugar levels can impair blood flow and wound healing, making it difficult for cuts and wounds to heal properly.

Secondary effects of diabetes

Diabetes can lead to a number of serious secondary effects:

Condition	Description
Heart disease and stroke	High blood sugar levels can damage the blood vessels, leading to atherosclerosis, a condition where plaque builds up in the arteries. This can increase the risk of heart attack and stroke. Additionally, diabetes can contribute to high blood pressure and high cholesterol, which are both risk factors for heart disease and stroke.
Nerve damage (neuropathy)	High blood sugar levels can damage the nerves throughout the body, leading to numbness, tingling, pain, and weakness. This can affect the feet, hands, and other parts of the body.
Foot problems	Nerve damage and poor blood flow to the feet can increase the risk of developing foot ulcers and infections. These infections can be difficult to treat and can sometimes lead to amputation.
Vision loss	High blood sugar levels can damage the blood vessels in the retina, leading to diabetic retinopathy. If left untreated, diabetic retinopathy can cause blindness.
Miscarriage and stillbirth	Diabetes can also affect pregnancy. Women with diabetes are at a higher risk of experiencing **miscarriage and stillbirth**. Diabetes can increase the risk of giving birth to a baby with birth defects. Good blood sugar control before and during pregnancy can help to reduce these risks.
Kidney problems	High blood sugar levels can damage the kidneys, leading to diabetic nephropathy. Over time, diabetic nephropathy can lead to kidney failure, which may require dialysis or a kidney transplant.
Sexual problems	Nerve damage can lead to erectile dysfunction in men and decreased sexual desire or arousal in women. In women, diabetes can cause vaginal dryness and infections. High blood sugar levels can affect hormone production, which can also contribute to sexual problems.

Recap questions

1. What is the primary function of insulin in the body?
2. What are the two main types of diabetes?
3. What are two risk factors for Type 2 diabetes?
4. What is insulin resistance?
5. How can high blood sugar levels affect weight?
6. What are two potential vision problems caused by high blood sugar levels?
7. Which symptom of diabetes can be caused by dehydration?
8. What is one common effect of fluctuating blood sugar levels?
9. Why can high blood sugar levels lead to fatigue?
10. What is one potential complication of poor wound healing in people with diabetes?

Body systems affected by diabetes

Diabetes can have wide-ranging effects on other body systems, highlighting the importance of monitoring and maintaining blood sugar levels.

Endocrine system: Diabetes disrupts the endocrine system's ability to regulate blood sugar levels. The pancreas, a key organ in the endocrine system, produces insulin to control blood sugar. In people with diabetes, the pancreas may not produce enough insulin or the body may become resistant to its effects.

Cardiovascular system: Diabetes can damage blood vessels, increasing the risk of heart disease and stroke. High blood sugar levels can contribute to atherosclerosis, a condition where plaque builds up in the arteries, narrowing them and reducing blood flow. This can increase the risk of heart attack and stroke. Diabetes can also contribute to high blood pressure and high cholesterol levels, which are also risk factors for cardiovascular disease.

Nervous system: High blood sugar levels can damage the nerves throughout the body, leading to numbness, tingling, pain, and weakness. Neuropathy can affect the nerves in the feet, hands, legs, and other parts of the body. In severe cases, neuropathy can lead to foot ulcers and infections, which may require amputation.

Immune system: Diabetes can weaken the immune system, making individuals more susceptible to infections. High blood sugar levels can impair the function of white blood cells, which are essential for fighting infections. Diabetes can also damage blood capillaries, making it difficult for immune cells to reach the site of infections.

Digestive system: High blood sugar levels can slow down the digestive process, leading to constipation. Diabetes can damage the nerves in the digestive system, causing gastroparesis, a condition where the stomach empties slowly. This can lead to nausea, vomiting, and bloating.

Reproductive system: Diabetes can affect both male and female reproductive systems. In men, diabetes can lead to erectile dysfunction. In women, diabetes can cause vaginal dryness and infections. Diabetes can also increase the risk of complications during pregnancy, such as miscarriage and stillbirth.

Recap questions

1. How does high blood sugar increase the risk of heart disease and stroke?
2. What is neuropathy, and what are some of its symptoms?
3. What is diabetic retinopathy, and what are its potential consequences?
4. How does diabetes affect the immune system?
5. What is gastroparesis?

C1.6 Dementia

Dementia is a progressive brain disorder that causes a decline in cognitive function. It can affect memory, thinking, language, and behaviour. There are many types of dementia, but two of the most common are **Alzheimer's disease** and **vascular dementia**.

- Alzheimer's disease is caused by the buildup of abnormal protein deposits in the brain.
- Vascular dementia is caused by damage to the blood vessels in the brain, often due to stroke or other circulatory problems.

Causes of dementia

Alzheimer's disease is characterised by a buildup of abnormal protein deposits within and around brain cells. These deposits, known as **amyloid plaques**, disrupt the normal functioning of brain cells and lead to their death.

Vascular dementia is caused by reduced blood flow to the brain, often due to narrowing of blood vessels, strokes, or transient ischemic attacks (TIAs):

- **Narrowing of blood vessels:** Over time, the arteries that supply blood to the brain can become narrowed due to atherosclerosis, a condition where plaque builds up in the arteries. This narrowing can restrict blood flow and oxygen supply to brain cells, leading to damage and cognitive decline.
- **Strokes:** Strokes occur when a blood vessel in the brain becomes blocked or bursts, cutting off blood flow to a specific area of

the brain. This can cause significant brain damage and lead to cognitive decline.

- **Transient ischemic attacks (TIAs):** TIAs are mini-strokes that last for a short period of time. While they do not cause permanent damage, they can indicate underlying vascular problems and increase the risk of a full-blown stroke. Multiple TIAs can lead to cumulative brain damage and contribute to vascular dementia.

Primary effects of dementia

As dementia progresses, individuals may experience a variety of cognitive symptoms:

- **Memory loss:** often the first symptom of dementia and can involve difficulty remembering recent events, names, or faces. As the condition progresses, individuals may also have trouble remembering long-term memories.
- **Difficulty with problem-solving:** People with dementia may struggle to solve problems or complete tasks that they used to find easy. This can include difficulties with planning, organising, and sequencing tasks. They may find it challenging to plan ahead or follow through on tasks.
- **Language difficulties:** Dementia can affect language skills, making it difficult to find the right words, understand conversations, or follow complex instructions.
- **Changes in mood and behaviour:** As dementia progresses, individuals may experience changes in mood and behaviour, including irritability, anxiety, depression, or agitation. They may also become withdrawn or disoriented.
- **Disorientation:** Individuals with dementia may become confused or disoriented, particularly in unfamiliar surroundings. They may have trouble remembering where they are or how to get back home.

As their dementia progresses, individuals may require increasing levels of care and support.

Secondary effects of dementia

In addition to the primary effects of disrupted cognitive function, dementia can also cause:

- **Slowness of thought and confusion:** individuals may experience a decline in their thinking speed and ability to process information. They may become easily confused or have difficulty following conversations.
- **Memory loss:** In addition to short-term memory loss, individuals with dementia may also experience long-term memory loss, forgetting important events or people from their past.
- **Problems concentrating:** People with dementia often struggle to concentrate and focus on tasks. They may find it difficult to follow conversations or complete simple activities.
- **Severe personality changes:** Dementia can lead to significant changes in personality and behaviour. Individuals may become withdrawn, irritable, or anxious. They may also exhibit inappropriate or impulsive behaviour.
- **Depression:** The cognitive decline and emotional challenges associated with dementia can lead to feelings of sadness, hopelessness, and isolation. Individuals may lose interest in activities they once enjoyed or feel overwhelmed by their symptoms.
- **Incontinence:** Dementia can affect the body's ability to control bladder and bowel functions, leading to incontinence.
- **Difficulties swallowing or coughing:** Dementia can affect the muscles involved in swallowing and coughing, increasing the risk of choking or aspiration. This can lead to malnutrition and other health problems, such as aspiration pneumonia.

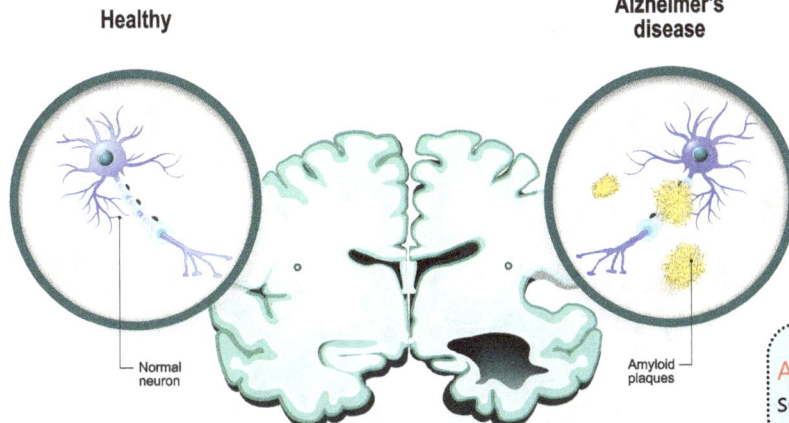

Dementia is caused by abnormal deposits around neurons

> **Aspiration** – The act of inhaling or drawing something into the lungs.

Body systems affected by dementia

Dementia can have a significant impact on other body systems, including:

- **Nervous system:** dementia can also affect the nervous system in other ways. For example, people with dementia may experience motor problems, such as difficulty walking, balance problems, or tremors. They may also have difficulty controlling their bladder or bowels.

- **Cardiovascular system:** Individuals with dementia are at increased risk of heart disease and stroke, which can be caused by factors such as high blood pressure, high cholesterol, and diabetes. These conditions can further damage the brain and accelerate **cognitive decline**.

- **Respiratory system:** Individuals with dementia may have difficulty swallowing or coughing, which can increase the risk of choking or **aspiration**. This can lead to respiratory infections and other complications. Dementia can affect the muscles involved in breathing, making it more difficult to take deep breaths.

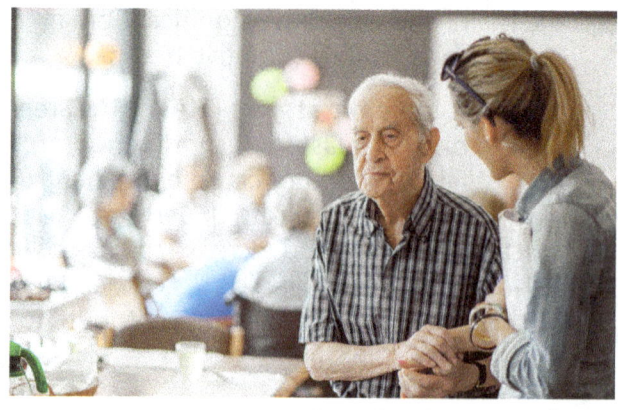

Recap questions

1. What are the two most common types of dementia?
2. What is Alzheimer's disease caused by?
3. What are TIAs and how can they contribute to vascular dementia?
4. Besides cognitive decline, what other physical challenges can individuals with dementia experience?
5. How can dementia impact the respiratory system?
6. How can dementia affect an individual's language skills?

Practice questions

1. Describe how asthma can increase the risk of pneumonia. [2 marks]
2. Discuss the potential long-term health consequences of asthma, considering both respiratory and cardiovascular systems. [6 marks]
3. Describe two ways in which diabetes can affect the nervous system. [4 marks]
4. Discuss the potential impact of diabetes on the endocrine, immune, and digestive systems. [6 marks]
5. Explain how dementia can impact the cardiovascular system. [4 marks]
6. Describe two cognitive symptoms of dementia. [4 marks]
7. Discuss the potential physical and emotional challenges that individuals with dementia may face. [6 marks]

C1.7 Acquired brain injury: traumatic and non-traumatic

Causes of injury

Acquired brain injuries happen when the brain is damaged after birth. There are two main causes of acquired brain injury: traumatic and non-traumatic.

- **Traumatic brain injury** occurs when the head is hit hard, like in a road traffic accident, during an assault, or as a result of a fall. The effects of a traumatic injury on the brain vary depending on the type of injury, location of the injury, and the severity of injury.

- **Non-traumatic brain injury** does not involve a physical blow to the head. Non-traumatic brain injuries can occur due to:
    * a person having a stroke
    * infections like **meningitis**
    * lack of oxygen (for example during drowning or suffocation)
    * disease e.g. tumours.

The brain typically uses about 20% of the body's total oxygen supply, so it is extremely sensitive to any changes in oxygen levels.

When a person suffers a stroke, a small area of the brain is starved of oxygen. This causes a localised effect, as only a small part of the brain loses oxygen.

Other causes of low oxygen include:

- cardiac arrest (when the heart stops working),
- respiratory arrest (when the respiratory system stops working),
- drowning.

These can lead to more widespread effects in the brain and body.

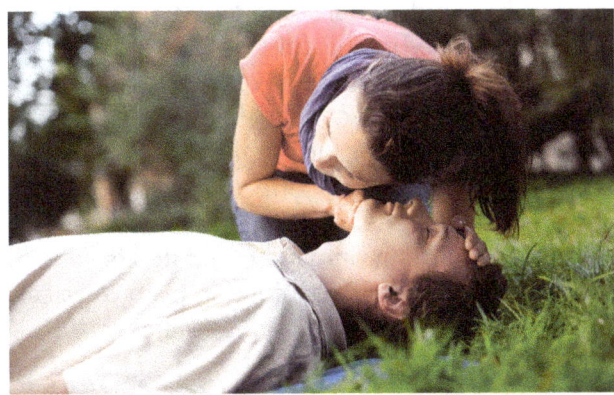

A brain injury can lead to unconsciousness

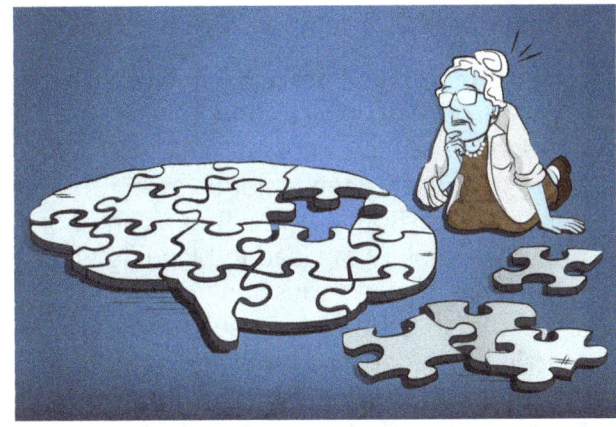

Primary effects of acquired brain injury

The primary effects of acquired brain injury will vary depending on the severity and location of the injury. The brain is responsible for all our emotions, feelings, thoughts, decisions, judgements, and physical actions. It is therefore no surprise that damage to the brain can impact every part of someone's life.

Primary effects occur immediately after the injury has happened. Common primary effects include:

- **Concussion** – A concussion is a result of mild traumatic brain injury. Concussions are often due to a blow to the head, a sudden impact, or violent shaking of the head and upper body. These cause the brain to be jolted or shaken inside the skull. A concussion causes the brain to experience a temporary disruption in its normal functioning.

- **Unconsciousness** – This is where a person is not aware of their surroundings and does not respond to an external stimulus like sound or lights. They will often look like they are sleeping.

- **Coma** – A coma is a deep state of unconsciousness where a person is completely unresponsive and cannot be wakened. A person in a coma, will have their eyes closed, and they will not show normal sleep-wake cycles. Comas can last for a few days to several weeks or even longer. Some people may recover fully from a coma, while others can experience long-term disability or remain in a persistent vegetative state.

- **Amnesia** – Amnesia is a partial or complete loss of memory. It can affect short-term memory, long-term memory, or both. Amnesia may be temporary or permanent.
- **Damage to blood vessels in the brain** – The force of physical trauma can cause blood vessels to rupture or tear. A stroke can be caused when a blood vessel ruptures in the brain. Both physical trauma and non-traumatic injury can lead to bleeding within the brain. This can cause an increase in pressure in the brain or result in parts of the brain being deprived of oxygen or nutrients.

Secondary effects of acquired brain injury

The secondary effects of a traumatic brain injury develop over the days and weeks following the initial injury. The secondary effects will vary depending on the severity and location of the injury.

A **traumatic brain injury** can cause **secondary effects** like:

- **Headaches and dizziness**: inflammation and swelling in the brain, as a result of the injury, can cause the person to suffer from headaches. Where there has been bleeding in the brain, this can result in increased pressure (increased intracranial pressure) which can press on nerves, brain tissue and blood vessels, causing headache pain and feelings of dizziness.
- **Memory loss**: memory loss is a common secondary effect. The frontal lobes and **hippocampus** are the areas of the brain responsible for processing memories. Damage to these areas could mean that the individual might have problems remembering past events or creating new memories.
- **Personality changes**: The brain is a complex organ that regulates emotions, controls behaviours and social interactions, it is understandable that any injury may cause changes to someone's personality. Damage to the frontal lobe can lead to impulsive behaviour, poor judgement, and irritability. Damage to the limbic system in the brain can result in emotional instability, mood swings and difficulty regulating emotions. In addition to the direct damage caused by the injury, the individual may be struggling to come to terms with changes to their social roles, relationships, and physical and mental abilities because of the damage.
- **Fatigue**: the experience of fatigue (tiredness) in individuals with traumatic brain injury can result from a combination of physical, cognitive, and emotional factors. Injury to the brain can result in normal processes like the sleep cycle and metabolism being disrupted. The injury might also have caused physical impairments like muscle weakness, paralysis, or coordination difficulties. Cognitive processes like attention, memory, and decision making may also be affected by the injury.

The brain uses a lot of energy coping with these effects of the injury, and this often leads to feelings of tiredness and exhaustion.

Both traumatic and non-traumatic injuries can cause the following secondary effects:

- **Secondary effects in children**: Both traumatic and non-traumatic injuries in children can lead to physical and developmental delays. Often in children, the full effects of the injury are not seen until the individual starts to use particular skills. Some fine motor skills, for example writing and drawing, develop between the ages of 4-6 years. A child with a brain injury that has occurred prior to this age might not show any effects until they start school. For other children, the secondary effects of brain damage could be life-changing injuries, resulting in both physical disabilities and learning disabilities.

Recap questions

1. What are the two main causes of acquired brain injury?
2. What is a traumatic brain injury, and how can it occur?
3. What are some examples of non-traumatic brain injuries?
4. Why is the brain particularly vulnerable to oxygen deprivation?
5. What are some common primary effects of acquired brain injury?
6. What is amnesia, and how can it be caused by brain injury?

- **Issues with balance and coordination**: The brain stem (**cerebellum**) are the parts of the brain responsible for coordinating movement. Damage to these areas of the brain will result in problems with balance and coordination. Nerve damage, muscle weakness and paralysis will also affect balance and coordination.

- **Cognitive impairments**: Cognitive processes include thinking, reasoning, and making judgements. An acquired brain injury can affect cognitive function in different ways. Someone with a brain injury may process information more slowly or find it difficult to stay focused on a task. The individual might have difficulties with speech, language, and communication. They may struggle with problem solving or decision making. All these changes will impact the person's daily life and their ability to maintain independence.

- **Sensory impairments**: Acquired brain injuries can lead to various sensory impairments, including changes in vision, hearing, taste, smell, and touch.

    * **Visual impairments** may involve changes to eyesight, double vision, or problems with spatial awareness.

    * **Hearing impairments** may range from mildly impaired to severe hearing loss and can affect the ability to hear different sounds or where the sound is coming from.

    * **Nerve damage** could affect the sense of touch by causing numbness and tingling.

- **Physical impairments**: Acquired brain injuries can result in nerve damage, muscle weakness, coordination difficulties and paralysis. Weakness and paralysis can affect the arms or legs and may limit mobility. Nerve damage may result in difficulty in coordinating movements resulting in them being jerky rather than smooth.

- **Irritability**: Irritability in people with acquired brain injuries could be due to

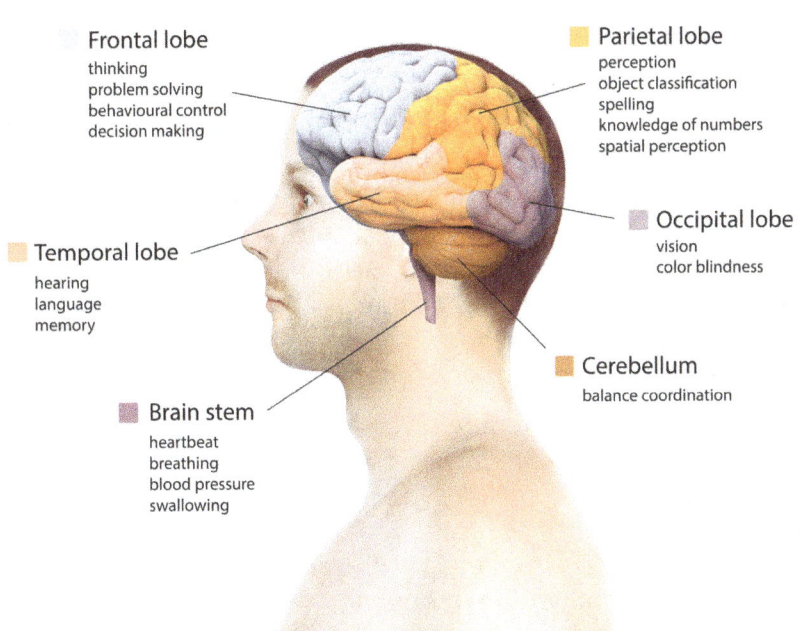

Brain lobes and their function

Cognitive – Relating to the mental processes involved in acquiring knowledge and understanding.

Metabolism – The chemical processes that occur within a living organism to maintain life, such as the conversion of food to energy.

several factors. Damage to the frontal lobes or limbic system can result in the individual being unable to process emotions correctly. Cognitive impairments may lead to frustration and anger at not being able to perform simple tasks. The person may also be struggling with physical pain and discomfort which could leave them feeling irritable.

- **Sleep disturbance**: Injury to the brain can result in normal processes like the sleep-wake cycle being disrupted. This could lead to the individual struggling to fall asleep, stay asleep or achieve deep sleep. Physical pain and discomfort as a result of the injury could also affect the quality of sleep. The individual may also be experiencing stress and anxiety because of their injury which could impact on their sleep.

Recap questions

1. How can a traumatic brain injury lead to headaches and dizziness?

2. Why can fatigue be a significant secondary effect of a traumatic brain injury?

3. How can an acquired brain injury affect a person's physical abilities?

Body systems affected by acquired brain injury

Acquired brain injuries can have wide-reaching impacts on other body systems.

Nervous system: the brain and spinal cord form the **central nervous system**. The **peripheral nervous system** is made up of all the other nerves in the body that are connected to sense organs and muscles.

The central nervous system receives nerve impulses from the peripheral nervous system and coordinates responses. Damage to the brain may result in some of the sensory impulses from the peripheral nervous system not getting through to the brain or prevent motor impulses from being sent to the muscles or glands.

Cardiovascular system: Cardiovascular disease occurs when fatty deposits build up in the arteries. This narrows the arteries, increases blood pressure, and can lead to blood clots forming within the vessels. A stroke is a type of cardiovascular disease that occurs in the blood vessels in the brain.

- An **ischaemic stroke** happens when a blood clot blocks the blood and oxygen supply to part of the brain. This is usually as a result of fatty deposits building up within the arteries in the brain (atherosclerosis).

- **Haemorrhagic strokes** happen when a blood vessel bursts inside the brain leading to bleeding in the brain. This is usually a result of high blood pressure which weakens the artery walls, making them more likely to burst.

- **Respiratory system:** Damage to the brainstem (which controls breathing) could lead to changes in breathing depth or could result in an irregular breathing pattern. The brain injury could cause paralysis in the breathing muscles (diaphragm and intercostal muscles), preventing the lungs from inflating.

- **Musculoskeletal system:** Acquired brain injuries can have a massive impact on the musculoskeletal system. Nerve endings are found in every muscle in our bodies at the neuromuscular junctions. Damage to the motor areas in the brain can lead to muscle weakness or paralysis, making it difficult to control movements.

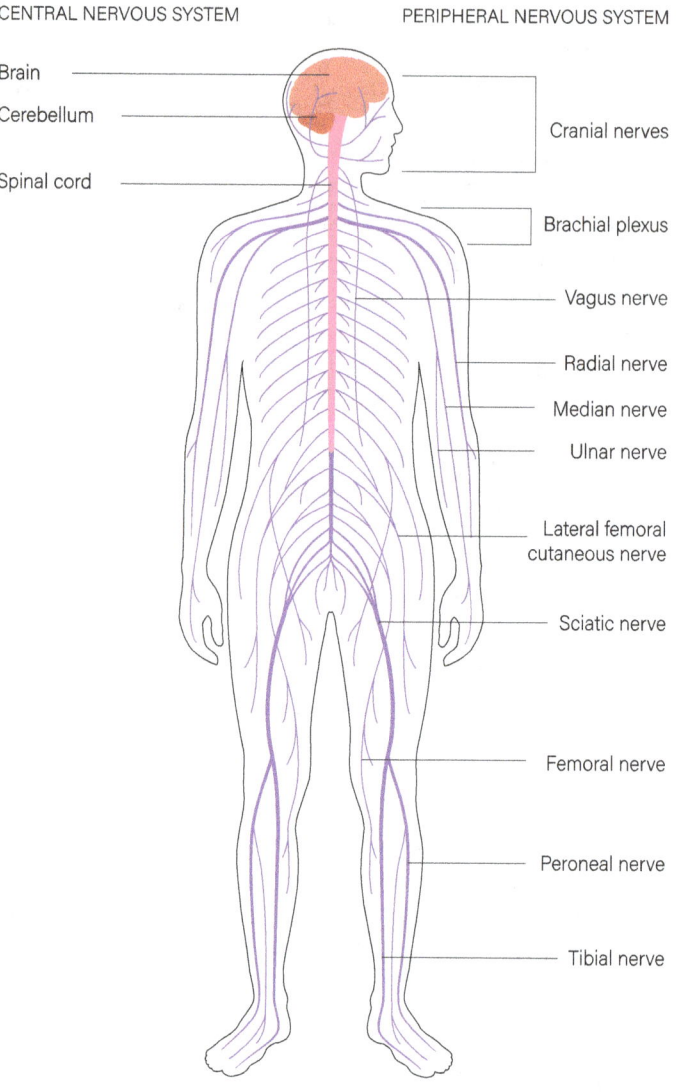

The nerves of the PNS

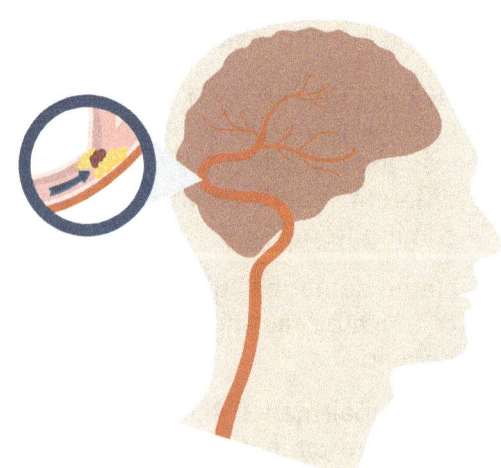

The site of an ischaemic stroke

Neuromuscular junctions – The site where a motor neurone transmits a nerve impulse to a muscle fibre.

Motor areas – Regions of the cerebral cortex responsible for planning, controlling, and carrying out voluntary movements.

Recap questions

1. What are the two main components of the nervous system?
2. How can brain damage affect the cardiovascular system?
3. What is the difference between an ischemic and a haemorrhagic stroke?
4. How can brain injury affect the respiratory system?
5. What is the role of the neuromuscular junction?
6. How can brain injury impact the musculoskeletal system?

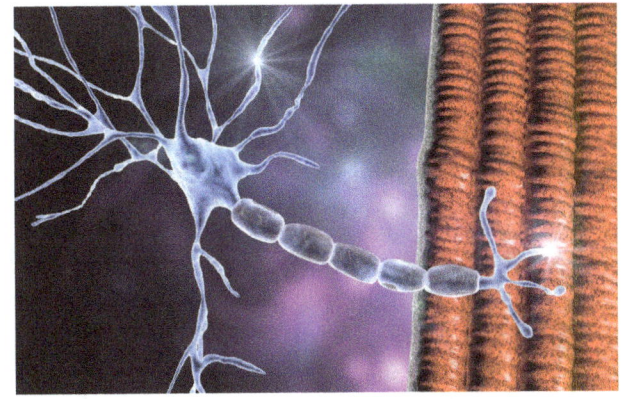

A motor neuron connecting to a muscle

C1.8 Cancer: breast, bowel and lung

Cancer is a disease where the cells of the body grow uncontrollably, and these abnormal cells then spread throughout the body. There are many types of cancer, affecting various parts of the body. Three of the most common types of cancer are **breast cancer**, **bowel cancer**, and **lung cancer**. Breast cancer affects the breast tissue, bowel cancer affects the large intestine, and lung cancer affects the lungs.

Breast cancer

Causes of breast cancer

Breast cancer is the uncontrolled growth of abnormal cells in the breast tissue. A combination of genetic, lifestyle, and environmental factors all play a role in the development of this disease.

- **Genetic factors:** Some women may have a genetic predisposition to breast cancer. This means that they inherit genes that increase their risk of developing the disease. These genes (BRCA genes) are known as **cancer-risk genes**. Women with mutations in these BRCA genes have a significantly higher risk of developing breast cancer.
- **Lifestyle factors:** Certain lifestyle factors can also increase the risk of breast cancer. These include:
    * **Alcohol consumption:** Women who drink more than two alcoholic beverages per day are at greater risk.
    * **Overweight and obesity:** Being overweight or obese after menopause can increase the risk of breast cancer. This is thought to be due to the production of excess oestrogen, a hormone that can stimulate breast cell growth.
- **Environmental factors:** Exposure to certain environmental factors may also contribute to the development of breast cancer. These include:
    * **Radiation:** Exposure to ionising radiation, such as from X-rays or radiation therapy for other cancers, can increase the risk of breast cancer.
    * **Oestrogen:** Oestrogen is a hormone that is essential for female development and reproduction. However, prolonged exposure to high levels of oestrogen can increase the risk of breast cancer. Women who have undergone menopause and use hormone replacement therapy may have a slightly increased risk of breast cancer due to oestrogen in the medication.

Primary effects of breast cancer

Some of the primary effects of breast cancer include:

- **Changes in size or shape of one or both breasts:** One of the most common symptoms of breast cancer is a change in the size or shape of one or both breasts. This can include swelling, lumps, or a feeling of fullness/heaviness.

- **Discharge from nipples:** Discharge from the nipples - clear, bloody, or occurring without squeezing - can be a sign of breast cancer.
- **Swelling in armpits:** Swelling or lumps in the armpit can be a sign of breast cancer, as lymph nodes in the armpit can be affected by the disease.
- **Dimpling on breast skin:** The skin on the breast may become dimpled or puckered, resembling the surface of an orange peel. This is often caused by the cancer invading the underlying tissues, so is usually a sign of advanced breast cancer.
- **Change in the appearance of the nipple:** The nipple may become inverted or flattened, or there may be a change in its texture or appearance.

Secondary effects of breast cancer

Breast cancer can also have significant secondary effects on other body systems. One of the most serious complications is **metastasis**, which occurs when cancer cells spread from the breast to other parts of the body. In metastasis, the cancer cells break away from the primary tumour, they then enter the bloodstream or lymphatic system, and travel to other organs. Once they reach a new location, these cells can invade surrounding tissues and grow into secondary tumours, known as metastases, in organs such as the bones, lungs, liver, and brain.

Metastasis (also known as Stage 4 cancer) can have a devastating impact on a person's health and can ultimately lead to organ failure and death. For example, if breast cancer spreads to the lungs, it can interfere with breathing and lead to respiratory failure. If it spreads to the liver, it can damage the liver and impair its ability to filter toxins from the blood. This can lead to liver failure. If it spreads to the brain, it can cause neurological problems such as seizures, headaches, and cognitive decline.

Bowel cancer

Causes of bowel cancer

Bowel cancer is a type of cancer that begins in the large intestine. Like breast cancer, a combination of genetic, lifestyle, and environmental factors is believed to play a role.

- **Genetic factors:** Some individuals may

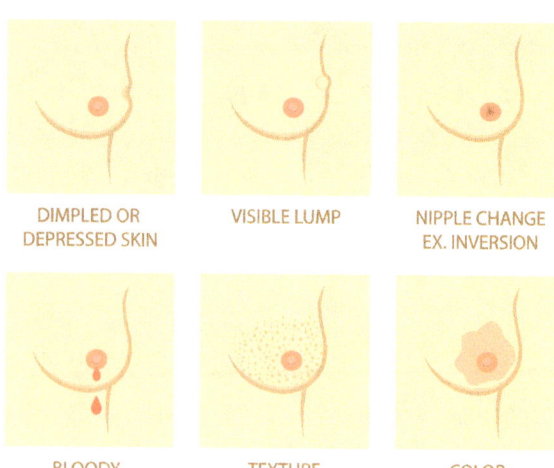

SYMPTOMS OF BREAST CANCER

DIMPLED OR DEPRESSED SKIN   VISIBLE LUMP   NIPPLE CHANGE EX. INVERSION

BLOODY DISCHARGE   TEXTURE CHANGE   COLOR CHANGE

Recap questions

1. What are the BRCA genes, and how are they related to breast cancer risk?
2. List two lifestyle factors that can increase the risk of breast cancer.
3. What is metastasis, and how can it affect a person's health?
4. Name two common symptoms of breast cancer.
5. What is the role of oestrogen in the development of breast cancer?
6. What is one environmental factor that can increase the risk of breast cancer?

have a genetic predisposition to bowel cancer. This means that they inherit genes that increase their risk of developing the disease. Individuals with mutations in these genes have a significantly higher risk of developing bowel cancer.

- **Lifestyle factors:** Certain lifestyle factors can also increase the risk of bowel cancer. These include:
  * **Smoking:** Smoking is a major risk factor for bowel cancer.
  * **Consumption of red and processed meat:** Eating large amounts of red and processed meat has been linked to an increased risk of bowel cancer.
  * **Alcohol consumption:** Excessive alcohol consumption can also increase the risk of bowel cancer.

- **Weight**: Being overweight or obese can increase the risk of bowel cancer.
- **Inflammatory bowel disease**: Individuals with inflammatory bowel disease, such as Crohn's disease or ulcerative colitis, have a higher risk of developing bowel cancer.

Primary effects of bowel cancer

Some of the primary effects of bowel cancer include:

- **Changes in faeces**: One of the most common symptoms of bowel cancer is a change in bowel habits. This may include changes in the consistency of stools, such as becoming thicker, thinner, or more watery. Individuals may also experience changes in the frequency of bowel movements, such as constipation or diarrhoea.
- **Changes in occurrence of defecating**: there may be changes in the timing of bowel movements. They may become more frequent or less frequent than usual.
- **Bleeding from the anus/blood in stool**: Blood in the stool is a serious symptom of bowel cancer The bleeding can be bright red, or dark and tarry.
- **Pain in the abdomen**: Abdominal pain or discomfort is another common symptom of bowel cancer. This pain may be in the lower left or right side of the abdomen.
- **Bloating**: bloating or a feeling of fullness in the abdomen can be another symptom.
- **Weight loss**: Unexplained weight loss can be a sign of bowel cancer.

Secondary effects of bowel cancer

Bowel cancer can have significant secondary effects on other body systems.

- One of the most common secondary effects is on the cardiovascular system. Internal bleeding or bleeding from the anus can lead to anaemia, a condition in which there is a decrease in the number of red blood cells. This can cause symptoms such as fatigue, weakness, and shortness of breath. Anaemia can also affect the heart, leading to heart failure in severe cases.
- Another secondary effect of bowel cancer is on the musculoskeletal system. The body may experience a loss of bone and muscle mass due to the cancer itself, the effects of treatment, or changes in diet and activity

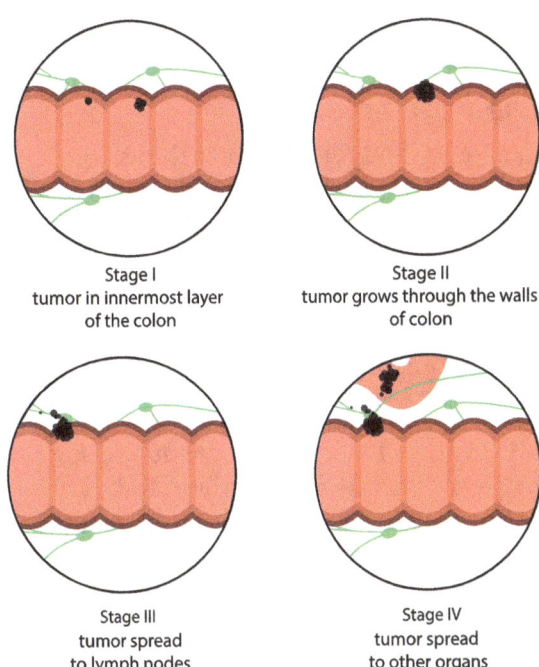

The stages of bowel cancer

levels. This can lead to weakness, fatigue, and an increased risk of fractures.

- Metastasis is another serious complication of bowel cancer. This occurs when cancer cells spread from the bowel to other parts of the body. These secondary tumours can affect various organs, including the liver and lungs. Metastasis can lead to organ failure and death. For example, if bowel cancer spreads to the liver, it can cause liver failure. If it spreads to the lungs, it can cause respiratory problems and difficulty breathing.

Recap questions

1. List three lifestyle factors that can increase the risk of bowel cancer.
2. What is a common symptom of bowel cancer that involves changes in bowel habits?
3. What is anaemia and how can it be a secondary effect of bowel cancer?
4. What is metastasis and what are two organs that bowel cancer can spread to?
5. What are two secondary effects of bowel cancer on the musculoskeletal system?

Lung cancer

Causes of lung cancer

Lung cancer is a type of cancer that begins in the lungs and is characterised by the uncontrolled growth of abnormal cells, which can form a tumour and potentially spread to other parts of the body. Like breast and bowel cancer, a combination of genetic, lifestyle, and environmental factors are believed to play a role.

- **Genetic factors**: Some individuals may have a genetic predisposition to lung cancer, meaning they inherit genes that increase their risk of developing the disease. Individuals with mutations in these genes have a significantly higher risk of developing lung cancer.

- **Lifestyle factors**: Certain lifestyle factors can also increase the risk of lung cancer, including smoking cigarettes and tobacco use. Smoking is the most significant risk factor for lung cancer and can significantly increase the risk of developing the disease. The longer you smoke and the more cigarettes you smoke, the higher your risk of lung cancer.

- **Environmental factors**: Exposure to certain environmental factors may also contribute to the development of lung cancer, including:
    * **Passive smoking**: Exposure to second-hand smoke can increase the risk of lung cancer, even if you do not smoke yourself.
    * **Exposure to certain chemicals and substances**: Exposure to chemicals and substances, such as arsenic and asbestos, can increase the risk of lung cancer. These substances are used in several occupations and industries, including mining, construction, and manufacturing.

Primary effects of lung cancer

Some of the primary effects include:

- **Persistent cough**: A persistent cough that does not go away is one of the most common symptoms of lung cancer. This cough may be dry or productive (produces phlegm).

- **Recurrent chest infections**: Individuals with

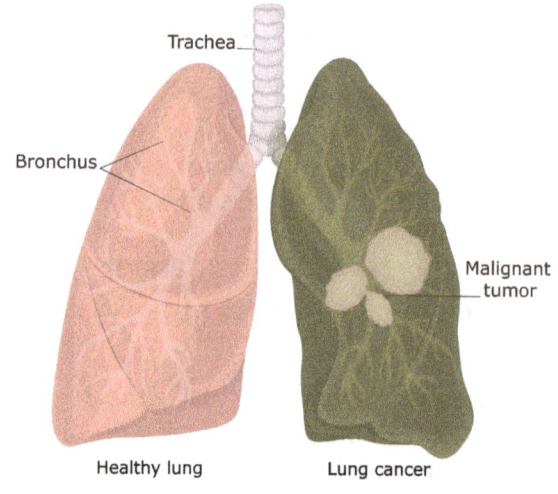

Lung cancer

lung cancer may experience recurrent chest infections, such as bronchitis or pneumonia. This is because the cancer can weaken the lungs' ability to fight off infections.

- **Coughing up blood**: Coughing up blood is a serious symptom of lung cancer. This can occur when the cancer grows into the airways and causes bleeding.

- **Pain when breathing or coughing**: Lung cancer can cause pain when breathing or coughing, especially if the tumour is pressing on nerves or other structures in the chest.

Secondary effects of lung cancer

Lung cancer can have significant secondary effects on other body systems:

- **Cardiovascular system**: One of the most common secondary effects is on the cardiovascular system. Internal bleeding or coughing up blood can lead to anaemia, a condition in which there is a decrease in the number of red blood cells. This can cause symptoms such as fatigue, weakness, and shortness of breath. Anaemia can also affect the heart, leading to heart failure in severe cases. Additionally, lung cancer can increase the risk of blood clots, which can lead to stroke (blood clots in the brain) or pulmonary embolism (blood clots in the lungs).

- **Digestive system**: Individuals with lung cancer may experience a loss of appetite and weight loss, which can lead to malnutrition and weakness. This can be caused by the cancer itself, the effects of treatment, or changes in diet and activity levels.

- **Musculoskeletal system**: The body may experience a loss of bone and muscle mass due to the cancer itself, the effects of treatment, or changes in diet and activity levels. This can lead to weakness, fatigue, and an increased risk of fractures.
- **Metastasis**: This occurs when cancer cells spread from the lungs to other parts of the body. These secondary tumours can affect various organs, including the brain, bones, liver, and adrenal glands. Metastasis can lead to organ failure and death. For example, if lung cancer spreads to the brain, it can cause neurological problems such as seizures and cognitive decline.

Recap questions

1. What are the three main categories of factors that can increase the risk of developing lung cancer?
2. Name two lifestyle factors that significantly increase the risk of lung cancer.
3. What is the most common symptom of lung cancer?
4. How can lung cancer affect the cardiovascular system?
5. What is metastasis, and how can it impact the body?
6. Besides smoking, list two other environmental factors that can increase the risk of lung cancer.

Apply your understanding

Zara is a 12-year-old girl who recently received a diagnosis of Type 1 diabetes. She enjoys playing netball, and badminton. Since her diagnosis, Zara has been learning how to manage her blood sugar levels through insulin injections and regular blood glucose monitoring. She is adjusting well to her new routine but finds it challenging to keep up with her active lifestyle while managing her diabetes.

Explain the causes of Type 1 diabetes. Discuss the importance of regular blood glucose monitoring and insulin treatment in managing the condition. Finally, outline the potential consequences if blood glucose levels are not effectively regulated.

Practice questions

1. Describe two possible secondary effects of breast cancer. [4 marks]
2. Discuss the role of both genetic and environmental factors in the development of breast cancer. [6 marks]
3. Explain how lifestyle factors can contribute to the development of breast cancer. [4 marks]
4. Explain how excessive alcohol consumption can increase the risk of developing bowel cancer. [4 marks]
5. Discuss the relationship between lifestyle factors and the development of bowel cancer. Include at least three specific lifestyle factors in your answer. [6 marks]
6. Explain how both genetic and environmental factors can contribute to the development of lung cancer. [4 marks]
7. Explain the importance of early detection and treatment in improving the outcome for individuals with lung cancer. [6 marks]

End of Unit Questions

1. .The diagram shows the structure of an animal cell. Label the structures A, B and C in the diagram. (3)

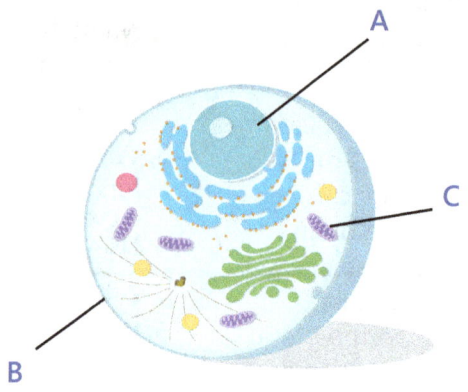

2. Identify one type of connective tissue. (1)

A simple

B cartilage

C striated

D sensory

3. Describe the process of catabolism. (1)
4. Describe the differences between aerobic and anaerobic respiration (4)
5. Give the definition of homeostasis (2)
6. Describe the role of the hypothalamus and the blood vessels in regulating body temperature (4)
7. Explain how the pancreas regulates blood sugar levels (4)
8. Explain one way that a non-traumatic cause can lead to brain injury (3)
9. Rob is a 52-year-old who has recently had a stroke. He is now experiencing muscle weakness and dysphasia. Discuss how the effects of a stroke on the brain can affect Rob's other body systems. (9)
10. White blood cells are known as:

A erythrocytes

B thrombocytes

C leukocytes

D antibodies.

11. Describe the role of phagocytes in protecting the body against pathogen. (2)
12. Maya is a 15-year-old girl. She was diagnosed with asthma when she was 10 years old. Maya is often short of breath and suffers from frequent chest infections. She uses an inhaler to help with her breathing. Using your knowledge of asthma, explain why Maya is often short of breath and why she is more likely to get a chest infection. Describe how an inhaler helps Maya in her everyday life. (9)

13. Name two common irritants that can trigger an asthma attack. (1)
14. Name one psychological impact of living with chronic asthma. (1)
15. State one potential consequence of sleep apnoea for individuals with asthma. (1)
16. Name the primary cause of coronary heart disease. (1)
17. Name one common symptom of a heart attack. (1)
18. State the medical name for high blood pressure. (1)
19. Discuss the impact of CHD on the cardiovascular, respiratory, and digestive systems. (6)
20. Name the two main types of stroke.
21. Describe what is meant by dysphasia.
22. Discuss the potential consequences of a stroke on the cardiovascular and nervous systems, including the long-term implications for an individual (9)
23. State the primary risk factor for developing lung cancer. (1)
24. Name one way in which lung cancer can affect the digestive system. (1)
25. Describe two secondary effects of lung cancer on the body, other than those affecting the cardiovascular system. (4)
26. Discuss the potential impact of lung cancer on an individual's quality of life, considering both physical and psychological effects. (6)
27. Describe two ways in which a traumatic brain injury can affect the respiratory system. (4)
28. Describe two secondary effects of a traumatic brain injury on an individual's personality. (4)
29. Discuss the impact of acquired brain injury on the musculoskeletal system, including the role of the motor areas of the brain. (6)
30. Explain the difference between ischemic and haemorrhagic strokes, including their causes and potential consequences. (6)
31. State one way in which obesity can increase the risk of breast cancer. (1)
32. A woman is concerned about her risk of developing breast cancer. Explain the steps she could take to reduce her risk, considering both lifestyle and medical options. (6)
33. State one genetic factor that can increase the risk of developing bowel cancer (1)
34. Name one primary effect of bowel cancer that relates to changes in bowel movements. (1)
35. Describe two secondary effects of bowel cancer on the cardiovascular system. (2)
36. Explain the potential impact of bowel cancer metastasis on the body. Include examples of specific organs affected and the potential consequences. (6)

Unit 3 Principles of health and social care practice

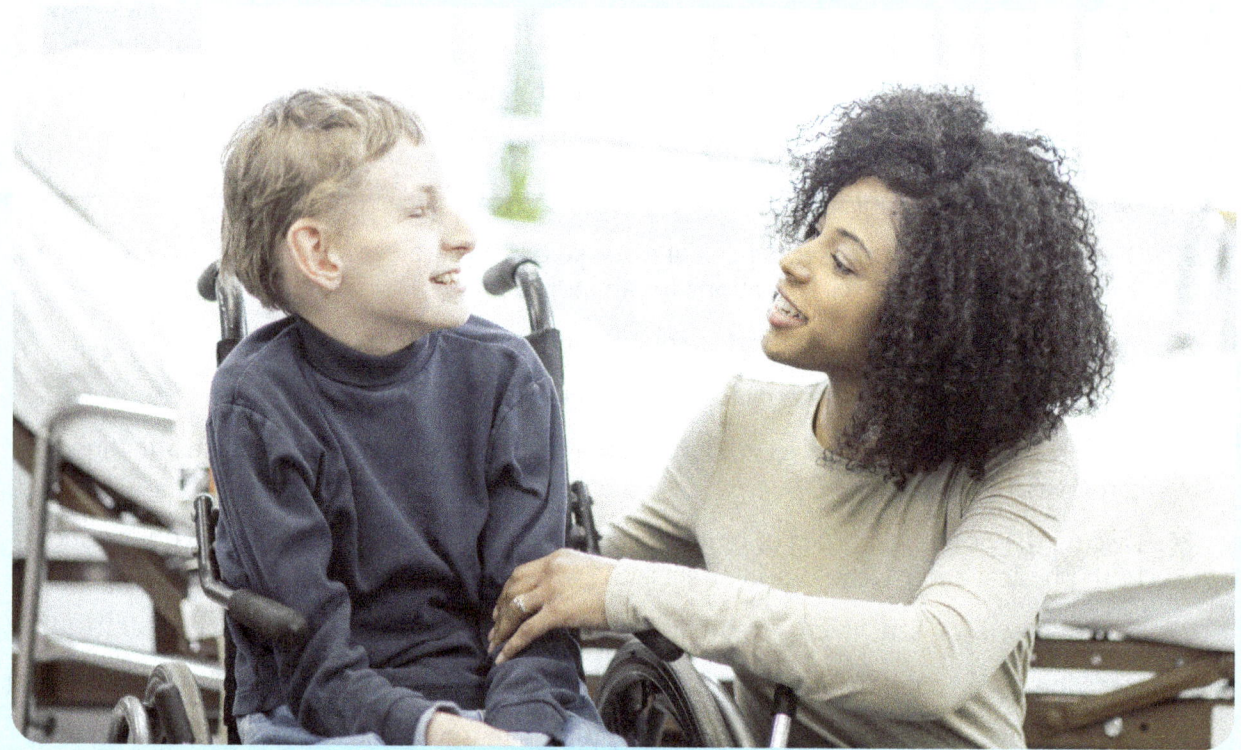

In this unit you will learn about the principles that underpin health and social care practice. You will learn about:

- The values, skills and principles that are needed to support people's care needs.
- The organisation of care practice.
- Laws, regulations and guidance.
- The social determinants of health, and the importance of equality, diversity and inclusion.

How will I be assessed?

In this unit you will be assessed through an internal assessment consisting of a series of tasks, covering Learning Aims A, B and C. The assignment is set by the awarding body and marked by your tutor.

Learning Aim A: Understand the principles of health and social care practice which underpin meeting the care and support needs of individuals

Learning Aim B: Examine how organisations, legislation and guidance inform practice in health and social care

Learning Aim C: Examine how social determinants affect the health status of individuals and the importance of equality, diversity and inclusion in practice

Learning Aim A: Understand the principles of health and social care practice which underpin meeting the care and support needs of individuals

A1 Values essential to health and social care practice

NHS Core Values

Professionals that work in the NHS are expected to demonstrate these six core values when delivering care.

Working together for patients

This means ensuring that **professionals work together** so that the patient always comes first and that they feel like all their needs are being met. It involves listening to the patient, to determine what they need in order to have a positive experience during their care. For example, it could include things such as adhering to an individual's religious beliefs during their time in hospital or ensuring an individual's dietary requirements are met. Working together for patients helps to promote the health and recovery of an individual.

Respect and dignity

During a patient's experience in an NHS service, they must be treated with respect and dignity. Professionals should ensure they value every person, listen to them, and treat them as individuals. Professionals should seek to understand the differing priorities, needs, views, abilities, and limits of an individual, and take these into account. In practice this can mean:

- Ensuring patients and their family are **actively involved** in their own personal care plan, so that they are included in decisions about their care or treatment.
- Providing patients with **appropriate choices** regarding the treatments available or the options of services offered to them.
- Promoting **independence** during a stay in hospital
- Making necessary **adaptations** within someone's home, such as ramps or a chair lift, to further promote independence.

Professionals must **never** be rude or patronising, behave arrogantly or humiliate patients.

Commitment to quality of care

Professionals working in the NHS should always demonstrate a commitment to:

- Providing high-quality care.
- Always trying to improve the quality of care.

This means getting the patient experience right each time by ensuring their needs are met consistently, and adapting care to ensure they receive a positive and effective experience.

One way of meeting this value is for services to gain feedback from both staff and patients. This can highlight areas of care that are working well and areas that need improving. This is something all professionals should always be striving for as part of their commitment to their work.

Compassion

Compassion means having **empathy** for patients – for example, having the ability to understand how a patient and their family might be feeling in that moment.

A professional should respond to individuals in their care with humanity and kindness throughout. For example, professionals should provide emotional support to individuals to try to alleviate any distress they might be feeling.

Improving lives

The NHS takes a holistic approach to their patients' lives and endeavours to **meet all the**

121

needs of an individual – not just their physical health. For example, an individual admitted to hospital with a physical health condition may also suffer some mental health issues. The NHS needs to be able to respond to each need of an individual in their current situation.

The NHS also takes a proactive approach to improving lives through preventative health campaigns to promote individuals making positive healthy lifestyle choices. For example, the NHS quit smoking campaign 'Stoptober' that runs every October.

Everyone counts

The NHS takes an anti-discriminatory approach when providing services and treatments for service users. The NHS must ensure all services are available for any and all individuals. This core value can be associated with a piece of legislation called 'The Equality Act 2010' where nine key protected characteristics were identified to promote anti-discriminatory practice across the UK. It is illegal to discriminate an individual with one or more of these characteristics.

> Service user – Refers to an individual that attends a service as a patient.
>
> Respect – Treating people well and having a good understanding of another person's feelings, wishes and needs.
>
> Dignity – Valuing a person's feelings, experiences and views, and ensuring they feel important and listened to.
>
> Commitment – Being dedicated to an individual's care.
>
> Holistic – Being considerate of all the needs of a service user. Including their physical, emotional, social, and spiritual needs.
>
> Anti-discriminatory approach – Methods to ensure the equality of all individuals.
>
> Protected characteristics – It is illegal to discriminate against anyone because of their: **age**, **disability**, **gender reassignment**, **marriage** and **civil partnership**, **pregnancy and maternity**, **race**, **religion or beliefs**, **sex**, and **sexual orientation**.

Activity

Consider and answer the following questions.

1. What is the overall aim of the NHS Core Values?
2. Write a list of five ways the NHS can improve the lives of individuals.
3. Sarah is looking for residential care for her mother who is 80 years old. Consider a list of things she should look out for while visiting and looking around residential homes that would indicate whether these person-centred values are being followed.

Recap questions

1. What type of approach does the NHS take to improving lives?
2. Which piece of legislation helps to promote the core value of 'everyone counts'?
3. How can dignity be promoted?
4. How can a professional adapt the quality of care being provided?
5. Which NHS core value requires empathy?

Skills for Care Values

Skills for Care is a workforce development and planning body for adult social care in England. Professionals delivering adult social care must be able to demonstrate the following.

Dignity and respect.

Dignity and respect is about ensuring a service user feels valued, listened to, and has a feeling of positive self-worth throughout their time in a service. Professionals who continuously treat people with dignity and respect create a trustworthy environment between patient and professional. This helps to create a culture of high-quality care.

A good example is being respectful of a patient's decisions and choices. For example, if a patient requests a female practitioner, then this should be respected.

Learning and reflection

An important skill for any professional is **reflecting on their own practice**. This means looking back on behaviour, attitudes and interactions with colleagues and patients, to see what went well and what could be improved. This can aid future decisions and improve quality of care. It is important that professionals consider feedback from patients, families, and staff to highlight areas for growth and to implement appropriate changes.

It is also essential that professionals continually **learn and improve** their practice. For example, this could be:

- Taking part in continuous professional development (CPD).
- Keeping up to date with the latest developments in technology or treatment.
- Learning new skills - for example, learning how to administer vaccinations.

Working together

The skill of working together is underpinned by the notion that 'patients come first.' Professionals in multi-disciplinary teams must follow certain strategies to work together successfully. These include:

- Effective communication
- Respect for each other
- Flexibility
- Adaptability

These strategies help teams work together collaboratively for the benefit of the service users.

Commitment to quality care and support

Professionals must be committed to maintaining and delivering **high-quality care** and support to every patient. This means following the standards and guidelines outlined

> CPD – Continuous professional development. Updating training in a particular area or learning a new skill to enhance expertise.
>
> Multi-disciplinary team – A group of healthcare professionals from different disciplines that work together to meet the needs of one individual.
>
> Communication – The exchange of information by speaking, writing or other means.
>
> Flexibility – Having a willingness to change or compromise.
>
> Adaptability – Being able to adjust or change in new situations.
>
> Competency – Being able to do something successfully and well.

in their service's policies and procedures, to ensure consistency in the care being delivered.

Professionals can also demonstrate commitment by always seeking to **improve their services and practice** to meet the demands and needs of the communities they serve. For example, professionals may set up services such as 'quit smoking' groups in a local area with high smoking rates. This would support individuals in the local area to make healthier life choices and avoid future health complications.

Professionals should also commit to improving their competency throughout their career. This could be through regularly practicing and refining skills, as well as learning new ones.

Recap questions

1. Which Skills for Care Value requires a professional to look back at their behaviour?
2. Which Skills for Care Value supports patients' autonomy over their care?
3. Name two strategies needed to work together successfully.
4. What is CPD?
5. How does CPD demonstrate commitment?

Activity

Consider and answer the following questions.

1. Which of the Skills for Care Values do you think is the most important when delivering care? Justify your decision.
2. Eva is a student nurse and has just been introduced to the Skills for Care Values. Considering these values, which one should Eva work towards first. Explain your choice.

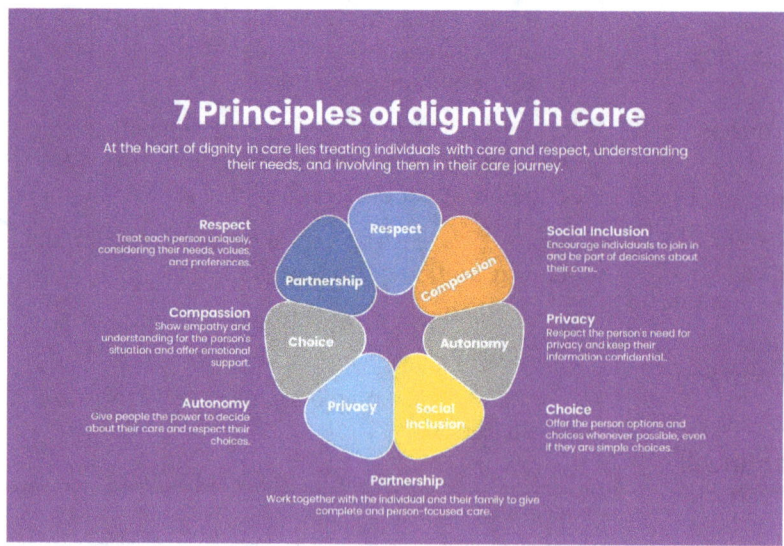

The 6Cs

In 2012 NHS England made six key values central to all nurses and midwives' practice. These care values, known as **the 6Cs**, are now a mandatory part of the introductory Care Certificate for healthcare support workers and adult social care workers.

Care

Care is at the heart of health and social care professionals. Their primary aim is to ensure that **care is provided to all** service users and that the **care is accurate and appropriate** for everyone, taking a person-centred approach. Providing effective care not only supports everyone's health, it also promotes the overall health of the community. Care can be demonstrated by:

- ensuring service users are comfortable
- addressing their needs promptly
- treating them with dignity and respect throughout their care.

Compassion

Compassion must be upheld for service users by remaining empathetic throughout an individual's care. Professionals can demonstrate compassion by **actively listening** to their patients' needs and wishes, acknowledging their feelings, and **providing them with support**. This support goes beyond that of their medical treatment.

Competence

Competence is about ensuring professionals remain up to date with their knowledge and skills, so that they can deliver care effectively. This can be demonstrated through regular CPD, to refresh themselves in a particular area, such as safeguarding, or to gain new knowledge and skills. Competency is important for all 6Cs.

Communication

Communication is vital for upholding a positive caring relationship with service users and their families. Professionals need to be able to **listen to service users** and be able to **communicate the next steps** in their care. The NHS has adopted the idea of 'no decision without me,' which means service users must be at the heart of any decisions made about their care. This can further be demonstrated by empowering service users in the decision-making process for their care plans, allowing them to maintain their independence.

Courage

Courage allows professionals to be advocates for their patients, striving to always do the right thing for service users and to speak out if there are concerns. For example, professionals have a duty of care to safeguard patients from malpractice and need to report any concerns they have about malpractice – poor working practices or ethical misconduct.

Person-centred approach – Treats service users as unique individuals and places them at the heart of the service. This approach considers the holistic and differing needs of individuals, which the service aims to meet.

Advocate – A person who speaks on behalf of someone else. This may be because they lack the capacity to do this. For example, an individual with a severe learning disability may be unable to speak for themselves and make informed decisions.

Safeguard – To protect all individuals who attend a service from harm.

Malpractice – Behaviour or actions that go against a service's policies and procedures. Legal action can be taken against individuals or services that are demonstrating malpractice.

Commitment

Commitment of professionals means that the holistic needs of service users are consistently met throughout their care. Professionals uphold this value through a dedication to high-quality care and striving to always improve quality of care. Commitment can be demonstrated by incorporating the other key values in their professional practice. For example, upholding their competency and effectively communicating with service users to ensure they fully understand the information provided to them.

Recap questions

1. Which of the 6Cs adopts the ideology of 'no decision about me without me'?
2. Which care value allows for advocacy?
3. How can the care value of compassion be demonstrated by professionals?
4. Which of the care values underpins all the 6Cs?
5. How can professionals demonstrate the care value of competence?

Activity

Consider and answer the following questions.

1. To what extent do you think the 6Cs are important when delivering care?
2. Which care value is being demonstrated in these situations. Explain your answers.
   - A healthcare professional attending a training session on moving and handling patients.
   - A physiotherapist supporting a patient with their mobility, despite the patient displaying anger towards the professional.
3. Health and social care professionals must be able to effectively communicate with their patients. Consider a list of things professionals could do to ensure they meet this care value successfully.

Apply your understanding

Jeremy is a 45-year-old man with a complex medical history, including type 2 diabetes, hypertension, and obesity. Jeremy has arrived at his local GP surgery with pain in his abdomen. Dr Patel takes the time to listen to Jeremy's concerns and explains probable causes of the pain in a compassionate and empathetic manner. Dr Patel makes a recommendation for Jeremy to be referred to the local hospital for further tests as he suspects Jeremy might have acute pancreatitis.

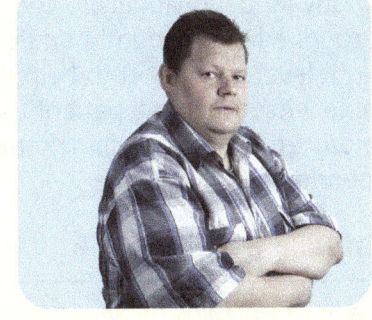

1. How is the skill of dignity and respect demonstrated in Jeremy's situation?
2. Which other key skill is demonstrated in this scenario? How do you know this?

A2 Person-centred care and approaches

In this section you will learn about how health and social care professionals can use a range of skills to promote effective care that includes empowering an individual.

Standard of care

In health and social care settings, professionals must work towards a standard of care that includes promoting **individuality, choice, independence, rights** and **privacy**. The overall aim of providing an effective standard of care is to **empower** individuals with their care/support needs.

Individuality

Individuality refers to the acceptance of an individual's personal characteristics and preferences. Professionals are expected to recognise and respect an individual's qualities. Professionals that can accept individuality are better equipped to provide effective care and are more likely to create positive relationships with the individual.

Choice

Choice in health and social care settings means providing individuals with more than one option linked to their care or support needs. For example, providing a range of food choices to meet different dietary requirements or providing choice over which medical professional is involved in the care planning process.

Independence

Independence means completing daily tasks or making decisions on your own. People who are unwell or who need additional support may not have full independence. However, it is the job of health and social care professionals to promote an individual's independence wherever possible. This can be done by encouraging and motivating individuals to complete their daily routine independently, and providing the right level of support to help them. For example, encouraging a patient to stand up every day after surgery will help them to shower independently again.

Rights

Rights are principles of what people are allowed to do or are entitled to have. Health and social care professionals and providers must consider a range of different types of rights when delivering care.

- **Legal rights**: Some rights are enforced in law. For example, the Human Rights Act 1998 sets out fundamental rights that all people have, including the right to life, autonomy and dignity. Other important legal rights are covered in the Care Act 2014 and the Equality Act 2010.

- **Other rights**: Organisations will have their own policies and procedures which may include rights above and beyond the legal rights. These extra rights can be considered

> Empathy – The ability to understand the needs and feelings of others from their point of view.
>
> Preferences – Having a greater liking for a particular thing or way.
>
> Respect – Considering the needs and preferences of another and accepting these.
>
> Autonomy – Having independence in the decisions and choices you can make away from external influences.
>
> Dignity – Having a sense of pride in yourself.
>
> Morally right – Beliefs about what is considered right and wrong.
>
> Sensitivity – The ability to respond to another person's feelings or needs in a kind and considerate manner.

to be morally right, and can include skills such as **empathy** and sensitivity. For example, leaving the room when an individual wants to wash themselves or use the toilet, if they are able to do so, demonstrates respect and dignity towards an individual, and allows them some level of independence.

Privacy

Privacy refers to:

- **Personal privacy**: Service users may have to undergo embarrassing or intimate procedures. Ensuring their privacy is maintained as much is possible is really important – for example, making sure doors are closed, that only necessary people are in the room, ensuring there is a curtained area for undressing.

- **Privacy of personal information**: Service users have legal rights for their personal information to be kept confidential. **GDPR** (General Data Protection Regulation) is a legal requirement that services and professionals must follow. It covers what data can be collected, for how long, and how it should be stored. For example, paper documents must be locked away and online files should be password protected.

> **Activity**
>
> Consider and answer the following questions.
>
> 1. How important is it for professionals to follow these standards of care?
> 2. What are the possible implications of not following the standards of care?

> **Recap questions**
>
> 1. Which standard of care considers a person's human rights?
> 2. Which standard of care ensures a patient can get dressed without others present?
> 3. Give an example of something a professional can give a patient choice over.
> 4. How can individuality be promoted?
> 5. What is the difference between 'independent' and 'dependent'?

Empowering individuals

A person-centred care approach is best met through **empowering** individuals to become stronger and more confident in controlling their own lives.

This can mean providing an individual with **choices** over their care and the opportunity to have some level of **independence** in their life.

It is important when promoting empowerment to value individuality, and to consider an individual's opinions, feelings and ideas about their own care.

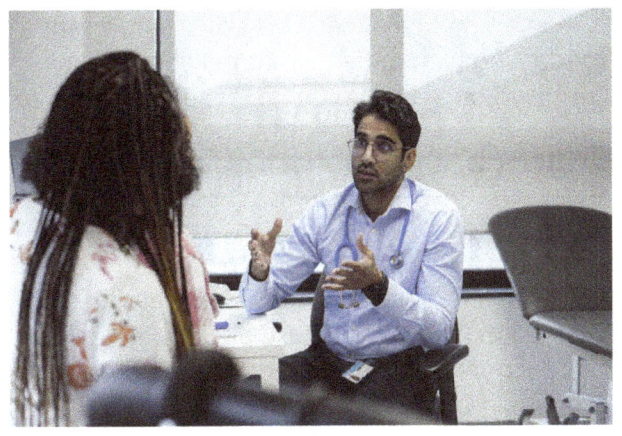

Focus on needs-led care

After considering an individual's opinions and feelings to empower an individual, professionals must then ensure their needs are met within the care planning process. Needs-led care is where professionals consider an individual's holistic needs, such as their physical, emotional and spiritual needs, before delivering care. The needs of an individual will help determine the type of care and support they require. For example, considering a person's dietary requirements or religious practices helps determine the treatments that can be offered.

Inclusive practice supports needs-led care. **Inclusive practice** refers to giving individuals access to an environment that is respectful and responsive to a diverse range of needs. For example, ensuring an individual with a physical impairment has appropriate access to services – this could include ensuring there is wheelchair access or adequate seating areas to support wait times.

People skills

When providing person-centred care professionals must use a variety of skills to deliver effective care. These include:

- empathy
- patience
- engendering trust
- flexibility
- sense of humour
- negotiating skills
- honesty
- problem-solving skills.

Empathy

Empathy is the ability of an individual to understand another's situation and how that person may be feeling. This allows professionals to build a positive rapport with the patient which supports better outcomes for the patient. This is important because showing a level of empathy can help to reduce patient anxiety, increase patient participation in their care and build trust between professionals and patients.

Patience

Patience is a skill that can be developed over time. It allows professionals to listen carefully to patients' concerns about their symptoms or worries they might have. By taking the time to listen, and consider their thoughts and feelings, professionals are more likely to give better explanations, which further fosters positive relationships and supports patient satisfaction. Acting with patience means professionals can take time to offer thoughtful and attentive care in a timely manner. This skill is important for dealing with patients that may be anxious, confused or easily dismissive of support.

Engendering trust

Engendering trust refers to the way professionals should behave to develop trust from service users. This is an essential skill for professionals. Without trust, all the other skills can become difficult to enact. When service users trust the service providers it can increase the quality of care and the care outcomes, because patients are more responsive to those they trust.

Honesty

Honesty goes hand in hand with engendering trust, as an important part of building trust comes from being honest. This means professionals and services are transparent and clear regarding their diagnosis, treatment options and outcomes. Being honest throughout a patient's care allows them to make informed and realistic decisions based on accurate information. Furthermore, honesty also allows professionals to be accountable for their actions, so that a level of **competency** is maintained.

Flexibility

Flexibility refers to how adaptable a professional can be when meeting the differing needs of individuals. Professionals must be able to quickly adapt to individual circumstances and needs. Care should be person-centred – not one size fits all – and tailored for each individual. It is important for

> Responsive – Reacting to individuals' needs in an appropriate and timely manner.
>
> Diverse – Working with a variety of individuals that come from differing cultural and social backgrounds.
>
> Rapport – A positive relationship between two people with a mutual understanding of each other's feelings.
>
> Patient satisfaction – A measure of how happy a patient is with the care they have received.
>
> Attentive care – Care that meets the needs, wishes and circumstances of an individual.
>
> Dismissive – To ignore a person's feelings or to deem someone unworthy of care.
>
> Not one size fits all – The same thing is not always applicable or appropriate for everyone.

professionals to develop a flexible approach as it allows them to handle unexpected challenges as they arise, such as a sudden change in a patient's health condition or to accommodate the needs of a patient's family without causing conflict.

Sense of humour

A **sense of humour** can help develop a rapport between a professional and service user. It can help reduce anxiety and make some uncomfortable conversations more manageable for patients and staff. For some individuals, a sense of humour can be a coping mechanism in difficult situations, and this should be addressed in a sensitive manner by the professional.

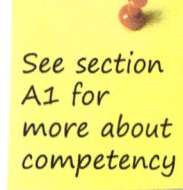

See section A1 for more about competency

However, it is important for professionals to consider the appropriateness of humour. For some it can help to ease tension, but for others it can cause misunderstandings which could then lead to offence or conflict. Therefore, it

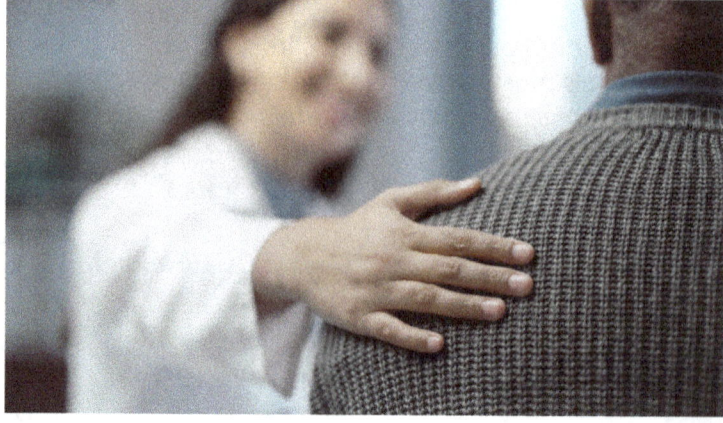

is pivotal that professionals take care when displaying humour and to consider the context of any jokes or comments.

Negotiating skills

Negotiating skills are needed whenever two parties want different things. Professionals use them to achieve a reasonable outcome for everyone. Negotiating skills are needed, for example, when:

- There is conflict between patients and staff decisions regarding treatment
- There are difficult or unrealistic family expectations
- Professionals in different teams have different workloads or financial or time constraints.

Problem-solving skills

Professionals will be regularly required to diagnose effectively, develop personalised care plans, and navigate lots of difficult situations. All of this requires some level of problem solving.

Effective problem-solving requires a professional to:

> **Conflict** – A disagreement or argument between individuals.
>
> **Multi-disciplinary working** – Involves professionals from different areas of work, that are knowledgeable in different fields, that can then support the needs of one individual.

- be knowledgeable about a topic
- think critically about situations
- evaluate all possible options
- then select one that is most likely to give the best outcomes in that particular situation.

For example, understanding the available treatment options for a diabetic individual but also being aware of the individual's context, including dietary requirements, which could hinder the effectiveness of treatments available to them.

In some cases, problem solving requires more than one professional, which demonstrates commitment to individualised care and maintains a level of teamwork through multi-disciplinary working.

> **Recap questions**
>
> 1. What is the difference between honesty and trust?
> 2. What does the term 'negotiate' mean?
> 3. Which people skill means 'to be adaptable'?
> 4. How can empathy be demonstrated?
> 5. Which people skill means 'to listen carefully to an individual no matter how long it takes'?

> **Activity**
>
> Consider and answer the following questions.
>
> 1. Which people skill do you think is the most important when delivering care? Justify your decision.
> 2. Consider a list of scenarios within the health and social care sector of when a sense of humour might not be appropriate.

Care/support plans & electronic health records (EHR)

Both a **care/support plan** and an **electronic health record** (EHR) are integral to providing person-centred care, and are required in all health and social care environments, but both serve different functions.

Care plan

A **care plan** is a detailed and individualised overview of the medical and supportive care a patient has received and needs to manage their health conditions. It includes:

- the aim of treatment
- interventions or actions to be taken
- and a timeline for achieving these aims.

The plan should be updated at regular intervals by professionals based on the patient's progress. For example, a cancer patient's plan will outline how often chemotherapy is to be administered and the outcome from each session based on test results.

In addition to all this information, the care plan will also inform professionals of the patients' preferences, needs and values. For example:

- their dietary requirements
- whether they require a male or female professional.

Patients should be, wherever possible, involved in the planning process and should be given the opportunity to amend the plan at any point. This is important as it **empowers** the patient to report any changes to professionals and to commit to the plan, with the intention of achieving a desired outcome.

Electronic health record

Electronic health records (EHR) are digital version of a patient's paper chart. They contain all information regarding a patient's medical history, diagnoses, medications, treatment plans, vaccination dates, allergies, scan results and lab results such as blood test results.

This record is made accessible to any health care provider that is caring for a patient on a need-to-know basis and provides methods on the EHR for different professionals to communicate information to each other regarding a patient's care. For example, an EHR can be shared amongst professionals using a shared digital system, where each professional has their own login with permissions that allow them to access EHRs for specific patients.

> Preferences – The things that someone likes or wants to do.
>
> Needs – Requires something that is essential or important for an individual's health.
>
> Values – A person's own judgement of what is important.

See page 123 for more information on empowerment.

It is important for the EHR to be up-to-date, so that different professionals are updated on a patient's care. For example, within a busy healthcare setting there will be regular shift and staff changes across multiple teams. Each member of staff needs to have the latest and most accurate information on a patient's progress.

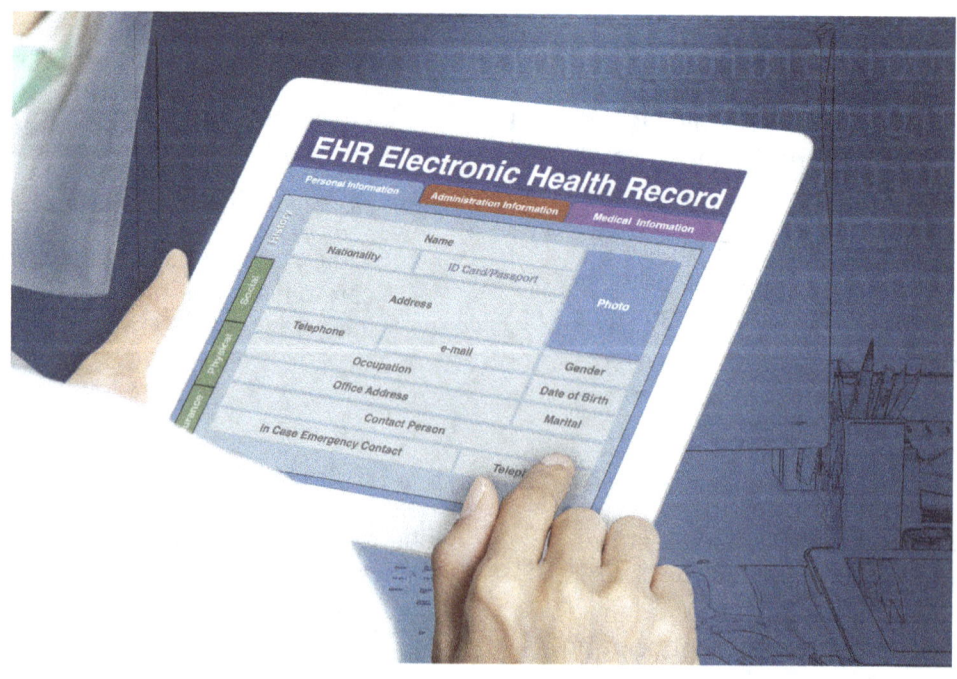

Raising concerns

Another aspect of person-centred care involves clearly outlining to patients the varying **channels of support** that a service can offer. This includes how to:

- contact the service/professionals
- file a complaint
- raise a concern
- seek advice from advocacy services.

See Unit 6 for more on raising concerns.

These channels should be explained when a care plan is being created. Making these channels accessible will help individuals to feel confident and **empowered** to address any issues with their care.

Possible reasons why a patient may raise a concern include:

- Safety concerns
- Inadequate communication
- Medication errors
- Neglect
- Lack of respect
- It is important for any concerns that have been raised to be addressed by services and professionals, as soon as possible, to prevent problems from escalating.

Advocacy – Speaking on behalf of another individual as they are deemed incapable.

Accessible – To make a setting easy to get to or into.

Escalating – Getting worse very quickly.

Activity

Consider and answer the following questions.

1. What are the possible implications of not ensuring a care plan or EHR are up to date?
2. How does a care/support plan empower individuals?
3. Create your own summary of both a care plan and an electronic health record (EHR).

Recap questions

1. Identify two pieces of information that should be present in a care plan.
2. Identify two pieces of information that should be present in an electronic health record (EHR).
3. Give an example of a reason why a patient may choose to raise a concern.
4. What is the difference between a care plan and an EHR.
5. Why is it important for an EHR to be kept updated?

A3 Communication in health and social care

In this section you will learn about the different types of communication, including digital communication. You will also gain an understanding of how and why communication is important, and the impact both effective and poor communication can have on individual outcomes.

Types of communication

- **Verbal** – the use of words to transmit ideas, thoughts or feelings across to another person.
- **Non-verbal** – the sharing of information without using words. This can include facial expressions, body language and eye contact.
- **Written** – a method used to create and maintain records; written information should be presented in a clear way for others to be able to read and understand.
- **Digital** – information that is shared between people using online tools.

Supporting person-centred care

When communicating with patients and their relatives it is important to consider how good communication can support **person-centred care**, for instance by:

- Providing accurate information
- Supporting privacy and dignity
- Using listening skills

> Considerate – To show careful thought about someone else's feelings or situation.
>
> Advocate – A person that can speak on behalf of another.

- Avoiding **jargon, slang and acronyms**
- Providing empathy and emotional support

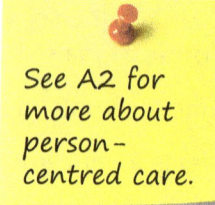

See A2 for more about person-centred care.

Respect and patience

Communication is not just limited to professionals and patients but also includes relatives, carers, friends, colleagues and all members of multi-disciplinary teams.

Communication between all these individuals should always demonstrate **respect** and **patience**. This means being considerate of what another person is saying throughout a conversation, and listening without interruption. This is important as it demonstrates to the patient and others that you, as a professional, **care** about their wellbeing and are **committed** to supporting a positive outcome for them.

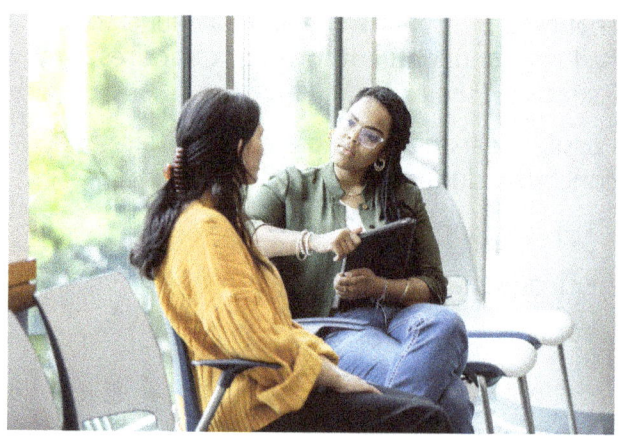

Effective communication between colleagues

There are several reasons as to why communication is important between colleagues and other professionals. This includes:

- **Collaboration** on the care being provided through the sharing of ideas.
- **Coordination of responsibilities** such as delegating areas of duties for a shift.
- **Shared decision making** on the treatment plan for a patient or on the discharge conditions.
- **Shared responsibilities** for planning and problem solving.

Adapting communication

It is important that professionals can **adapt** their communication methods based upon an individual's needs, such as **learning disabilities**, **dementia** or **hearing impairments**.

Professionals may also have to consider how they communicate with advocates of these individuals, so that information can be relayed back to individuals correctly and so the right decisions are made that benefit the individual.

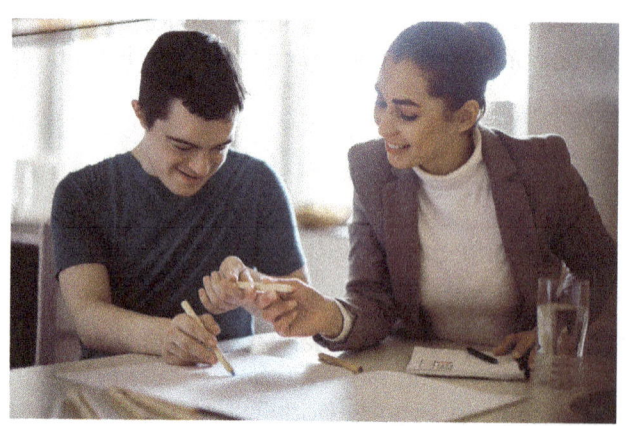

People with learning disabilities

When communicating with anyone with additional needs it is important that the message being given is clear and understood. Individuals with a learning disability may be unable to comprehend complex information. Therefore, messages should use simple and straightforward language that avoids **jargon**, **slang** or **acronyms**.

It is also important to consider how information is passed on to individuals with a learning disability. Professionals should ensure information is broken down into smaller, more manageable chunks, giving the individual time to process it before moving on. Throughout a conversation the professional should demonstrate **patience** and allow extra time for individuals to respond to information, or to ask further questions.

Professionals must always maintain the skill of active listening so that the individual feels valued and heard. When caring for individuals with a learning disability it is also crucial to check their understanding. This can be done by asking them to repeat back information or to explain their understanding in their own words. This helps the professional to confirm the message has been understood and communicated well.

People with dementia

Communication with an individual with **dementia** should use clear, simple language, delivered in a slow and calm manner.

It is also important to focus on one idea at a time, again avoiding complex language – this will help to minimise any anxiety or frustration.

Dementia patients can become easily distressed because they are unable to process information as well as they once could. Using shorter sentences and repeating key points can help them to recognise key information.

Professionals should also consider their **non-verbal** cues when communicating, such as their facial expression or body language. Tone of voice should also remain friendly and reassuring.

Any conversation with a dementia patient is best in a quiet and calm environment, to prevent distractions and make it easier for the patient to focus and engage in the conversation.

People with a hearing impairment

Individuals with a **hearing impairment** have some level of difficulty understanding audible information. This means that professionals must ensure their face is clearly visible so that patients can use lip reading techniques to understand what they are saying. Speaking clearly and at a moderate pace, so that patients can follow along, is also crucial.

It is important to not shout as it can distort speech and the way individuals interpret lip movement, which can cause misunderstandings. Non-verbal methods are also a vital element because hand gestures and facial expressions can also give clues about the message being conveyed.

Sign language is a common method of communication for individuals with a hearing impairment. Not all professionals are trained in BSL (British Sign Language), therefore services should consider having an interpreter present as.

As with dementia patients, conversations should be had in quiet environments to avoid distractions, and professionals should also check an individual's understanding of the conversation to avoid misconceptions about treatments or diagnosis.

Other forms of communication, such as visual aids (pictures or diagrams) can also be effective in supporting individuals in their understanding of information.

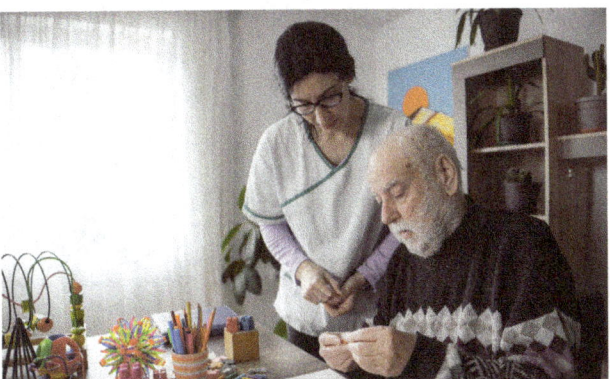

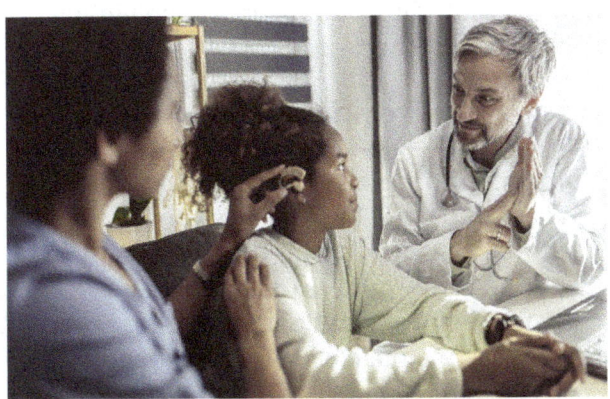

Impact of good and poor communication

Good communication can impact outcomes for individuals within health and social care settings. Good communication can:

- Cause individuals to **share more information with professionals**
- Mean that staff within teams have a good understanding of information as it has been **communicated in a clear and understandable way**
- Motivate individuals **to follow treatment plans**
- Cause individuals to **take on board advice** and act upon it, such as living a healthy lifestyle
- Have a positive effect on **mental wellbeing**

> **Audible information** – Information that we hear.

However, poor communication can also impact outcomes for individuals. It can:

- Lead to **increases in harm, length of stay** and **resource use**
- Negatively affects **staff morale**
- Mean that professionals do **not have the most correct and up-to-date information**
- Lead to **delays** in implementing **effective treatment or care**
- Lead to **inconsistent and inaccurate records**
- Mean that **issues can remain unresolved**.

Activity

Consider and answer the following questions.

1. To what extent do you think non-verbal communication is effective when delivering care? Justify your answer.
2. What would be the difference in health outcomes between:
   - A service user who has a hearing impairment and uses BSL, but the professional does not know BSL
   - A service user with a hearing impairment who receives a professional that does understand BSL.

Recap questions

1. Give two examples of non-verbal communication.
2. Identify two benefits of good communication.
3. Identify two ways poor communication can impact on outcomes for individuals.
4. How could communication be adapted for an individual with dementia?
5. Give a reason for why communication is important between colleagues.

Digital communication

Digital technology is used in the health and social care sector in a variety of ways. Currently, practices use digital tools such as **home monitoring**, **virtual wards** and **video consultations/check-ups**.

Home monitoring devices

Home monitoring devices can be given to patients who need to regularly monitor specific health issues, such as high blood pressure (hypertension). They are used to ensure a patient's safety and wellbeing whilst at home, so they can maintain a level of independence.

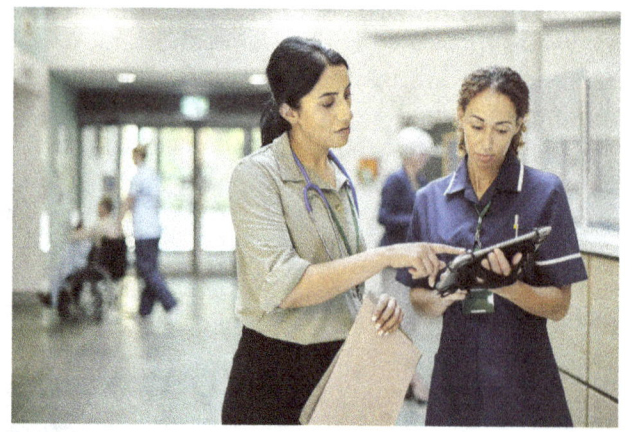

They can be used for individuals suffering from conditions that affect day-to-day functioning, such as dementia, or can be used for individuals in later adulthood that have become a fall risk due to issues with mobility, such as osteoarthritis.

- They can pass everyday data readings to health services. Common examples include blood sugar levels for people with diabetes and oxygen in the blood for people with respiratory problems.
- They can alert a call centre, carers or the emergency services if an individual needs immediate help.
- Motion sensors can be used to detect movement in the home for older people. A lack of movement could indicate a fall.
- A **personal alarm** can be carried or worn, for example around the wrist like a watch or as a necklace. It can be used in emergencies to alert relevant services to a problem.

Virtual ward

A **virtual ward** is when a patient receives care in the comfort of their own home so that patients can continue to have some independence and autonomy over their lives.

A virtual ward provides hospital-level care to patients but in their home. The aim of a virtual ward is to free up beds in hospitals for other patients, and to support a quicker recovery.

A patient receiving care through this method would still have access to a multi-disciplinary team (MDT) and would receive care from the relevant professionals within the home, including regular visits by clinical staff either in person or through a **video consultation**, to conduct tests and treatments.

Virtual wards make good use of technology to support a patient, including apps, wearable

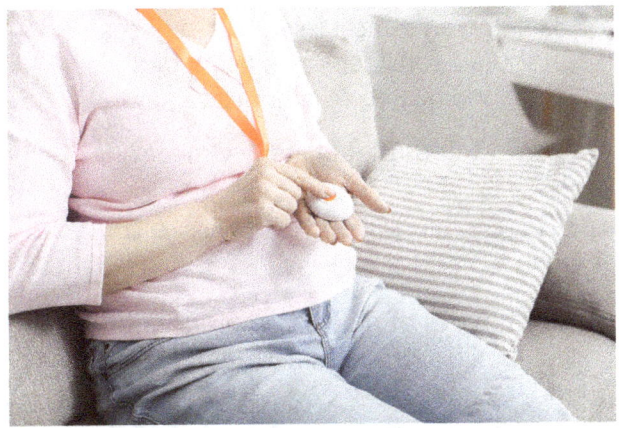

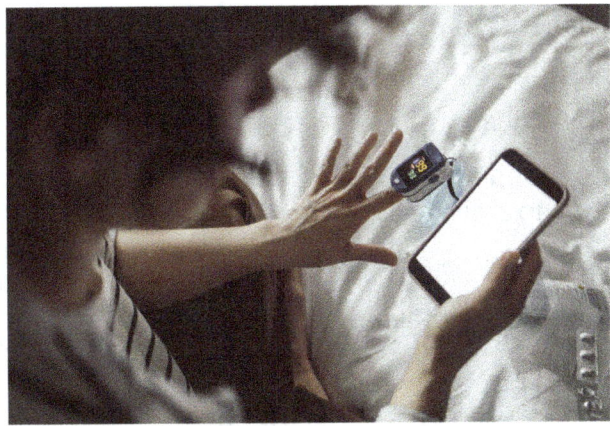

devices (such as personal alarms) and other medical devices for staff to easily check and monitor a patient's recovery.

Video consultations

The COVID-19 lockdown in 2020 led to the need for **video consultations** and **check-ups**. This is an appointment with a medical professional over the internet, using a video camera.

This method of consultation is still widely used to support patients who may be unable to travel, due to illness or the location of a service.

A video appointment is very similar to a face-to-face appointment, where you can:

- discuss any issue, you have with a professional,
- be diagnosed with some conditions/ illnesses,
- be prescribed medication
- be referred on to further services (referrals).

However, a video call does require access to a good internet connection, which not everyone has. It also requires people to have access to a smartphone or computer. Therefore professionals do aim to make a phone call to patients instead, if a video call cannot take place.

Benefits of digital communication

There are several benefits of digital communication. These are explained in the table on the next page.

Benefits to professionals	Benefits to individuals
• Time efficient	• Increases access to services and professionals
• Enhances face-to-face engagement	• Provides health information and education
• Opportunities to provide reassurance to individuals	• Improves confidence in managing own health
• Develop and maintain relationships	• Improves independence
• Catch problems/changes early	• Improves experience of service provision
	• Does not require interpretation services

Considerations of digital communication

However, there are some things professionals and services should consider when implementing digital communication in their practice. This includes:

- **The cost to individuals** – some equipment is not always funded by the NHS due to individuals not always meeting the criteria for financial support.
- **Ethical issues** – services need to consider how issues such as informed consent and confidentiality are addressed when communicating online.
- **Safety of information shared** – services need to ensure they meet cybersecurity legislation and professionals must meet these standards and understand what to do if they have an online security breach.
- **Digital literacy** of staff and individuals – not all individuals are able to access technology or understand how to use this. Therefore, digital communication must be simple and easy to use.

Autonomy – Having independence in the decisions and choices you can make away from external influences.

Hospital-level care – Care that provides specialised medical attention and treatment for individuals.

Multi-disciplinary team – A group of healthcare professionals from different disciplines that work together to meet the needs of one individual.

Clinical staff – Refers to staff who work within a medical setting that provide direct care to patients.

Referrals – Referring or sending a patient for further review or treatment to another health care professional/service.

Informed consent – Permission gained from patients with their full knowledge and understanding of the potential consequences.

Confidentiality – Ensuring an individual's information remains private.

Cybersecurity legislation – The umbrella term for four main legislation schemes that outline cybersecurity and data protection.

Find out more

www.eboru.com/BTEC-HSC-links

BSL. Virtual wards.
Cybersecurity legislation. Video consultation.
Home monitoring.

Recap questions

1. Identify an example of a digital tool.
2. How does digital communication improve person-centred care?
3. Identify **two** benefits of digital communication to either professionals or individuals.
4. Name an ethical issue that services should consider when using digital technology to communicate.
5. What does digital literacy mean?

Activity

1. Why might digital communication be particularly useful for people with English as an additional language?
2. Which types of digital communication would allow professionals to detect changes early?

A4 Confidentiality

In this section you will learn about what confidentiality means along with how it can be maintained and the possible consequences of failing to adhere to confidentiality policies.

Keeping information confidential

In health and social care settings **confidentiality** is an important **ethical and legal requirement**. Professionals and service providers must protect service users' and staff members' personal and sensitive information.

Any piece of information obtained by a service must be done so with that person's **permission**.

- This means they have given consent for their details to be stored by the service.
- Consent must also be given for any personal or sensitive information to be shared with family, friends or carers. This is typically logged in the 'permissions' section of an individual's file.

It is vital for permission to be obtained in order to adhere to GDPR laws and to ensure trust is maintained within a service.

Services hold a large amount of data about both staff and service users, so it is of great importance that this information is stored in the correct way to avoid data breaches.

Any sensitive information, or information that could identify an individual, should be:

- password-protected if stored on a computer
- locked away in a filing cabinet or filing room if it is paper-based.

Access to this information should then only be given to relevant staff on a need-to-know basis. This means information about a particular individual should only be shared when it is required to provide safe and effective care.

Sharing confidential information

When sharing information between staff, confidentiality should still be maintained. Before sharing any confidential information you should consider whether it is:

- **Necessary** – it needs to be shared.
- **Proportionate** – only the necessary amount of information is to be shared.
- **Relevant** – only information that is needed in order to give high-quality care.
- **Accurate** – the information must be up to date.
- **Timely** – information to be shared only when it is needed.
- **Secure** – information should only be shared in a safe way, where it could not be accessed by unauthorised people. For example, sending confidential information in an unprotected Word file over email is not secure. All files and electronic devices should be password protected.

Policies and procedures

Professionals in the health and social care sector must follow organisational policies and procedures to protect data. For example, organisations will have a **confidentiality policy** for those that work with person-identifiable and sensitive information. The policy will outline:

- When and how to share records.
- How to report concerns about the recording of information.
- How to store records.

It will also include details about **whistleblowing**. Whistleblowing means that staff have a legal right to raise any concerns they have about poor practice or malpractice within a setting.

In relation to confidentiality, this could be because a service or user is not storing patient records securely. More generally, whistleblowing can be related to any malpractice in a service.

Breaching confidentiality

The confidentiality policy will also outline the consequences for breaching confidentiality. This can include:

- **Disciplinary action** – this can include loss of reputation or loss of employment.
- **Criminal charges** – a data breach can be seen as a form of theft and could lead to large fines or imprisonment.

GDPR – Legislation that covers how organisations can use and store people's personal information.

Need to know basis – Only telling someone the facts they need to know about an individual to provide adequate care.

Policies – A set of actions proposed by an organisational setting. These can follow legislation.

Procedures – How a set of actions should be conducted.

Activity

Consider and answer the following questions.

1. What are the benefits and limitations of whistleblowing?
2. How does maintaining confidentiality establish trust between the service user and professional?

Recap questions

1. What is confidentiality?
2. How does consent link to confidentiality?
3. Identify a consequence of breaching confidentiality.
4. What does person-identifiable information mean?
5. How should personal and sensitive information be stored?

Find out more

www.eboru.com/BTEC-HSC-links

Find out more about the NHS's confidentiality policy.

A5 Duty of care

In this section you will learn about professionals' legal responsibilities when caring for service users. You will also gain an understanding of how to manage difficult situations using relevant policies and procedures.

Legal obligations

Within the health and social care sector professionals have a **duty of care** to:

- provide **safe practice** for all individuals that access a service,
- to **protect** individuals
- to **prevent** harm.

Duty of care is otherwise known as a **legal obligation** to always act in the **best interests** of the individual and their family/carers that are using a service. This means that professionals are always **committed** to ensuring individuals receive high-quality care that considers their needs and wishes.

Acting in a person's best interests also means questioning any choices/decisions they make if you think it might put the individual at risk of harm. However, a professional can only prevent someone from doing something if:

- they have gained consent from the individual themselves,
- the individual has been deemed to lack the capacity to make effective decisions.

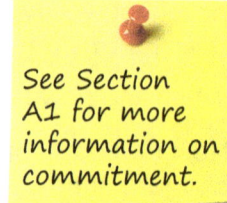

See Section A1 for more information on commitment.

Record keeping

Another aspect of duty of care is the maintenance of an individual's records. Professionals must ensure records are **up-to-date** and **accurate.** This means updating records with relevant information that is needed to support an individual. This could include relevant health checks or personal preferences. To meet their duty of care, staff should also share records with relevant teams and professionals on a need-to-know basis.

Standards of care

For professionals to meet their legal obligation they must also adhere to the agreed national standards of care that have been outlined by regulators. The national standards of care were updated in April 2018 and are relevant across all services within the health and social care sector. They are underpinned by five key principles, including dignity and respect.

The standards also outline five headline outcomes they want to ensure service users experience:

- I experience **high-quality care** and support that is right for me.
- **I am fully involved** in all decisions about my care and support.
- I have **confidence in the people** who support and care for me.
- I have **confidence in the organisation** providing my care and support.
- I experience a **high-quality environment** if the organisation provides the premises.

Codes of conduct and ethics

Regulators also outline **codes of conduct** and **codes of ethics** that professionals must follow. This now includes **nurses & midwives, allied health professionals** and **social workers.**

A code of conduct is what is seen as 'best practice' within a service and outlines the behaviours and attitudes professionals require when providing a service. Each service/set of professionals will have its own code of conduct set out by regulators although most codes are very similar. A code of ethics outlines expected moral behaviours, such as telling the truth.

Dignity, compassion and respect

Another aspect of a professional's duty of care is to ensure the treatment of service users encompasses **dignity, compassion and respect.**

- **Dignity** can be maintained by ensuring an individual's self-respect stays intact. For example, ensuring a patient remains clean and neatly dressed will help a patient to remain dignified during their stay in a service.
- Professionals that demonstrate **compassion** go out of their way to alleviate any discomfort an individual may be experiencing. This can also support an individual's dignity as by removing/reducing the cause of discomfort it helps to keep their self-worth in place.
- **Respect** is also an important aspect of duty of care as all individuals have a right for their individuality to be respected. Respect should be given for all individual's needs, wishes, **circumstances,** beliefs, lifestyle and experiences.

To not treat a service user with dignity, compassion or respect can create negative outcomes for their health and wellbeing, such as the avoidance of services leading to further ill health.

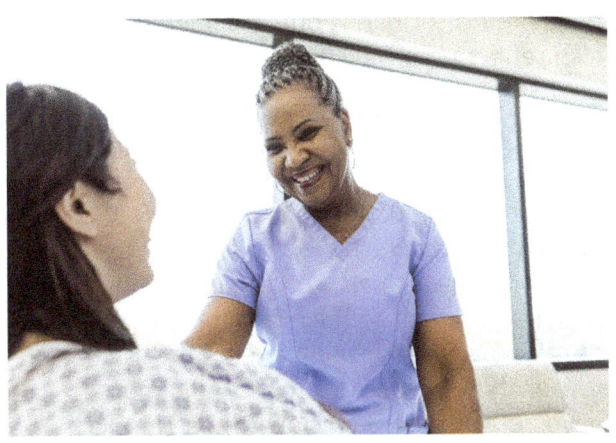

Appropriate services

It is important that individuals receive **services that are appropriate** to their age and life stage. For example, children are directed towards health care in the paediatric department and the elderly to the geriatric department.

It is also important that individuals receive services appropriate to their **individual circumstances**. This can include their health or living situation. This means professionals must be compassionate towards their circumstances and direct them to the most appropriate service.

For example:

- an individual displaying symptoms of psychosis will need access to a mental health team rather than a standard ward
- an individual living in poverty and unable to purchase their prescriptions may need support from the NHS Business Services Authority (NHSBSA) so that their circumstances can be assessed to determine if they are eligible for additional funding for their health or social care needs.

> **Need to know basis** – Only telling someone the facts they need to know about an individual to provide adequate care.
>
> **Moral behaviours** – What a society determines as acceptable behaviour to allow individuals to live in harmony with each other.
>
> **Life stage** – A period an individual goes through and will experience certain types of development in each life stage. For example, infancy or early adulthood.
>
> **Paediatric department** – A hospital department that specialises in caring for children.
>
> **Geriatric department** – A hospital department that specialises in caring for older people.
>
> **Psychosis** – A symptom of some mental health conditions that causes a disconnect between an individual and reality, affecting thoughts and feelings.

Rights and choices

A professional's duty of care must adhere to the legal rights they have.

For example, everyone has legal rights outlined in the Human Rights Act 1998. This legislation must be followed by all professionals so as **not to deprive any individual of their basic rights**.

For example, all individuals have a human right to not experience discrimination. If professionals do discriminate against an individual, they are therefore neglecting their duty of care.

Ensuring all rights of an individual are met means they can live as independently as possible and are empowered to **make choices** and **take appropriate risks**. For example, having the freedom to decide whether to participate in a research project for a new drug.

Personal conduct

Duty of care is not just about a professional's **personal conduct** during working hours but also about how their personal lives must also meet expected professional standards. Any behaviour or opinions outside of work should also reflect positively on the professional.

For instance, having images or videos posted on social media after a night out with friends could reflect poorly as a professional if these show your conduct to be unprofessional or inappropriate for your job role. Therefore, it is vital for professionals working in the health and social care sector to maintain **confidentiality** of their own personal information. This means that any use of social media must have appropriate **privacy settings enabled** to prevent confidential information being leaked to members of the public, which could compromise a professional's position in their job.

However, it is important to note that, even with personal privacy settings enabled, professionals should be very cautious in their use of social media, as they must still demonstrate respect for individuals, carers, families and colleagues. No information about anyone you have a professional relationship with should ever be posted on social media.

To be disrespectful on these platforms, in any manner, could lead to investigations into a professional's conduct in the workplace.

Managing dilemmas

On occasion, dilemmas can arise about duty of care and it is important that professionals understand how to manage these appropriately. Ways to manage dilemmas include the following.

Following policies and procedures.

Policies and procedure are in place to ensure the protection of individuals, self and colleagues - for example, following procedures such as how to implement COSHH regulations, or understanding an organisation's safeguarding policy. It is vital that all policies and procedures outlined in a service both adhere to the legal obligation of duty of care and to ensure the safety of all involved.

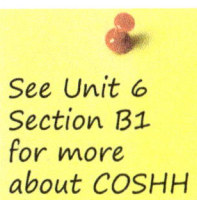

See Unit 6 Section B1 for more about COSHH

Mental capacity assessments (MCA)

- **Mental capacity assessments (MCA)** are made for those who may be unable to make effective decisions independently, due to specific circumstances such as conditions like dementia or schizophrenia. Capacity refers to an individual's ability to be able to make appropriate decisions that will benefit their own care. An MCA is conducted to determine how well an individual can make decisions, so that professionals can support them to still have some level of independence about their own care and support.

Taking positive risks

- Occasionally service users need to be supported to take **positive risks.** A positive risk can benefit users when trying to address their needs. For example, when deciding on a course of medication for an illness, an individual is told that the side effects could worsen their symptoms but has a good chance of relieving those symptoms. Professionals can help the individual see the positive risks of taking the medication, as the chances are that it will help them.

> COSHH – Control of Substances Hazardous to Health. A regulation that protects staff and others from hazardous substances in the workplace.
>
> Capacity – When an individual is deemed capable of making informed decisions for themselves.
>
> Line manager/shift leader – An individual who oversees a group of people during a shift or during their career in a health and social care environment.
>
> Safeguard – Ensuring individuals safety from risks such as neglect or abuse in a health or social care

Reporting procedures

- If an event was to occur that can cause harm or distress to individuals within a health or social care service, it is imperative that professionals follow the relevant **reporting procedures** to manage the dilemma effectively. This can include things such as reporting concerns about working conditions or faulty equipment as soon as possible. If professionals do need to report any concerns such as concerns about wellbeing, abuse, neglect or professional misconduct, they must follow the services reporting procedure. This often means **reporting any incidents** to their line manager or shift leader as soon as possible.

It is crucial that **any concerns of this nature are reported immediately** to safeguard the individuals involved and protect them from any further consequences.

Activity

1. Which aspect of a professional's duty of care do you think is the most important?

2. How does a professional's personal conduct in their personal lives impact upon their career in the health and social care sector?

Recap questions

1. What is 'duty of care'?
2. Identify two methods of managing a dilemma in health and social care.
3. Define the term 'dignity'.
4. Which piece of legislation supports the rights of all individuals?
5. What is a code of conduct?

A6 Working with vulnerable children and adults at risk

Vulnerabilities

The **Applying All Our Health (2022)** document outlines clear definitions of **vulnerability** and how specific individuals may be deemed as vulnerable. It states that being vulnerable is 'defined as in need of special care, support, or protection because of age, disability, risk of abuse or neglect'. This can apply to both children and adults over the age of 18 years. The document gives professionals an understanding of what vulnerabilities are and how they can be addressed to prevent negative consequences for individuals.

> Designated safeguarding lead (DSL) – A professional responsible for the care and safety of individuals within their setting.

Safety and safeguarding

Within health or social care settings professionals have a legal obligation (duty of care) to protect individuals' rights.

Individuals have rights to **live in safety**, both at home or within a service, that is **free from abuse and neglect.** This means children and adults should not be subjected to:

- any form of neglect such as not being fed
- any form of abuse, whether that is physical or mental abuse.

This, of course, applies to all children and adults.

A professional has a duty of care to keep vulnerable users safe by preventing harm and reducing the risks of abuse and neglect. To do this effectively, professionals must always follow all safeguarding policies and procedures.

- Each service will have its own policy about how to safeguard adults and children at risk from harm, but all will adhere to legislation such as the **Human Rights Act 1998**.
- Services that work closely with children will adhere to **The Children's Act 2004**, which outlines information on how to safeguard children, and the relevant authorities and services that support this.

Vulnerable users should still be empowered to make appropriate and effective choices about their care to still have some control over the way they choose to live their lives. For example, a vulnerable child may need support in terms of housing, health or social care needs and necessities but they should still be able to make choices over what they wear, food choices, personal space and their identity.

Following policies and procedures when reporting and documenting safeguarding concerns

It is important that professionals understand their role and responsibility in adhering to policies and procedures about documenting and reporting safeguarding concerns.

Knowing about and following the policies and procedures in place for raising safeguarding concerns, means that services meet legal requirements, ensures each concern is addressed, keeping children and adults safe from harm.

For example, schools have a rigorous system of reporting concerns through online platforms that lead straight to designated safeguarding leads (DSL), so that they can then follow up with concerns as appropriate. The DSLs then take over the safeguarding and protecting of children by involving the necessary individuals or services for the individual's needs.

Multi-agency working

Multi-agency working is the collaboration of professionals from a range of specialisms to support individuals. It is an important aspect of supporting vulnerable individuals, as it allows adequate care to be provided from a range of services and skilled professionals. This is particularly important for vulnerable individuals with complex needs.

Effective multi-agency teams support individuals through **good communication between different professionals**. This promotes good outcomes for individuals as gaps between care services are reduced, ensuring that the holistic needs of individuals are met, and care is tailored to meet those needs.

Find out more

www.eboru.com/BTEC-HSC-links

The code for nurses & midwives:

The code of ethics for social workers:

Vulnerabilities according to the Applying All Our Health (2022).

Recap questions

1. What does vulnerability mean?
2. What does safeguarding mean?
3. What does multi-agency working involve?
4. Which document outlines vulnerabilities of service users?
5. Identify a characteristic that is protected under this document.

Activity

1. What are the possible consequences of not following relevant policies and procedures for both professionals and vulnerable service users?
2. What could happen if multi-agency working fails?

End of Learning Aim Practice Activity

Look at these two case studies.

Case study 1: Nurse Thompson works in a busy hospital ward and has been caring for two individuals with vastly differing needs. **Mr Smith** is an elderly gentleman who has been diagnosed with dementia. He often chooses to sit quietly in the communal room and look out into the garden area. Nurse Thompson finds that each day she needs to support Mr Smith with his day-to-day routine prior to sitting in the communal room. This includes providing personal care and guiding him through meals and his medication schedule, whilst providing a level of comfort, as Mr Smith can often become confused and distressed.

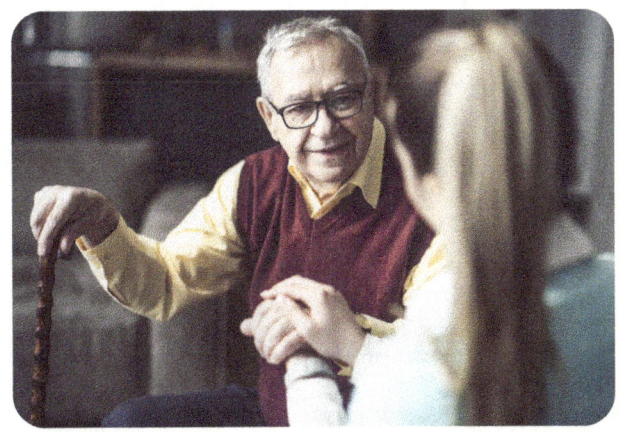

Case study 2: Nurse Thompson has also been caring for **Ms Patel**, a young woman who has recently experienced a traumatic spinal cord injury which has left her paralysed from the waist down She uses a wheelchair. Nurse Thompson has been working with Ms Patel to assist her in daily exercises and providing her with encouragement and reassurance with each movement. Nurse Thompson often finds herself engaging in her conversation with Ms Patel and notices a shift in her emotional state during these conversations. Ms Patel can also be quite vocal when Nurse Thompson does something with which she does not agree. Nurse Thompson then finds herself being very reflective on her practice to better support Ms Patel in the future.

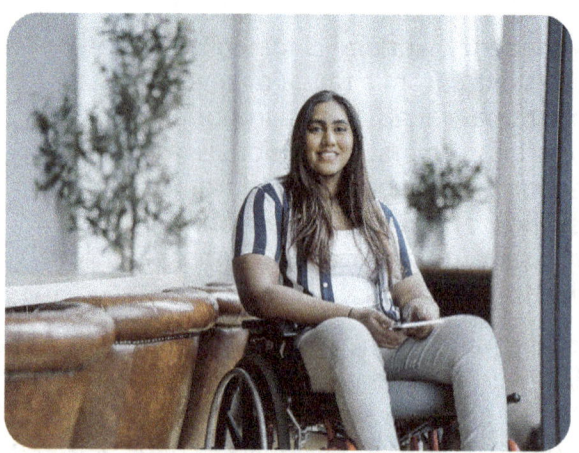

--

For each case study you need to think about the ways in which Nurse Thompson can overcome challenges in order to provide person-centred care to Mr Smith and Ms Patel.

You can write down your ideas about the following:

- What values do you think are essential for Nurse Thompson so she can provide person-centred care?
- What kind of methods could she use with each of them when building relationships and establishing trust? Will the methods be the same for both people?
- How could Nurse Thompson use effective communication to establish trust?
- What is Nurse Thompson's duty of care? How might she overcome barriers and manage dilemmas for both Mr Smith and Ms Patel, relating this to her duty of care.
- Why it is important for Nurse Thompson to balance individual right and choices of Mr Smith and Ms Patel?.

This practice task will help you prepare for the following assessment criteria:

A.P1 Explain the values and skills necessary for professionals caring for two individuals with different needs.

A.P2 Explain how effective communication can be used by professionals to build relationships with two individuals with different needs.

A.P3 Explain the implications of a duty of care in health and social care practice.

A.M1 Assess the impact of factors on service provision and the potential challenges to providing appropriate care to meet the needs of two individuals.

A.D1 Evaluate the challenges of providing an appropriate care environment for two individuals

Learning Aim B: Examine how organisations, legislation and guidance inform practice in health and social care

B1 Organisations, legislation and guidance affecting health and social care services

In this section, you will learn about various organisations and legislation within health and social care, that help govern the day to day running of services.

You should note that these organisations and legislations are subject to change, and you must refer to the most up-to-date versions in your assessment.

Roles and responsibilities of key organisations

Department of Health and Social Care

The **Department of Health and Social Care** is one of the main organisations that govern overall practice in the health and social care sector. It is responsible for the implementation of policies and legislation for hospitals, family practitioner services, community health and social services. It is a government department, led by the Health Secretary, who is a government minister.

Its primary aim is to promote and protect the population's health and wellbeing. It also has a key role in policy and legislation.

Here are some of the department's key responsibilities:

- To support and advise ministers in creating and delivering policies that adhere to the government's objectives.
- To lead the nation in improving global and domestic health issues.
- Remaining accountable for services that meet the agreed plans.
- Continuous assessment of health and social care frameworks, to ensure they work and are fit for purpose and.
- To take necessary action to resolve complex issues.

NHS England

NHS England is another key organisation that governs overall practice with a primary focus on delivering 'high-quality services for all'. NHS England is an organisation that implements the day-to-day running of health and social care services under the National Health Service. This includes ensuring staff employed by NHS England have the necessary skills and expertise to perform their job effectively. NHS England is also responsible for carrying out research to provide new ways of treating patients, as well as organising money to continue providing productive and efficient services.

Here are just some of the services the NHS governs:

- GP Practices
- Hospitals
- Pharmacies
- Mental health services
- Dental practices
- Urgent and emergency services
- Opticians

NICE

National Institute for Care Excellence (NICE) has responsibilities for health and social care services in both England and Wales and its recommendations can be used by any organisation financed by the government that provide a health or social care service. Their primary aim is to both provide and update guidance on best practice in health and social care services, to support individuals with healthier outcomes. They are also in charge of evaluating new health technology before its use in NHS services, to ensure the effectiveness of the equipment so that taxpayer money is spent well, and that services and individuals are receiving value for their money.

Social Care Institute for Excellence (SCIE)

Social Care Institute for Excellence (SCIE), established in 2001, is an independent organisation that prides itself on making improvements to social care practice. They take a 'people-focused' approach where they ensure that staff working in social care with both children and adults understand what good practice looks like and can safeguard its service users well. Whilst independent, they work with partners such as the Department of Health and Social Care.

Key roles of the SCIE:

- To support policy development.
- To drive forward social care outcomes through embedding practice which works, in order to improve quality of care.
- To work alongside individuals with relevant experience in the care and support system.
- To support staff with continuous professional development and coaching.

Care Quality Commission (CQC)

Care Quality Commission (CQC) is responsible for the inspection and monitoring of health and social care services in England. Their priority is to ensure that all services in England are delivering high-quality care in a safe and effective manner. The CQC have this responsibility so that vulnerable service users, such as those with poor mental health, can have their rights protected whilst involved with a service.

Their role is to:

- Register care providers
- Monitor, inspect and rate services
- Act against services that fail to meet their duty of care
- Publish information about any quality issues within health or social care services

The CQC will inspect and monitor all registered care providers and this can include:

- Care homes
- Services in your home including domiciliary care
- Clinics such as family planning and weight loss clinics
- GP services
- NHS Trust hospitals and independent hospitals
- Dentists
- Community services such as day centres
- Mental health services

The CQC gives a rating against five key questions, and an overall rating for the service. See the diagram below:

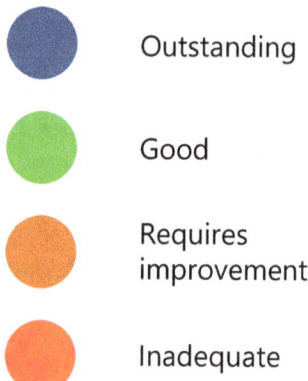

- Outstanding
- Good
- Requires improvement
- Inadequate

1. Is the service safe?
2. Is the service effective
3. Is the service caring?
4. Is the service responsive?
5. Is the service well-led?

CQC inspection ratings

Recap questions

1. Which organisation is responsible for inspecting healthcare services?
2. Outline the role of the National Institute for Care Excellence (NICE).
3. Which organisation oversees care for social services?

Regulatory bodies

Within health and social care services there are other regulatory bodies, with their own codes of practice.

Regulatory body	Who they work with and what do they do?	Code of practice
Nursing and Midwifery Council (NMC)	Nurses and midwives in the UK. The NMC has the authority to investigate misconduct allegations and the power to restrict a nurse's practice.	• All nurses and midwives must be registered with the NMC. • Nurses and midwives are required to provide evidence of continuous learning and training. • Individuals' needs are assessed and responded to. • Uphold a patient's dignity.
Social Work England	Social workers. Main purpose is to ensure users receive high-quality support through a people-focused approach.	• Promote the rights, strengths and wellbeing of people. • Establish and maintain trust of people. • Accountable for their own practice. • Actively participating in CPD.
Health and Care Professions Council (HCPC)	Regulates a wide range of health and social care professionals and is underpinned by the Health and Social Care Act (2012). Professions include physiotherapy, occupational therapy, social workers and paramedics. To be an approved HCPC member professionals must have achieved relevant qualifications. Responsible for investigating complaints or concerns.	• Respect confidentiality. • Report concerns about safety. • Honest and trustworthy.
General Medical Council (GMC)	Organisation that registers and regulates doctors. The GMC is responsible for overseeing medical education and training, deciding which doctors are qualified to work in the UK and for setting the standards doctors must adhere to in their professional practice. The GMC can also investigate concerns about a doctor's behaviour or professional practice, and can stop doctors from practicing in serious cases.	The GMC has several standards to account for different areas or people a doctor may work with. These can include: • Confidentiality. • Maintaining professional boundaries. • Protection of children and young people. • Identifying and managing conflicts of interest.

Before an organisation can provide adequate support to its professionals, they must first be supported by organisations to support practice and workforce development. This includes **Skills for Health** and **Skills for Care**.

Skills for Health

Skills for Health is a health care body that was established in 2001 and aims to develop the skills, roles, and capabilities of healthcare professionals across the UK to support better patient outcomes. They are also responsible for recruitment into the healthcare sector, including apprenticeships.

Skills for Health outlines the frameworks, standards and qualifications needed to enter this job sector and then provide the necessary support for individuals to access their desired career.

Skills for Care

Skills for Care also established in 2001 and supports the workforce development for those working in the adult social care sector. They also liaise with government and relevant partners to maintain high standards of those working in social care. This includes ensuring they have the appropriate skills and knowledge to deliver high-quality care and support. They too provide guidance on best practice through data driven evidence of what good practice looks like.

Professional Standards Authority (PSA)

The **Professional Standards Authority (PSA)** was set up under the Health and Social Care Act (2012) to help protect individuals by improving the way health and social care professionals are regulated and registered. This includes doctors, nurses, pharmacists, social workers and paramedics. The PSA supports regulators such as the General Medical Council (GMC) to conduct performance reviews each year to assess how well the standards are being met. The standards outline underpin different areas that should be reviewed, including education and training, registration and fitness to practise.

The PSA's overall key responsibilities are:

- To review decisions made by regulators about a professional 'fitness to practise'.
- To accredit voluntary registers that meet the standards and suspend or remove accreditation if necessary.
- To give policy advice to ministers.
- To encourage research to further improve regulation of professionals.

Key legislation that informs practice and its purpose

Legislation	Purpose	Services	Impact on services
Health and Social Care Act 2008	To improve the quality of health and social care services. This legislation established the CQC and provides power to the CQC to act against services not meeting the standards. Introduced the registration of health and social care services. Outlines standards of care. Encourages multi-agency working. Aims to protect vulnerable service users.	GP surgeries. Dentists. Opticians. Mental health services. Care homes and residential care services. Domiciliary care providers. Community health services. Ambulance services. Hospices and palliative care services.	Services are regularly inspected by the CQC and given ratings. Services must adhere to the standards of care. Services are legally accountable for the services provided. Services must ensure safeguarding procedures are met and maintained. Services should ensure staff are trained, qualified and competent in their role. Services must take a person-centred approach.

Legislation	Purpose	Services	Impact on services
Care Act 2014	Promotes the wellbeing of those in need of care and puts a legal duty on local authorities. To prevent individuals' needs from escalating by arranging the necessary services or resources. Introduced a national eligibility threshold. Introduced carers rights which gives them formal recognition of their role. Promotes collaboration between NHS, local authorities and other providers. Instructs local authorities to provide access to information and advice about care services. Introduced a framework for adult safeguarding.	Local authorities. Residential and nursing homes. Supported living schemes. Domiciliary care services. NHS Health care services Day centres.	Services must adhere to frameworks for safeguarding and service quality. Services are to work more closely with other services. Services must deliver high-quality care whilst also balancing administrative and financial restrictions.
General Data Protection Regulations (GDPR) (2018)	To protect individuals' personal data and to give service users control over how the information is used. Sets out the rules for how services should collect, store, process and share data. Regulates the transfer of personal data outside of the UK. Established penalties for non-compliance.	All services that handle personal information of individuals must adhere to GDPR. Hospitals – NHS and private. GP practices. Dentists. Pharmacies. Mental health services. Social care services.	Services must have strict procedures on the handling and storing of personal data. Requires services to notify data protection authority if a data breach occurs. Services must appoint a data protection officer (DPO). Services will have to pay penalty fines for failing to comply to GDPR laws.
Freedom of Information Act (FOIA) (2000)	Allows the public access to information held by public authorities. Holds public authorities accountable about their decisions, spending and activities. They must provide information about these as requested. Encourages better data management systems. Increases public engagement.	Central government departments. Local authorities. Health authorities. Educational institutions. Police forces. Fire and rescue services. Regulatory bodies (CQC).	Services must disclose information when requested. Services must disclose their spending and budget information. Services must implement effective systems for managing records. Services to avoid legal action or penalties by ensuring their practice meets FOIA standards.

Legislation	Purpose	Services	Impact on services
Safeguarding Vulnerable Groups Act 2006	Protects individuals (children and vulnerable adults) who are at risk of harm or abuse. Introduced a framework for background checks for those who wish to work or volunteer with vulnerable individuals. Created the Disclosure and Barring Service (DBS) check. Safer recruitment procedures when hiring staff. Created a system for reporting concerns. Established a legal framework for managing risks when working with vulnerable individuals.	NHS trust hospitals and health care services. GP practices. Care homes. Domiciliary care services. Children's services. Residential children's homes. Foster care agencies. Social work services. Mental health services. Community support services. Educational institutes.	Staff must complete a DBS check before being allowed to work with vulnerable individuals. Services must train staff on their safeguarding policies and procedures.
Mental Health Act 2021	This Act replaced the 1983 Mental Health Act. Ensures patients' rights and preferences are considered in their care plans. Outlines clear guidelines for medical detention and restraint of patients. Promotes the involvement of family and carers in care planning and decision making. Aims to ensure equitable access to care for all demographic groups. Promotes early intervention to prevent mental health issues escalating.	NHS mental health services. Private mental health services. Community mental health services. Psychiatric units. Crisis intervention services. Rehabilitation services. Social services. GP practices. Youth services.	Services must prioritise patients' rights. Services are encouraged to improve their quality of care. Staff should receive training outlined by the Act. Services are to effectively communicate with families and carers. Multi-agency working.

Legislation	Purpose	Services	Impact on services
Mental Capacity Act 2005	Provides a framework for making decisions for individuals who lack the capacity to do this for themselves. Safeguards vulnerable individuals. Gives a clear legal definition of mental capacity and how this can be assessed. Encourages individuals to appoint trusted individuals as power of attorney. Outlines and encourages the use of mental capacity advocates.	NHS health services. Mental health services. Social services. Residential care homes. Domiciliary care services. Supported living services. Hospices and palliative care services. Advocacy services. Legal services (assist in organising power of attorney).	Staff must be trained on assessing mental capacity. Services must take a person-centred approach. Services and staff must communicate effectively with families, advocates and power of attorney. Staff should have a comprehensive understanding of completing the necessary documentation.
Deprivation of Liberty Safeguards	Introduced under the Mental Capacity Act 2005. Provides a clear legal framework for authorising the deprivation of liberty. Outlines criteria for protecting individuals from being detained without proper assessment or authorisation. Established a review system to ensure legality of services.	Care homes. NHS hospitals. Mental health services. Domiciliary care services. Supported living services. Social services. Community services. Advocacy services.	States that staff in care settings should be trained on the deprivation of liberty principles. Services should adhere to changes in policies and practices to meet lawful requirements. Implementation of assessment processes to determine if a deprivation of liberty is necessary. Services should regularly review deprivation of liberty safeguards.
Equality Act 2010	Introduced to strengthen anti-discriminatory laws in the UK. Outlines protected characteristics and prohibits discrimination against them. Promotes equal opportunities in settings such as the workplace, education and public services. Supports services to take positive action for disadvantaged groups. Encourages inclusivity.	All organisations: Healthcare services. Education providers. Employers. Social services.	Services must ensure their practices comply with the Equality Act. Services must train staff in anti-discriminatory practice. Services should develop and implement equality and diversity policies.

Legislation	Purpose	Services	Impact on services
Human Rights Act 1998	Safeguards basic human rights. Established a legal framework for seeking justice for human rights violations. Ensures fair treatment of all.	All services that work with people. Healthcare services. Social services.	Services must ensure their practice aligns with the rights outlined in the Act. Staff should be trained in human rights principles. Services to adopt practices that promote human rights. Services are to address forms of discrimination to ensure an inclusive environment is maintained.

Family practitioner services – A service that provides one-to-one support to families during hardship or challenging moments in their lives.

Ministerial – Relates to government ministers that are responsible for the execution of laws.

Global and domestic health issues – Global refers to worldwide health issues such as COVID-19 and domestic refers to issues that occur in a particular area or household.

Accountable – A service is required to justify their actions or decisions.

Safeguard – A measure taken to ensure protection from harm.

Multi-agency working – The co-ordination of services that respond to the needs of a service user by working together.

Palliative care – Care given to improve an individual's quality of life during a life-threatening illness (end of life care).

Person-centred approach – Services should have a central focus on the individual by ensuring all aspects of care are tailored to the individual's needs, wishes and circumstances.

Local authorities – Otherwise known as a local council. An elected body that provides services for a particular local area.

National eligibility threshold – A framework that assesses an individual's needs and if they can be given support from the local authority for no additional costs.

Non-compliance – Failing to act in line with a law or an individual's needs.

Data breach – When personal information is accessed or disclosed without permission.

Data protection officer – An individual that is responsible for managing and organising implementation of data protection within a service.

Public authorities – A body that performs duties that is reliant on public funding, such as local maintained schools.

Vulnerable – A person who needs special care, support or protection due to the risk of harm being greater because of a particular characteristic such as age or disability.

Disclosure and barring services – A check that potential workers must go through to ensure that they are safe to work with vulnerable service users.

Medical Detention – The keeping of a person in a medical facility for assessment as they are deemed to be a risk to themselves or others because of their mental health.

Restraint – When a professional must use strategies to prevent an individual from harming themselves or others, this can sometimes involve physically holding an individual.

Demographic groups – Characteristics of individuals within a population. For example, age, race, gender and religion.

Lack the capacity – An individual's mind is impaired in some way which means their ability to make appropriate decisions is compromised.

Power of attorney – A legal authorisation that allows a person to act on behalf of another person because they lack the capacity to make effective decisions.

Recap questions

1. Identify the regulatory body responsible for nurses and midwives.
2. What is the difference between skills for care and skills for health?
3. Outline the role of the General Medical Council.
4. Which organisation is responsible for the inspection of different health and social care services?
5. Outline the role of the Department of Health and Social Care.
6. Which legislation is responsible for ensuring data is handled and stored correctly?
7. Which legislation outlines protected characteristics that should not be discriminated against?
8. Identify two protected characteristics outlined by this legislation.
9. What is the difference between an organisation and legislation? Outline the role of the Care Act 2014.
10. Outline the role of the Professional Standards Authority.

Activity

1. What are the potential impacts on service users if the Human Rights Act (1998) is not adhered to by services?
2. Why is it important to regularly review and update key legislation?

Find out more

www.eboru.com/BTEC-HSC-links

The Department of Health and Social Care

NHS England

NICE

Social Care Institute for Excellence

The CQC

Nursing and Midwifery Council

Social Work England

Health and Care Professions Council

General Medical Council

Skills for Health

Skills for Care

Professional Standards Authority

B2 Organisations of health and social care services

In this section, you will learn about the function of different types of health and social care services. You need to understand how the services are organised and structured.

The National Health Service (NHS) structures its services in the following ways:

Primary care

Primary care is typically the first place an individual will go to for healthcare support, as individuals are able to self-refer to these. For example, GP practices, dentists, opticians and pharmacies.

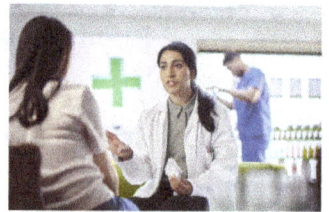

Primary care service	Function
General Practice (GP)	• Diagnose illness • Prescribe medication • Professional referrals to secondary or tertiary services • Vaccination programmes • Health education and advice
Pharmacy	• Prepare medication for dispensing • Dispense medication to service users • Store and manage drug inventory • Health education and advice
Dentistry	• Diagnose and treat problems relating to teeth, gums and mouth • Health education and advice • Promote good dental hygiene

Secondary care

Secondary care services are those that an individual has had a professional referral to, often through their GP. This is usually because further tests or treatment are required. Most hospital services, mental health services and community health services are examples of secondary care. Other examples include physiotherapists, psychologists and occupational therapists.

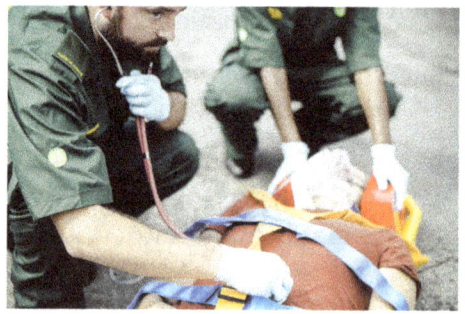

Secondary care service	Definition	Function
Urgent and emergency care including physical and mental health	Urgent care involves any non-life-threatening illness or injury that needs attention quickly. Emergency care involves life-threatening illness or injury that needs immediate treatment from paramedics or accident and emergency.	• Provide immediate medical attention • To prioritise patients based on the severity of their condition • To be available 24/7 • Multi-disciplinary team working • Health education and advice • Provide immediate relief for acute pain and symptoms
Planned or elective care	Medical care that has been planned for in advance, known as elective care.	• Diagnostic testing and scans • Provide outpatient care • Surgery • Treatments for conditions such as cancer

Tertiary care

Tertiary care provides highly specialised care for service users with complex needs. For example, neurosurgery, transplants, spinal injury units and secure forensic mental health services.

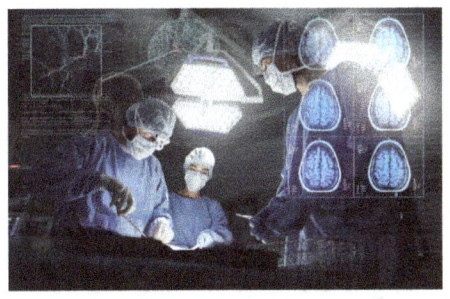

Tertiary care services	Function
Neurosurgery	To prevent, diagnose and treat conditions linked to the brain, spine and nervous system.
Transplants	The removing of key cells, tissues or organs from a body or person to another to save a life and restore essential functions.
Secure forensic mental health services	Individuals attend this service when there are concerns about their mental health. The service aims to support people in their recovery to return to the community as safe citizens. Individuals from court, prison, community, psychiatric hospitals and units and secure hospitals attend this service.

Community health

Community health focuses on supporting individuals with their physical and mental wellbeing within a local area and can provide this care from birth to end of life. This can include clinics such as weight loss programmes, sexual health clinics, quit smoking groups and health visitors.

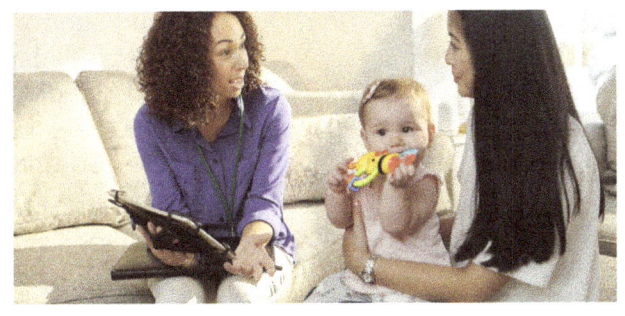

Community health services	Function
Sexual health clinics	• Provide contraceptive methods • Diagnose and treat sexually transmitted infections • HIV care • Education and advice about safe sex • Support individuals with their sexuality and promote healthy sexual relationships
Smoking cessation clinics	• Provide information and advice about the risks of smoking • Provide easy and affordable treatments • Offer one-to-one appointment • Offer drop in services • Offer group sessions • Ongoing support for individuals to quit smoking
Health visitors	• Provide early health intervention • Information and advice to parents and families • Monitor and support the health and development of babies and children up until 5 years old • Support parents and families in raising a healthy child

Social care

Social care services provide support to individuals that have some level of difficulty completing daily life due to differing needs, including disability or mental health issues. Social care services can provide support such as personal or practical care that encourages independent living.

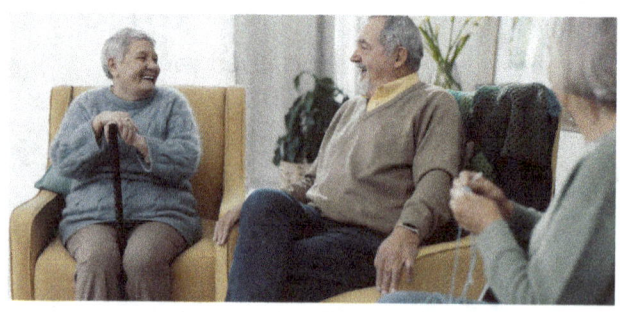

Social care services	Function
Care homes	• Residential care homes support individual needs and independence • Nursing homes provide complex medical care with qualified nurses on duty 24/7 • Provide accommodation • Provide personal care • Implement activities for residents • Provide good quality food • Support residents and family members
Home care (domiciliary)	• Provide daily/weekly/monthly visits or live-in care • Provide household assistance • Assess the home care needs of individuals • Implement the necessary resources/support needed for individuals to live independently • Medication support from qualified nurses • Personal care • Companionship
Rehabilitation services	• Aims to improve an individual's function or skill after an illness or injury or to support individuals' recovery from addiction (drugs/alcohol) • Promotes independence through activities • Assistance to improve or recover • Support and referrals for mental health

Palliative and end-of-life care

Palliative care is highly specialised medical care that can be given to individuals at any stage of a life-threatening illness and is provided by the necessary professionals.

End of life care is given to individuals with a prognosis of 6 months or fewer to live, and aims to improve the quality of life for a patient and their family by managing symptoms and side effects so that patients are comfortable and have their dignity as they approach end of life.

The function of palliative care and end of life care is to consider an individual's needs and wishes throughout their care. This includes meeting wishes such as where an individual would like to die. End of life care can be provided in a person's home, a care home, hospice or a hospital.

Learning disabilities care

Learning disabilities care is for individuals that have:

- difficulty understanding complex information
- difficulty learning skills
- or issues with looking after themselves or living alone.

Care for those with learning disabilities varies depending on the severity of the learning disability. Services can include occupational therapy and special education with the option for respite or residential services. The overall function of these services is to provide individuals with the necessary support so that they can be somewhat independent at home and to support families in supporting individuals. This support can be seen in many forms, such as personal care, practical support, education or respite care.

> Multi-disciplinary team – A group of professionals that work together to meet the needs of a patient.
>
> Outpatient care – Care that is given on the same day and without an overnight stay, meaning individuals can leave the service the same day.
>
> Cessation – Something that is coming to an end.
>
> Prognosis – How long a medical condition may last.
>
> Respite – A short-term break from caring for a person, or for the patient to have a rest away from carers.

Virtual wards and virtual hospitals

A **virtual ward** is when patients can receive care in their own home rather than in hospital but still receive the same hospital-level care. Patients that are on a virtual ward still have multi-disciplinary team care that provide tests and treatments that are reviewed daily via home visits or through digital technology.

The function of a virtual ward is to support the recovery process in an individual's familiar environment, which then supports the freeing of hospital beds for other patients.

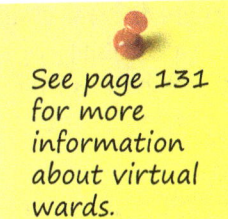

See page 131 for more information about virtual wards.

Virtual hospitals are facilities that function completely online and connects patients to medical professionals through digital technology. Virtual hospitals were introduced to provide more accessible and cost-effective care and were more commonly found after COVID-19 which saw the nation unable to attend in-person appointments, causing a shift to remote working.

Using technology allows for patients to be monitored remotely which can then alert relevant professionals to intervene when necessary. It has also improved patient satisfaction as it has removed the stresses of having to attend in person appointments.

Activity

1. Discuss whether virtual wards and hospitals always effective? Give reasons for your answers.
2. Why is it important to provide end of life care for patients?

Recap questions

1. Give an example of a primary care service.
2. What type of care provides highly specialised care?
3. What term is used to describe care that can be given in an individual's home?
4. What is the function of a health visitor?
5. What is the difference between a virtual ward and a virtual hospital?

B3 How health and social care services are organised to benefit the population

In this section, you will investigate integrated care systems that are related to the services previously discussed in B2. You will need to understand how services link together and the two components that make up integrated care systems, as well as their purpose.

Integrated care systems

Integrated care systems (ICS) were implemented to provide joined-up care, where different services come together to form a **partnership** to support outcomes for service users in a particular area. These partnerships can be between NHS organisations, social care services and local authorities. They work together to support services and its users.

ICSs have a **collective responsibility** for planning relevant services that can help improve outcomes either nationwide or locally. This is important as the needs of the general and local population are forever changing. They also share the responsibility of **reducing inequalities** within services by ensuring services are inclusive of all demographic groups.

A key responsibility of ICS's is the **implementation and accelerating of digital priorities** including electronic patient records (EPRs), digital social care records and shared care records (ShCRs). These priorities have been outlined by NHS England as a clear expectation of ICSs to ensure these digital methods are used in services and are regularly reviewed and improved upon to further support individuals in their care.

See page 126 and 277 for more information about electronic patient records.

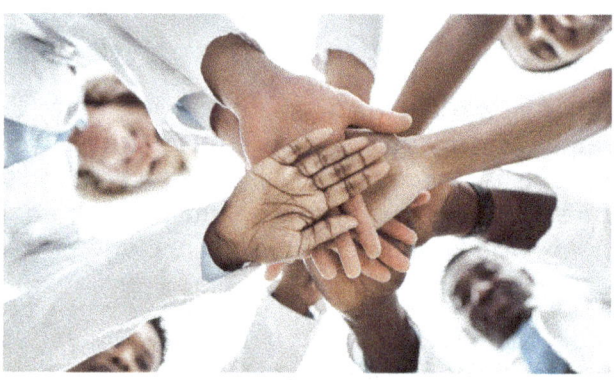

Purpose of ICSs

The main purpose of ICSs:

- To bring health and social care organisations together.
- To organise the use of collective resources so that users can receive care that is quick and appropriate for their needs.
- To improve overall health outcomes.
- To reduce inequalities in outcomes, experiences and access to services.
- To be supportive of individuals need to stay healthy and independent, particularly those with multiple needs, mental health issues and long-term conditions.

Components of an ICS

There are **two components of an ICS**:

- **Integrated Care Partnership** (ICP) which is a committee of individuals and services that have the responsibility for improving the care, health and wellbeing of the local population. An ICP must create a long-term plan for the local area that aims to improve health and social care services which will then benefit individuals' health and wellbeing. An ICP is made up of representatives from NHS organisations, local authorities, social care providers, voluntary and community organisations.

- **Integrated Care Board** (ICB) occur in each ICS area. These are NHS organisations with responsibility for the planning and funding of most the NHS services within that local area. The board will also develop a plan that outlines how the NHS will contribute towards the ICP's strategy.

> **Recap questions**
>
> 1. Identify a responsibility of an integrated care system.
> 2. Identify two representatives that make up an integrated care partnership.
> 3. Which component of ICS is responsible for the planning and funding of NHS services?
> 4. State two purposes of an ICS.
> 5. What digital priorities does an ICS have?

> Electronic patient records (EPR) – A system to manage patient information.
>
> Digital social care records – A replacement of paper records to an electronic way of managing, storing and sharing patient information.
>
> Shared care records – A collection of patient information that is stored in a central location for different care providers to contribute towards and access.
>
> Committee – A group of people working together for a specific function or need, often to encourage a change or make improvements.

> **Activity**
>
> 1. Discuss how effective integrated care systems are for meeting the needs of the local population.
> 2. Explain the possible consequences of not planning the funding of NHS services.

B4 Using critical thinking skills to draw valid conclusions

In this section, you are asked to use your critical thinking to analyse and evaluate the effectiveness of services in meeting the needs of individuals. You are required to break information into parts to establish relationships and connections so that you can identify key strengths and weaknesses of information. By doing all of this it will allow you to draw valid conclusions with justifiable reasons.

Questioning relevance of information and challenging own biases

You must be able to question how relevant content is for the individual in the case study. For example, are the strategies and policies relevant and up to date and able to effectively meet the needs of the individual. To challenge your own biases, you should be reflective on your own personal assumptions about scenarios in health and social care as your subjective ideas and experiences could influence your analysis of the information. You are encouraged to use additional sources to support your understanding of the scenario.

Breaking information into parts and identifying relationships and connections

You need to ensure you have understood all the information presented to you in your internal assessment, particularly that outlined in the case study. This will allow you to break down information into parts or sections, so that you can easily identify relationships and connections. For example, are there connections in terms of the services being used, do they make up an integrated care system? By identifying this it will then allow you to begin to pick out key strengths and weaknesses of the systems described.

Identifying strengths or weaknesses of information and why information is significant

You need to be able to critically identify whether information in the case study is wholly relevant to the task outlined in the Pearson Set Assignment. You will then be able to determine strengths or weaknesses of the content and link this to the case study so that your points are valid and justified. To determine if information is significant, you should be explicitly linking points to the issues outlined in the case study. If you deem information not significant this can then make a weakness of the information.

Drawing conclusions supported by structured reasoning

To produce a valid conclusion you must restate the key points outlined throughout the task through a summary which is linked to the case study. You must also justify your reasons by providing evidence for your ideas or acknowledging counter ideas to show you have critically thought about both sides of an idea. Your conclusion should also link to the wider themes or aims in health and social care. For example, do your points support the aim of improving the patient outcomes outlined in the case study?

> Biases – Putting your own opinion or thoughts onto a situation or idea.

Activity

You have been asked to analyse information and sources provided by the Care Quality Commission (CQC) and how these support the regulation of other health and social care services. You have been given access to a variety of sources, including the CQC website, independent reviews and articles, and reviews on social media.

Relationships and connections:

- What is the relationship between an independent review and social media reviews?

Strengths and weaknesses:

- Identify a strength of the CQC creating independent reviews.
- Explain how these could highlight biases by the CQC.
- How could these biases be challenged?
- Identify a weakness of relying on social media for information about an organisation.

Conclusions:

- Create a conclusion that explains the relevance and effectiveness of sources provided by the CQC.

End of Learning Aim Practice Activity

In this practice activity you will consider how health and social care services can work together to meet people's needs.

Carlos is a 78-year-old retired construction worker who lives alone after his wife recently passed away. Carlos suffers from arthritis and poor mobility which makes it difficult for him to perform daily tasks and maintain a tidy and clean house. Carlos and his wife did not have any children and he does not have any relatives to support him. He has expressed to his GP that he often feels lonely and has anxiety about how he can afford the weekly food shop due to his limited pension.

Jemima is a 28-year-old mother of two young children and lives in a temporary housing unit in a city after leaving an unsafe home environment. She has recently got a job cleaning in a local museum and is keen to find her own flat. Jemima has also recently been struggling with her youngest child's diagnosis of Cystic Fibrosis. After attending a recent appointment, where staff made assumptions about her as a single mother, she has been reluctant to go back to the service. This is beginning to negatively impact her child's health.

--

You need to consider the effectiveness of services working together to meet Carlos and Jemima's needs.

Write down your ideas about the following:

- Which health and social care services are likely to be important for Carlos and Jemima? You will need to think carefully about each of their specific circumstances and needs.
- Which organisations from section B1 affect these services? Which legislation affects these services?
- How are these different health and social care services organised? You will need to think about integrated care systems.
- How can these different health and social care services work together to meet Carlos and Jemima's differing needs?
- What impacts will all of this have on meeting the specific needs of Carlos and Jemima?
- How effective do you think these services working together can be for Carlos and Jemima?

This practice task will help you prepare for the following assessment criteria:

B.P4 Explain the influence of organisations, legislation and guidance on practice within health and social care services.

B.P5 Explain how different health and social care services work together to meet the care and support needs of two individuals with different needs.

B.M3 Analyse the impact of organisations, legislation and guidance on health and social care services working together to meet the needs of two individuals with different needs.

B.D2 Evaluate the effectiveness of health and social care services working together to meet the care and support needs of two individuals with different needs.

Learning Aim C: Examine how social determinants affect the health status of individuals and the importance of equality, diversity and inclusion in practice

C1 The effect of social determinants on individuals' health status

In this section, you will learn about a range of factors/social determinants that can affect an individual's health status and health outcomes in either a positive or negative way.

A **social determinant** refers to the condition in which people live their life. Factors such as work, and age can influence this as they can determine the level of resources, wealth and education a person or group of people have.

Health status factors

Health status can be defined as how healthy or unhealthy a person, group or population are. This considers both physical and mental health.

- **Physical** refers to the state of the body and any illness, injury or disease that effects it.
- **Mental** refers to the state of wellbeing, or otherwise, of the mind.

Health status of individuals is determined by the following factors.

Underlying health

The underlying health of a person, group or population has a clear impact.

Access to care

Access to care is how readily available a service is to individuals.

- **Timely** – Are individuals given appointments that allow them to access services at a convenient time for them? For example, after work or during school hours whilst the children are being cared for.
- **Appropriate** – Are services relevant to meet an individual's needs? For example, an individual displaying symptoms associated with dementia may be referred for further tests by a neurologist.
- **Easy to get to and use** – Are services in an accessible place for most of the population to access? Are they located close to public transport services so all individuals can get to services and use them?

> **Neurologist** – A doctor with a specialism in the diagnosis and treatment of the brain, spinal cord and nerves.

- **Available services meeting the choice and needs of an individual** – Services that an individual does access should ensure they are meeting the health needs of the person as well as considering their choices regarding their care. For example, actioning the request for a woman to have a female nurse present during an intimate examination.

Quality and experience of care

All service users are entitled to receive **high-quality** care with qualified and competent professionals. This ensures that professionals are **experienced** in delivering care, which means all needs of the individual are being met and therefore the status of their health is addressed and improved.

If service users experience poor quality care, with inexperienced staff, it causes distrust within the service which is then detrimental to the overall health status of the local population. If individuals distrust a service, the reputation of this service can be negatively affected, causing a snowball effect of individuals not accessing the service which leads to poor overall health.

Behavioural risks

The choices individuals make can have positive and negative impacts upon the status of their health.

- In the UK 11.6% of adults over the age of 18 **smoke** tobacco products. This reduces the health status of the population and puts significant strain upon NHS services. Smoking is the leading cause of health inequalities, as evidence suggests smoking is prevalent in less affluent communities. The risks associated with smoking are different types of cancer including, lung and throat cancer, increased risk of heart disease, risk of lung infections such as pneumonia, infertility and the effects on appearance, such as discolouration of the skin, teeth and nails.
- **Poor diet** or **malnutrition** is one of the leading causes of poor health within the UK. In 2023, the government estimates that 64.0% of adults in the UK were considered overweight. This carries significant health concerns, for example, poor mobility, heart disease, type 2 diabetes and strokes.
- **Physical inactivity** refers to individuals not exercising regularly or at all. This could be because of a variety of reasons such as pre-existing health conditions, time constraints, lack of resources for exercising or simply because they choose not to exercise. This can negatively impact the health status of individuals as it can contribute towards obesity, high blood pressure and type 2 diabetes.
- **Harmful alcohol consumption** is when individuals consume more than the recommended 14 units of alcohol a week on a regular basis. As well as the long-term health impacts, this can also lead to people carrying out riskier behaviours whilst intoxicated, such as drink driving. Recent NHS evidence highlights that 1 in 10 visits to accident and emergency departments are linked to alcohol. This is because alcohol impairs a person's ability to make effective and appropriate decisions. Additionally, long-term abuse of alcohol can lead to poor health status and effects such as liver disease, bowel cancer and damage to the brain, particularly with regard to memory.

Wider determinants of health

Other conditions can also influence the health status of individuals.

- **Quality of housing** can impact upon health. Poor housing conditions include:
    * overcrowding
    * tiny rooms
    * cluttered conditions
    * low or high temperatures
    * damp.

Poor-quality housing is associated with health conditions such as respiratory diseases, poor mental health and infectious diseases.

- **Income** is based on how much a person earns. This can determine lots of other things, such as the quality of housing a person has access to and the diet they consume.
- **Processed food** is often cheaper than fresh ingredients, which has an impact on people's diets. Ultra-processed food is not good for us and can lead to issues with malnutrition and obesity.
- **Income** can also impact a person's ability to access services. For example, a person on a low income that does not have access to their own transport may be unable to afford public transport to get to the service
    * A person with a low income may be unable to afford some costs associated with their care, such as prescription costs or dental care. (Some costs are covered by the government for people receiving various benefits.)

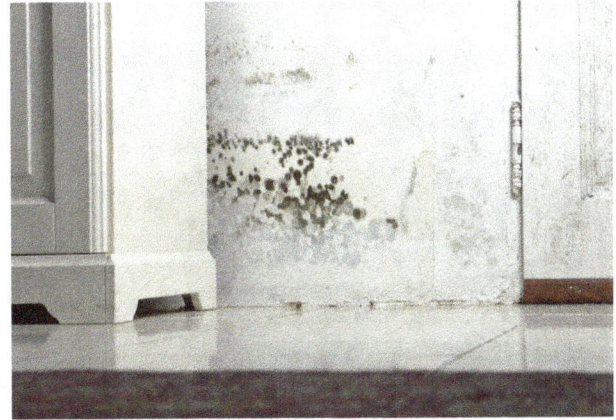

Damp and mould can have a serious effect on health

- The level of **education** an individual has can be important for overall health status. This is because the more awareness they have about health conditions, and their causes, the more individuals are able to make healthier behavioural choices. However, individuals with less education may not understand the risks or know how to change their behaviour. Some individuals may also lack education about the NHS's health and social care services and are unable to access support due to not understanding the system.

- Some individuals may have little **access to green space**, meaning they may not have their own garden or limited park areas. This may be particularly prevalent in more urban areas. This means some people may have limited opportunities for physical activity, leading to health issues that arise with lack of exercise.

- Access to **healthy food**. As discussed, diet can also be a determinant of health status. However, whilst this can be due to behavioural choices, it can also be due to the availability of certain types of food – for example, there may not be a shop within walking distance that sells healthier food. If you do not have access to transport, this could severely limit access to a healthy diet, and ultimately contribute towards ill health.

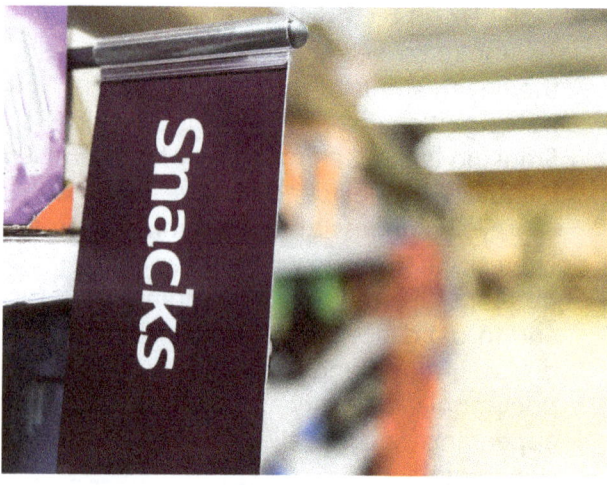

- **The work individuals do** can have a positive or negative impact upon other wider determinants of health that have been discussed. It might be linked to the level of income received from a job, but also be linked to health risks associated with the work. For example:

    * **Physical jobs** such as manual labour can be linked to health conditions such as arthritis and prone to accident and injury.

    * Jobs that involve **sitting down for long periods**, such as professional drivers, can impact on physical movement and diet.

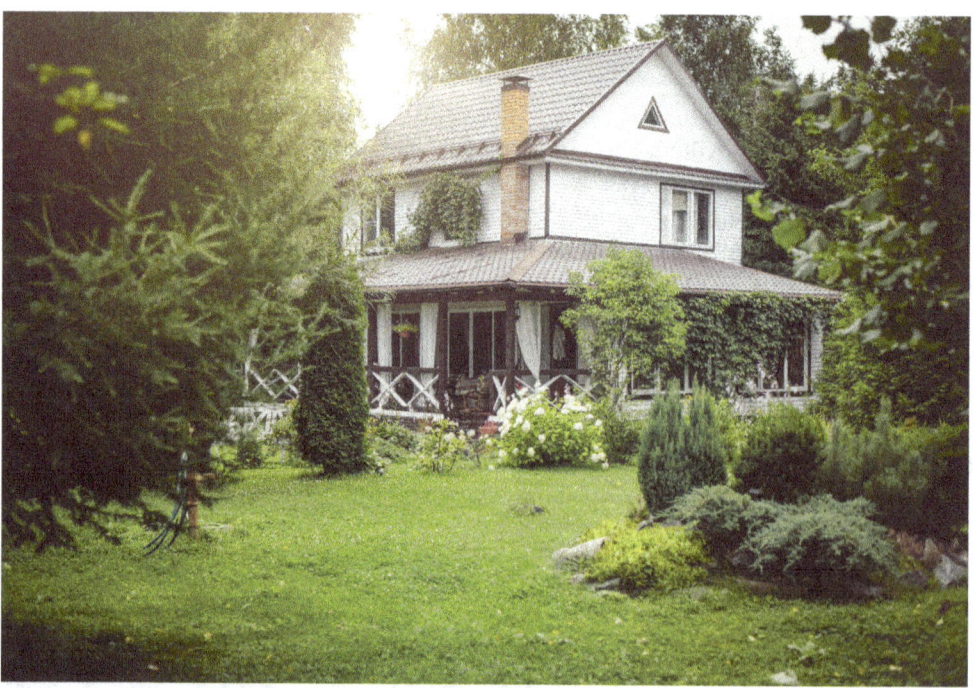

Someone with a higher income and access to green space, such as a garden, is more likely to have better health outcomes

Social and environmental factors affecting health status and health outcomes

Factor:	Description	Possible impacts
Socio-economic factors • Income • Deprivation	This links to the income a person or household earns from their job. The level of income can then influence if individuals experience deprivation or not. Deprivation can be seen in the form of materials (material deprivation).	• Limited access to health care services. • Poor nutrition – issues around obesity or malnutrition. • Mental health issues. • Reduced physical activity.
Geography • Regional differences • Urban or rural areas	Regional differences can impact an individual's ability to access services based upon a postcode lottery. Whether an individual lives in urban or rural areas can influence again the access to services but also to commodities such as green spaces or gyms.	• Limited access to services due to location. • Availability of services for the local area. • Opportunities for physical activity could be increased or limited.
Individual characteristics protected by law • Age • Disability • Ethnicity • Religion and belief • Sex • Sexual orientation • Gender identity • Pregnancy and maternity • Married or civil partnership • Neurodiversity • Education • Economic status	Protected characteristics outlined by the Equality Act 2010 (see page 147) are those that should not be discriminated against within services. There are some additional characteristics that should also be considered by services. For example: • Neurodiversity – This refers to neurological differences such as autism or dyslexia. • Education – Patience and further explanation may be required depending on a person's level of education. • Economic status – People could be discriminated against because of how much they earn.	• If discrimination occurs it may cause distrust, and an individual may choose not to access services. • Services being inclusive of all individuals.
Socially excluded groups • People experiencing homelessness • Asylum seekers • Refugees	In society there are some groups of people that are deemed excluded by societal norms as they don't necessarily fit society's expectations. Homelessness refers to an individual without a consistent and stable home, and can refer to someone living on the streets. An asylum seeker is a person or group of people that have had to leave their home country due to violence or war and are seeking protection in another country with the goal of being recognised as a refugee under international law. A refugee will then be unable to return to their home country as it has been deemed by law to be unsafe for them.	• Mental health issues such as extreme stress. • Chronic illness due to inconsistent health care. • Restricted access to services. • Infectious diseases. • Injury or violence.

Intersectionality of social determinants

Overall, as health and social care professionals, it is important to recognise the role of intersectionality of social determinants. This means professionals need to recognise that a person's identity can influence different social determinants.

For example, gender and income can impact the level of education a person has or their access to green space and healthy foods. This is important to acknowledge, as these different social determinants can then influence **health outcome**s of a population or individual as well as their **health status**.

The ability to see the connections between social determinants means professionals and services are more able to intervene to prevent future or further ill health. For example, identifying health needs of a local population are due to high smoking rates means services such as smoking cessation groups can be implemented.

Deprivation – When an individual is lacking something. For example, lacking material goods that are a necessity.

Postcode lottery – Differences in health care based on geographical location. For example, when an affluent region has more GP practices than a poorer region.

Urban area – More developed areas such as cities.

Rural area – Areas with lots of open land such as the countryside.

Neurodiversity – The differences in the way individuals think, learn and behave. A neurodiverse person could have a condition such as Autism or Dyslexia.

Education – Knowledge or skills gained through learning. Formal education results in qualifications from a school, college or university.

Norms – Societal expectations of behaviour that are considered 'normal'. For example, eating with a knife and fork.

Asylum seeker – A person who has left their home country to seek protection in another country.

Refugee – A person who seeks protection in another country as their home country is deemed unsafe.

Intersectionality of social determinants – The connection between social characteristics such as

Recap questions

1. Define the term health status.
2. Identify one behavioural risk to health.
3. State two characteristics that are protected in law but can impact an individual's health status.
4. What is the difference between an asylum seeker and a refugee?
5. How can quality of housing influence an individual's heath status?

Activity

1. Discuss which social determinant you think has the biggest impact upon health status? Why?
2. Describe why intersectionality is important for improving health outcomes. What are the possible consequences of ignoring intersectionality?

C2 Improving health outcomes in practice

Equality, diversity and inclusion

In this section, you will learn the definitions of equality, diversity and discrimination and how professionals can ensure their practice upholds inclusivity. You will also gain an understanding of how inclusivity can benefit both professionals in practice and for service users.

Equality in health and social care not only means individuals are fairly treated within services but that they also have equal opportunities for accessing services. Possible barriers are removed to ensure that equality can happen.

Diversity is about recognising and respecting differences between individuals based upon characteristics such as ethnicity, culture, gender identity and socio-economic status. It is important for health and social care professionals to understand individual differences, so that they can adapt their care accordingly.

Discrimination. Discrimination occurs when a group of people or individual receives negative actions towards them based on a preconceived opinion about a characteristic they may have. This can happen either directly or indirectly.

- **Direct discrimination** in health and social care is when an individual is openly treated less favourably than others because of a protected characteristic.

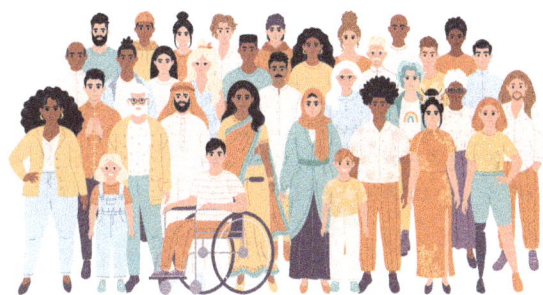

- Whereas **indirect discrimination** can prevent access to services for those with a protected characteristic. For example, not providing wheelchair access is indirectly discriminating against individuals who use a wheelchair.

Inclusion in practice

To be considered an **inclusive practice** professionals must ensure all individuals are included and able to access their services. A feature of inclusive practice is taking a **person-centred approach**, which means an individual is put at the centre or the heart of the care. For this approach to be effective professionals must **record and act upon the individual's unique needs, choices and preferences** about their care.

For example:

- Ensuring that their dietary preferences are noted and addressed during a hospital stay.
- Noting their preference for the pharmacy they use.

This is important because it promotes dignity, respect and autonomy for the individual, and allows service users to put their trust in the service or professional, which then supports health outcomes and satisfaction rates.

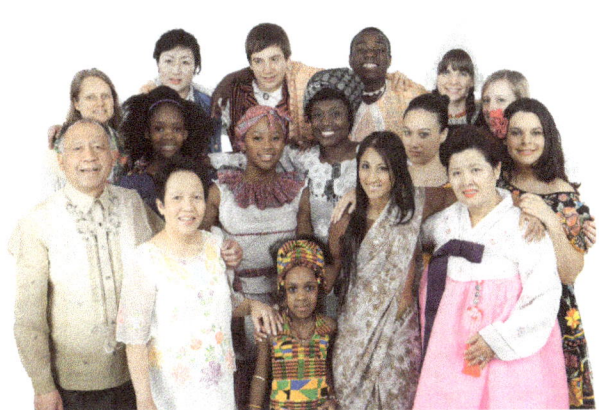

Generalisations and intersectionality

Professionals must remove any **preconceptions** or **generalisations** they have about an individual because of their visible characteristics. This means they should ignore any opinions or conclusions they might have about groups of people and must maintain neutral in their care approach.

Additionally, in order to provide high-quality person-centred care, professionals must have an **awareness of intersectionality**.

- This refers to the interconnectedness of social determinants and the influence these have on the overall health status of people.

- Professionals must have an empathetic understanding of how **individual characteristics can overlap** and how these are fluid and can change throughout the lifespan of an individual.

By having this level of awareness, professionals are better able to address individual needs and support them in improving their health status. This benefits the overall health outcomes of the population.

The importance of equality, diversity and inclusion for professionals in practice

Important for...	Description
Improving **efficiency** and the **effective running of services**.	If all individuals are included it allows a service to run effectively, meaning it is meeting the demands of everyone in the population without any hold-ups.
Increasing **levels of productivity**.	The ability to achieve more results within a time frame, which means more patients are being treated and effective patient outcomes are generated.
Improved **innovation**.	Understanding equality, diversity and inclusion means services can develop and implement new ideas, technologies and practices to support the diverse needs of the population. For example, using AI to help with translation.
Reduces **absence**.	Inclusivity allows service users to put more faith in the care profession. This helps motivate people to attend and reduces the number of missed appointments.
Recruiting and retaining a diverse workforce at all levels of employment.	Services that have a good understanding and awareness of equality and diversity ensure they employ people from diverse backgrounds. This helps to embed a **better understanding of different cultures** and **increases the representation of identities from the local community**. This helps to build trust between individuals and the services.
Demonstrating **cultural competence** in line with the Care Quality Commission (CQC) expectations.	To be **competent** means to have sound knowledge and understanding of something. To have **cultural competence** means to understand and respect the diversity of cultures, beliefs and values within the population. Culturally competent services are delivered in an inclusive manner and avoid bias and discrimination.
The continuation of **learning and development** about different cultures.	It is vital that all health and social care services keep up-to-date with the needs and preferences of different cultures. These needs and preferences, and appropriate language terms, may change over time. A big part of being able to deliver effective care is based around communication. This means services must acknowledge and have an understanding of differing language needs of the population. Different words have different meanings in certain cultures. It is important this is understood and addressed with respect. It is also imperative the professionals understand that some vocabulary associated with health and social care may not be familiar to all people. These words must be explained clearly.

The importance of equality, diversity and inclusion for individuals using services

Important for...	Description
Improving quality of care.	An inclusive setting means it is more likely that the needs and choices of service users are being met. This improves the overall quality of care that individuals experience. If an individual has all their needs and choices met it supports their engagement with the service, improving health outcomes and status.
Satisfaction levels.	Professionals that are respectful of an individual's diverse needs and characteristics will help to improve overall satisfaction levels for service users.
Meeting individual needs.	Inclusive services are more likely to meet individuals' needs, because services are then tailored to ensure they are **culturally sensitive** and appropriate.

Recap questions

1. Which key term is described as understanding the differences between individual characteristics?
2. Identify two reasons why equality, diversity and inclusion are important for professionals.
3. Which regulator of health and social care services outlines the expectations for cultural competency?
4. What type of approach is used by professionals and services when being inclusive?
5. Why are satisfaction levels important for positive health outcomes?

Activity

1. Discuss which factors are the most important for professionals when providing an inclusive practice? Why?
2. Why is it important that discrimination is discouraged by law, as outlined in the Equality Act 2010?

Dignity – The state of how worthy or respected we feel.

Autonomy – The state of having freedom of choice without external influence or control.

C3 Potential barriers to improving health outcomes in practice

In this section, you will learn about the **potential barriers** that can hinder a person's ability to access health care and improve health outcomes.

You will need a good understanding of discrimination and how this can be seen in health and social care practice and how this can then impact upon service users and their outcomes.

Discrimination

Discrimination can occur in many different forms. It is important that these are understood, and reasons why an individual might be discriminated against are recognised, so that they can be prevented. Forms of discrimination include:

Unconscious bias

- **Unconscious bias** is when someone unknowingly favours or disfavours a certain group of people or a person, due to preconceptions and biases they hold. This can then lead to stereotyping as decisions could be made that are influenced by false views. For example, a professional may assume that someone with a particular ethnic background lacks understanding of key vocabulary and therefore explains things more simply than is needed. This runs the risk of patronising a patient who might otherwise be quite confident with vocabulary. The 'unconscious' part of the bias in this example means that the professional doesn't even realise they are treating people from that ethnic background differently.

Othering

- **Othering** is the mistreatment of individuals or groups because they have been deemed as deviant against societies norms. This means they are not treated as part of society. This can often lead to individuals becoming marginalised. For example, referencing a group of people as 'they' or 'those people' suggesting that there is a divide between 'them' and 'us'.

Labelling

- **Labelling** is when someone assigns others with a 'label' that is based upon their characteristics, which may not be accurate. This is how stereotypes form about people, because society has attached labels to different aspects of an individual. For example, referring to an individual as 'a diabetic' detaches them from being a 'person with diabetes'. This can lead to assumptions about that person's lifestyle and behaviour, which can then impact the way they are then treated.

Prejudice

- **Prejudice** is a negative assumption or opinion about a person or group of people based on their characteristics but which does not have any justified reasons. For example, making assumptions about someone's abilities because of their age, such as believing an elderly patient is unable to complete certain exercises during their physiotherapy appointment, because it is assumed they are fragile and immobile.

Stereotyping

- **Stereotyping** is a fixed or over-exaggerated belief about a particular group of people based on certain characteristics. For example, having the belief that all patients with mental health issues are dangerous and aggressive so not including them in a group activity due to fear of a negative behaviour.

It is also important to understand that an individual can be discriminated against based on multiple characteristics. This includes the **protected characteristics** outlined in the Equality Act 2010.

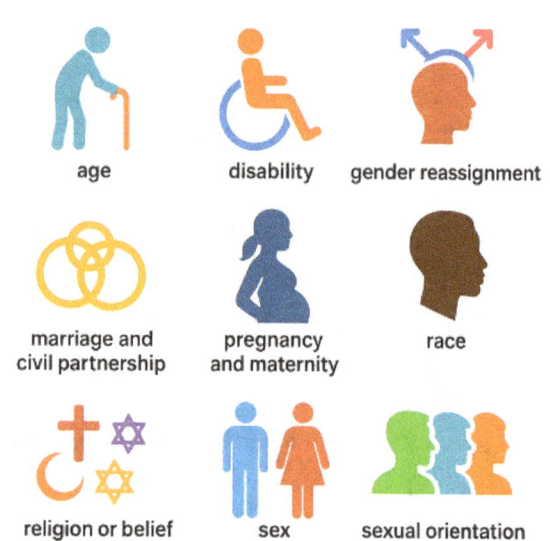

Deviant – Someone that does not meet the expected norms of society.

Marginalised – Someone that has been excluded from participating in society.

Challenge discrimination in practice

It is the responsibility of both services and staff to **challenge and prevent discrimination** in their practice. This is not only important from a legal perspective but also so that services can continue to run effectively with high-quality care that delivers positive outcomes and good levels of service user satisfaction.

Discrimination can be challenged in the following ways:

- By having an **awareness of intersectionality** and how this could lead to individuals being treated more or less favourably because of their characteristics and social determinants. This awareness means professionals can then ensure their practice remains neutral for all individuals.

- **Promote inclusion in the information** given to service users through the images used and resources. For example, including images of people from different ethnic backgrounds to promote inclusivity.

- Following the **organisation's policies and procedures** to report and challenge discriminatory practice. This means raising awareness of malpractice as it occurs so that it can be addressed quickly and efficiently.

- Support and encourage service users to **report discrimination** if it occurs, so that this can be challenged by the service provider.

The impact of pandemics on health outcomes:

A **pandemic** is defined as an outbreak of an infectious disease that spreads over a wide geographical area and impacts a high proportion of the world's population. The most recent example is the COVID-19 pandemic in 2019.

A pandemic can have significant impacts upon the health outcomes of different groups of individuals and populations.

Geographical differences

Individuals have different **vulnerabilities** across **different geographies**. This means that whilst people across the world can be subject to the same infectious disease, the impact it has can be very different.

For instance, for the COVID-19 pandemic:

- The disease was more dangerous for older people. So countries with older populations were more at risk. More economically developed countries (MEDC) tend to have older populations than less economically developed countries (LEDC), and were initially affected more by the disease.

- LEDCs do not generally have same levels of access to health care as MEDCs. So there was more support for people who fell seriously ill in MEDCs, although this support was seriously stretched in some countries such as the UK and Italy.

- Urban areas were initially affected more than rural areas, because people live closer together – and the disease spread due to close contact. However, rural areas often have far few medical resources, so the impact on rural areas was also high when it reached them.

- The disease spread more easily when people were indoors – so people in colder climates were more at risk.

Cultural differences

During COVID-19 there were also differences in **mortality rates** (death rates) across different cultures.

- In collectivist cultures like Japan and China they place stronger values on community than individualistic cultures like the United States. This meant that, for example, mask-wearing and social distancing were implemented in countries like Japan and

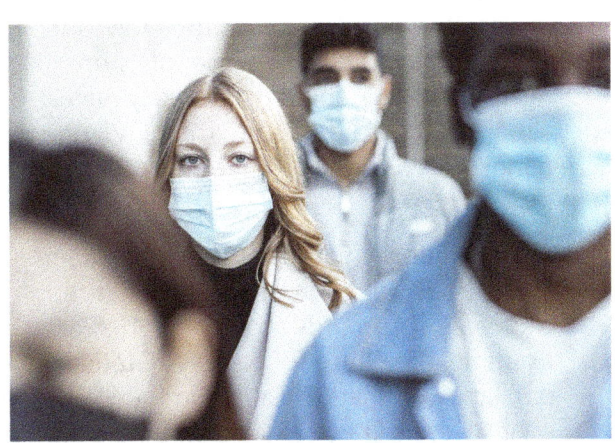

China without resistance from its citizens. In European countries and the United States there was some level of resistance from some of its citizens to these preventative measures, which then saw a spike in COVID-19 cases in these countries.

Examples of higher mortality rates across cultural groups

Mortality rates were higher for a number of different cultural groups. Some examples include:

- **Indigenous populations**, such as those in Brazil and Canada, probably due to limited healthcare and a mistrust of the government.
- **Roma**, **gypsy** and **traveller communities**, due to social exclusion as well as because of language and literacy barriers.
- **Migrant worker communities** in some countries across the world, because they lived together in large dormitories, were isolated from native populations and had far fewer rights.
- **Refugees** and **asylum seekers** living in overcrowded conditions were vulnerable to the disease. Those who were living in safer conditions may have been less willing to seek help or healthcare for fear of the authorities.

Effects on particular groups

Pandemics can also cause **significant effects upon different groups of people**. Some examples include:

- **Disabled people.** COVID-19 was more dangerous for people who had existing health conditions, and this disproportionately affected disabled people. If they were more vulnerable to the disease then they had to completely isolate, which has a big impact on people's mental health. Some disabled people may have already felt isolated before the COVID-19 pandemic, which became far worse during lockdown.
- **Ethnic minority communities.** It has been shown that some ethnic minorities in the UK were hit far harder by COVID-19. For example, the Office for National Statistics data showed that Black men in the UK were over twice as likely to die from COVID-19

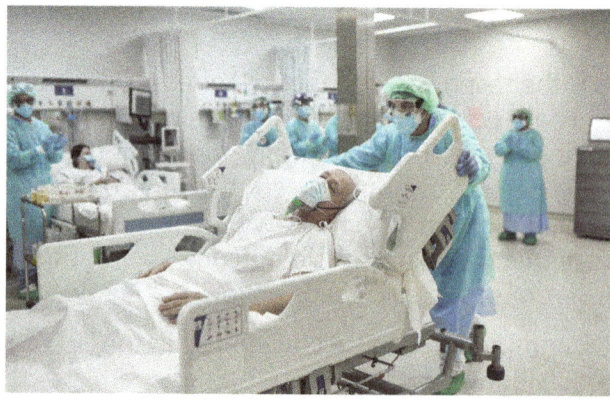

compared to White men. The reasons for this are complex but the COVID-19 highlighted the health inequalities that already existed and which we have touched on in Learning Aim C.

- **Care home residents.** Age and existing health conditions were major risk factors for COVID-19. People in care homes often fit into one or both of these categories, and had a much higher than average mortality rate. In addition, visitors were not allowed in care homes during lockdown, which had a major impact on mental health.
- **Prisoners.** Prisons are vulnerable to diseases such as COVID-19 because of close living conditions, being overcrowded and being confined indoors for most of the time. In the case of an outbreak, prisons may not have the resources or facilities to respond quickly. In addition, during lockdown visitors were not allowed, which led to complete isolation for some people and a decline in mental health. Where vaccinations are available during pandemics, prisoners are often a long way down the list to receive them, due to political reasons.

Deviant – Someone that does not meet the expected norms of society.

Marginalised – Someone that has been excluded from participating in society.

Collectivist culture – A country such as Japan or China that prioritises community and family and respect group decisions.

Individualistic culture – Many European countries such as the UK and the United States have a strong belief in personal freedom and independence over shared group goals.

Holistically – How different aspects of health and wellbeing are interconnected and can influence each other. For example, how social wellbeing can impact a person's emotional wellbeing.

- **Homeless people** are already socially excluded and find it hard to access health services. This was magnified during the COVID-19 pandemic. They are more likely to have underlying health conditions, which made this group more vulnerable to COVID-19. In addition, the disease easily spread through crowded homeless shelters. Homeless people tend to be more isolated, which was then heightened by the pandemic. On a positive note, the UK government led an initiative called Everyone In, where some 37,000 homeless people were moved into accommodation such as hotel rooms and emergency accommodation.

For all of these groups, pre-existing health inequalities led to increased mortality rates compared to the average in the UK. This is because systemic prejudices cause individuals to have disadvantaged health care support. During the pandemic these existing inequalities were magnified – but the pandemic was not the reason for them.

Significant life events

In a pandemic, the mortality rate normally increases. This means that, on average, people are more likely than normal to either:

- lose a loved one
- become seriously ill themselves, leading to end-of-life care.

In the case of COVID-19, the lockdown meant that bereavements, funerals and other culturally significant events were experienced without the support of close family and friends.

Contact with others

Because of the higher sickness rate, and emergency care provision, a pandemic may mean that people from different backgrounds or cultures are more likely to come into contact.

- This might lead to friction, misunderstanding and lower levels of empathy.
- It can make it more likely that people receive information in a language they do not understand.

- However, it could lead to a deeper appreciation of the things that many people have in common regardless of cultural background.

The COVID-19 pandemic also meant that many, many individuals had **less contact with others** than normal. It is important to recognise that health outcomes are not always related to physical health but can be considered more holistically. The mental health impacts of the COVID-19 pandemic are still being assessed.

Reprioritisation and restriction of services

Another major impact of a pandemic can be the **reprioritisation and restriction of services**. This means the government put measures in place to prioritise limited resources and prevent further spread of the disease. Although such restrictions are imperative for the controlling the spread of a disease, it can have many negative drawbacks, including:

- A high proportion of the population having health care needs that are not met.
- Increased mental health issues as a response to the pandemic.
- Education gaps if schools close.
- Loss of employment which then causes financial insecurity for many.

> **Find out more**
>
> www.eboru.com/BTEC-HSC-links
>
> COVID-19 related deaths by ethnic group.

Recap questions

1. Identify a form of discrimination.
2. Define this form of discrimination.
3. State two ways of challenging discrimination in practice.
4. What is a pandemic and give an example.
5. Why is it important to re-prioritise and restrict services during a pandemic?

Activity

1. Discuss whether you think the methods of challenging discrimination outlined are effective in their goal. Why? Are there any different ways of challenging discrimination?
2. Discuss the most important goal during a pandemic. Justify your answer.

End of Topic Practice Activity

In this practice activity you will consider the different factors that affect health and the importance of equality, diversity and inclusion.

James is 52 years old and currently lives in a small ground-floor flat in a large city. Many years ago, James suffered a spinal injury that left him unable to walk. He uses a wheelchair. He is also unable to work and relies heavily on disability benefits. After the injury James began smoking to cope with the pain and stress. This has become a habit James wishes to control better, as he was recently diagnosed with Chronic Obstructive Pulmonary Disease (COPD). He struggles to access his local smoking cessation group due to poor wheelchair access.

Amina is 45 years old and currently lives with her family in a large inner city after arriving in the UK as a refugee. She speaks very limited English. She has recently been diagnosed with type 2 diabetes and struggles to manage her condition due to the language barrier. She is reluctant to attend appointments after being discriminated against, as she felt dismissed and laughed at during her appointment with the diabetes nurse.

--

You need to consider the factors that affect the health status of James and Amina, and the impacts on them of inclusive working.

Write down your ideas about the following:

- Which health status factors from page 158-160 that might affect James and Amina? How?.
- Which social and environmental factors that might affect James and Amina's health? How?
- How could equality, diversity and inclusion help improve the health outcomes of James and Amina? Why is this important for each of them?
- How might inclusive working impact on the health, social and environmental factors that affect James and Amina? How might it affect the barriers that they face?
- How successful do you think inclusive working practices would be for James and Amina?

This practice task will help you prepare for the following assessment criteria:

C.P6 Explain the factors that may affect the health status of two individuals with different needs.

C.P7 Explain the importance of equality, diversity and inclusion in practice to improve the health outcomes of two individuals with different care needs.

C.M4 Analyse how working in an inclusive way in practice impacts on the factors and potential barriers that may affect the health outcomes of two individuals with different care needs.

C.D3 Evaluate the success of approaches to inclusive working practices on improving the health outcomes and overcoming potential barriers of two individuals with different needs.

Unit 4 Health, policy and wellbeing

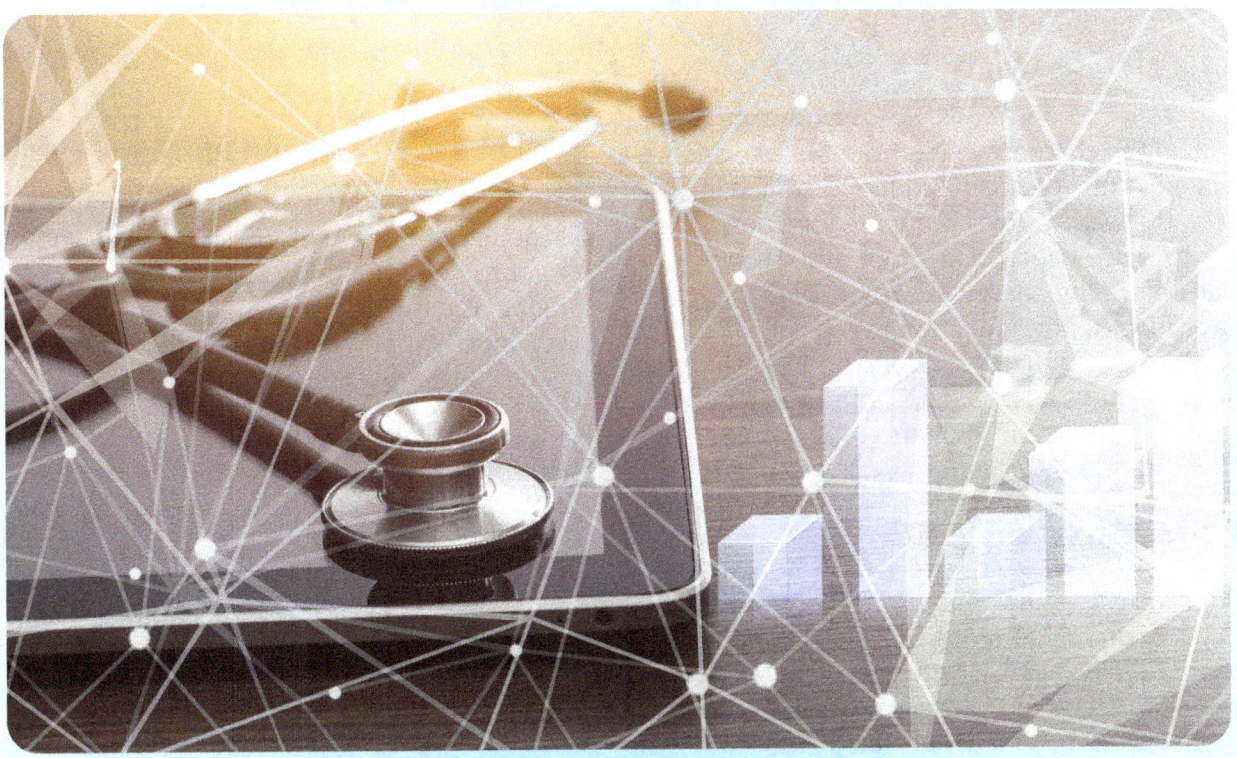

In this unit you will learn about the origins of public health policy and how these relate to current frameworks.

You will learn about:

- A range of factors that feed into public health practice.
- How these aim to improve the health of the public.
- A range of methods for promoting and protecting public health.
- Potential barriers to improving people's health-related behaviours.

How will I be assessed?

In this unit you will be assessed through an internal assessment consisting of a series of tasks, covering Learning Aims A, B and C. The assignment is set by the awarding body and marked by your tutor.

Learning Aim A: Understand the influence of social policy on public health

Learning Aim B: Examine the factors affecting public health policy and the impact of addressing these factors to improve public health

Learning Aim C: Examine the impact of social policy as a driver to improve outcomes in public health

Learning Aim A: Understand the influence of social policy on public health

A1 The origins and aims of social and public health policy

The origins of post-1948 public health policy

During the second world war, the government recognised that recovering from the war, and looking after soldiers returning to civilian life once the war was over, would require great efforts. They began planning for this recovery well before the end of the war. In 1942 the Beveridge Report identified five 'giant evils'. Beveridge said that we need to address all of these to thrive as a nation. These five giants were: want, disease, ignorance, squalor and idleness.

Access to free health

After the war a new Labour government wanted to move quickly to tackle these issues. They passed the National Health Service Act in 1946 and instructed the Minister for Health, Aneurin Bevan to set up a **National Health Service**. On 5th July 1948 the NHS came into being. It introduced:

- **Free medical treatment** for all British citizens
- Nationalised hospitals under the Ministry of Health
- Health centres to provide services like **vaccinations** and **maternity services**.
- An **emergency health service**.

The NHS has made healthcare accessible to all members of the public, which has had a massive impact on health. In 1951 the UK life expectancy at birth was 66.4 years for men, and 71.5 years for women. By 2021 this had risen to 79 years for men and 82.8 years for women.

We have also seen much lower rates of infant and maternal mortality. This has also been helped by:

- Advances in **birth control**.
- Better **maternity services**.
- At the same time, testing before babies are born (**antenatal testing**) means that health conditions can be spotted even before a child is born.

> **Activity**
>
> The language used in the Beveridge report is quite old-fashioned. These days we would refer to needs that must be met. Can you match the Giant Evils to more modern vocabulary that we would use to describe the needs Beveridge identified?
>
> | 'Giant Evil' | Need |
> |---|---|
> | Want | |
> | Disease | |
> | Ignorance | |
> | Squalor | |
> | Idleness | |
>
> Word list: **employment, quality housing, income, health, education**

Prevention and health education

Over the years since the NHS was founded, there has been an **increasing focus on preventing illness**, as well as treating people when they become ill. This includes educating the public about what helps people improve their own health and wellbeing through, for example, their diet and exercise.

It also includes **vaccination programmes** that mean that many dangerous childhood illnesses that used to be common, such as polio, diphtheria and measles, which can cause long-term health problems and disabilities, are now extremely rare.

Population health

Since 1948, public health policy in the UK has shifted from treating individuals with diseases or conditions, to thinking about the health outcomes for different groups. It also led to understanding what factors drive health outcomes and health inequalities, and what can be done to change this. This is known as population health.

Standardised approach

By bringing all health services together, there is now standardised training for doctors, nurses and other health care professionals. This means that the same standards of evidence-based approaches to diagnosis and treatment of illnesses are available to everyone.

Unemployment due to illness

Not only do all of these improvements benefit the health of individuals, but they also reduce the chances that people have to take time away from work when they are ill, boosting individuals' incomes and the economy more generally.

> **Vaccination** – A safe and effective way of protecting a person from getting a particular illness in the future, by giving them a small dose of a version of the virus or bacteria that causes the illness. Often the dose is already dead or weakened.
>
> **Life expectancy** – An estimate of how long a person is likely to live, based on a range of factors.
>
> **Infant mortality rate** – Out of every 1000 children who are born, how many die before they reach 1 year old.
>
> **Maternal mortality rate** – Out of every 100,000 women who give birth, how many die due to something going wrong with their pregnancy or labour.

The aims of public health policy

Social policy is any government action that is aimed at helping meet social needs. These needs are typically related to employment, education, healthcare, housing or substance misuse.

Social policy aims to **identify social or economic inequalities** between different groups and communities, and to reduce these inequalities.

Social policy mostly focuses on dealing with broad factors that have an impact on large groups of people. It may tackle issues that affect specific age groups, ethnic groups, people in specific locations or socio-economic groups. It should ensure that services are provided in ways that will see the most benefit for those who need them most.

The aims of public health policy include:

- **Identifying and reducing social and economic inequalities**, for example through providing income support or help with finding a job.

- **Promoting the health of the nation** to include reducing the rates of ill health, for example through public health advertising campaigns or work targeting groups identified as at risk of a particular health issue.

- **Protecting individuals, groups and communities from threats to health and wellbeing**, for example through vaccination programmes.

- **Empowering individuals to make healthy choices** and live a healthier lifestyle, for example through advertising campaigns giving information about healthier lifestyle choices.

- **Reducing health inequalities between groups and communities** in society, by monitoring which areas are suffering higher levels of a particular illness.

- **Addressing specific global and national health problems** over a period of time, such as the work done during the COVID-19 pandemic.

- **Working collaboratively on social policy** locally, nationally and in the international context.

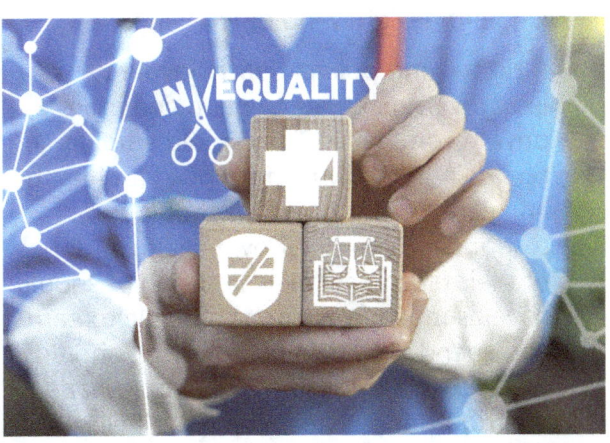

A2 Factors that influence policy making in health and social care

Since 1946 there have been many changes to the NHS and to the way health and care services are regulated in the UK. Each government has taken its own stance on the best ways to improve the health and wellbeing of the nation and the best way to run and fund these services.

For example, the **Care Act (2014)** aimed to simplify over 60 years of different laws that governed which adults were entitled to different types of care.

- The older laws put responsibility on **local government** and other organisations to provide certain levels of care. However, this meant that care was often focused on these services and organisations.
- The Care Act (2014) changed the perspective, beginning with assessing the focus of care onto needs of an individual, entitling them to care that will meet those needs. This is called the **personalisation of care**.

At present, the **Department of Health and Social Care** is the part of government with responsibility for the health of the nation.

- Working under the instruction of the Department of Health and Social Care, the **NHS** provides individual emergency and planned health care, for example through hospitals and GP surgeries.
- The **Office for Health Improvement and Disparities** focus on reducing differences in health outcomes between groups, so that whatever a person's background, they have the same opportunities to live a long and healthy life.
- The **UK Health Security Agency** works to prevent, prepare for and respond to infectious diseases and environmental hazards.

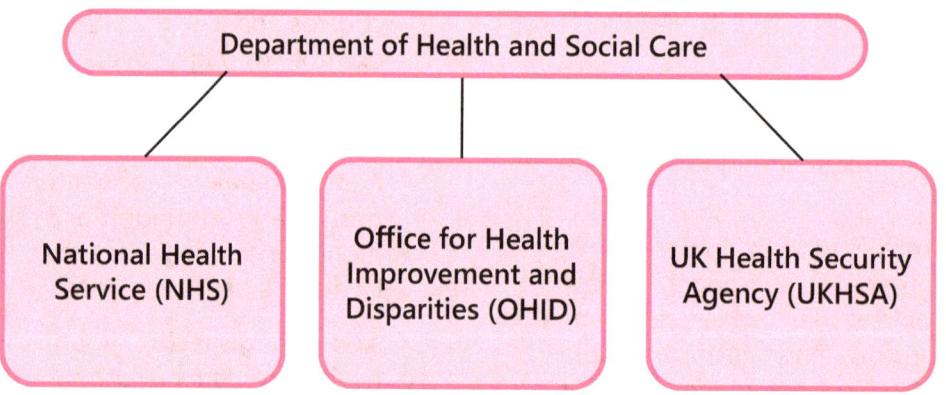

The effect of changes in government on social policy

Political ideology

Traditionally, political parties have been viewed as being either right wing or left wing.

- A **right-wing political party** favours less government intervention and more private companies. They would emphasise private and family responsibility for health and care, meaning people should take responsibility for their own health and that of their family members. Individuals should have as much freedom as possible to earn and spend their own money, taxes should be as low as possible and if people want to contribute to the health and wellbeing of others, they can choose to do this through volunteering or charitable donations, for example to food-banks.
- A **left-wing political party** emphasises collective responsibility for the health and wellbeing of all citizens. To achieve this, they are more likely to increase the size and scope of government organisations, and favour the public sector over private companies. Under this philosophy, society should look after the health and wellbeing of all, regardless of ability to pay. This should be funded by taxation, taking more from those with the most money, and less from those on a lower income.

In health and social care, when a left-wing government has been in charge there has been an increase in funding for health and social care services that are free for everyone, for example:

- Children's centres where expectant and new parents are given free guidance and support to provide the best start for all children.
- Increased funding to support students who are training to become healthcare professionals.

When a more right-wing government has been in power, there has been a greater reliance on the charitable and private sectors to provide services such as ante-natal classes, and social care, and health services have been instructed to make more efficient use of their resources so that taxes can be lowered.

State of the economy

However, in recent years the divisions between left and right-wing parties have become less clear, with both sides borrowing successful or popular policies from each other, and new parties joining the political arena. The **wider state of the economy** has arguably had a greater impact on social policy than ideological differences between political parties. For example, the **financial crisis of 2008** meant that **significant reductions were made** to the amount of money provided to fund health and social care. It didn't necessarily matter which political party was in power.

Previous experience

Social policy has also been **driven by lessons learned** from experience. For example, at times there have been significant failings in health and social care. Policy changes have come about afterwards, to try to prevent them happening again.

For example, between 2005 and 2008 there were significant problems at Stafford hospital. There were at least 400 more deaths than would have been expected, as a result of poor-quality care. When this came to light, a public inquiry was launched to investigate what went wrong. As a result of the inquiry, a number of changes were made to policy, including:

- More regulation of the training and roles of healthcare assistants
- Minimum staffing levels on hospital wards.
- A legally binding duty of candour to admit mistakes.

> Infectious diseases – Diseases that can be passed from one person (or animal) to another.
>
> Environmental hazard – Substances in the environment such as toxic chemicals, or events such as floods, that can negatively affect people, their homes or places of work.
>
> Ante-natal classes – Sessions where healthcare professionals educate expectant parents about staying healthy during pregnancy, the birth process and how to look after and feed a newborn baby.
>
> Duty of candour – A legal requirement that health and social care providers and staff must be open and honest when something goes wrong.

One of the changes that came from this experience was the introduction of the NHS 6Cs: care, compassion, competence, communication, courage and commitment.

Prevalent health and social care issues

Social policy is also driven by what are **the most pressing health or social issues** taking place at a particular time. For example, in 2020 many new policies rapidly came into force in response to the global COVID-19 pandemic.

Recap questions

1. What were the five 'giant evils' identified in the Beveridge report?
2. What is the role of the OHID?
3. Name one change that was introduced after the Stafford hospital scandal.

Activity

In this section, you have learned about a number of different changes to social policy agendas. Can you sort each of the changes below into the categories in the table?

Personalisation of care; Renaming and reorganising departments; Privatisation of services; Regulation of healthcare assistants; Duty of candour.

Different ways of planning care	Increased monitoring of health and social care teams and services	Restrictions on the types of care available for free

Changes to social policy agendas

Changes to social policies by different governments often focus on things such as:

- Different ways of planning and implementing care.
- Increased monitoring of health and social care teams.
- Increased restrictions in the types of care available in statutory service.

These changes might be for ideological reasons, because of costs and resource implication, or as a response to past poor-quality care.

Identification of health needs

In order to help the population we need to know what their needs are. This means we have to gather **data** that gives us **information about people's health**. This comes from a wide range of sources.

- Local hospitals, GP surgeries and other health services keep records of the people they see and treat.
- Local governments organise and keep records of social care provided in their local area.
- These local organisations will report information to regional and national bodies that use this information to monitor patterns of health and illness across the nations of the UK.
- Through the census, as well as birth and death certificates, the government keeps track of demographic data about the population.

When we look at these patterns of health and illness across populations, this is called epidemiology. Understanding how illnesses affect different groups, at different times and in different places helps us to plan care and support to match these needs. For example:

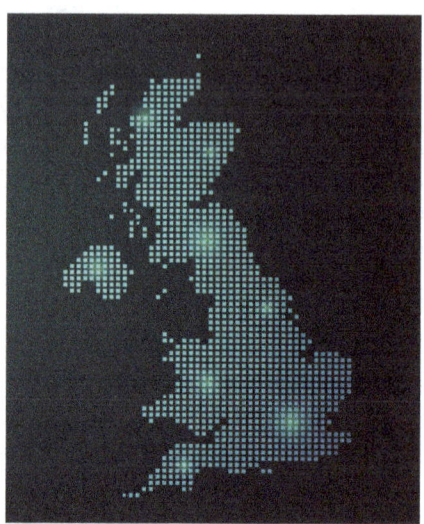

Health data trends

- Data about the number of measles cases in a particular city might identify an outbreak and lead to a local information campaign about prevention and vaccination.
- An outbreak of sickness might be linked to food poisoning and particular source of contaminated food or water.
- Long-term data might demonstrate the negative health affects of behaviour or substances.

Ethical Issues

It is important that individuals have personal choices about the way they receive care. This empowers individuals, as it means taking into account their unique needs and preferences.

Personlisation

Personalisation includes making sure that people are involved in decisions about their care, and leads to better health outcomes because people feel more in control of their health. At the same time, personalisation must be balanced against **safeguarding principles**.

The risks involved in any plan for care must be carefully considered, and there are times when a person's preferences may not be fully achievable.

For example, if someone with dementia, who lives alone, would prefer to stay in their own home, this must be balanced against how safe it is for them to continue living alone as their dementia progresses.

Maintaining confidentiality

Another ethical balancing act involves people's **rights to confidentiality**. Everyone is entitled to privacy, and information about them should be held confidentially. At the same time, **legislation and regulations** demand that sometimes information must be shared with other professionals. To not do so would be against the law.

Confidentiality can never truly be absolute, as it must be balanced with safeguarding.

Beliefs, values and sustainability

The **beliefs and values** of all service users must be **respected and honoured** as best as possible. However, not every preference can always be met, as there are limits to the resources available to meet everybody's needs.

We must consider how sustainable it is to put a large amount of resources into a case where there is a limited chance of success, when those same resources could be used elsewhere to support others. There is no easy answer, and each individual case must be considered on its own merits, but health policies and guidelines can support decision making.

Ethnic differences

Health policy must recognise that certain illnesses and health outcomes are more prevalent in specific ethnic groups. This could be due to a wide range of factors, such as:

- Variations in diet.
- Higher levels of economic hardship.
- Having had more negative experiences with health and social care services in the past, which can lead to a loss of trust.
- Health and social care professionals being less aware of how symptoms can appear differently in different ethnic groups. Similarly, they may also be less aware of how the effects of some medication may differ between different groups.

For example, black women in the UK are four times more likely to die in pregnancy or childbirth than white women. The reasons behind this are complex, but include a lack of awareness of how pregnancy-related illnesses present in black women. There is also evidence that black women's concerns are sometimes dismissed or not taken as seriously by healthcare providers.

Another example is how, during the early stages of the COVID-19 pandemic, Bangladeshi communities in the UK were twice as likely to die from the virus, compared to white people. Suggestions for why this was the case included higher rates of underlying health conditions such as diabetes, more crowded living conditions, and higher numbers of people in this community who worked in frontline jobs where they were more likely to be exposed to the virus.

Culturally competent healthcare means that health and social care professionals are aware of how the symptoms of certain illnesses present differently in different ethnic groups. For example, symptoms of a heart attack are slightly different in people of African, South Asian or white backgrounds.

Health policies should recognise these differences and make sure that steps are taken to build trust with all service users, and to improve outcomes for groups that have been let down in the past.

> Demographic data – Information about a population, such as age, gender, ethnicity, income, and education level.
>
> Epidemiology – The study of how diseases spread, who gets them, and why, helping to prevent illness and improve public health.
>
> Personalisation – Tailoring health and social care provision to an individual's specific needs, preferences, and circumstances to improve their wellbeing.
>
> Culturally competent healthcare – Healthcare that respects and understands different cultural beliefs, languages, and traditions, ensuring that everyone gets fair and appropriate treatment.

> **Apply your understanding**
>
> Marcy is 22 weeks pregnant when she begins to go into labour. She is rushed to hospital and given care to try to delay giving birth, to give the baby a better chance of survival.
>
> Since 2019, the guidance from the British Association of Perinatal Medicine is that doctors and nurses should discuss with parents and make a risk assessment about the chances of survival of a very premature baby. The result of the discussion will decide whether they will do everything possible to try to save the life of the baby. It may require invasive, painful and distressing treatments. The baby is likely to have multiple operations and be in hospital for many months. The alternative is to offer comfort-based care, to try to ensure that both Marcy and her baby are in as little pain as possible for the short time the baby will survive outside of the womb.
>
> In this discussion, health and social care practitioners must respect Marcy's beliefs and values. They must present evidence and information as neutrally as possible, so that Marcy fully understands the risks to her baby of long-term disabilities or other consequences of such an early birth.
>
> 1. Why is it so important to give Marcy a voice in this decision-making process?
> 2. Caring for a very premature baby takes specialist and expensive equipment, highly trained staff and a long time. Do you think this is justified if the chances of Marcy's baby surviving are very low? Can you explain why you think this?

A3 Groups that influence social and public health policy

Roles of national and international public health-related organisation that influence public health policy

There are a wide range of groups that influence the way public health policy is produced.

National groups

Within the UK:

- The **National Institute for Health and Care Excellence** (NICE) provides evidence-based guidelines and recommendations on care pathways, treatments and public health initiatives.
- The **Care Quality Commission** (CQC) regulates and inspects health and social care providers, similar to the way Ofsted inspects education providers. They identify areas where improvements are needed, and produce reports that guide policy makers.
- **NHS England** oversees the delivery of NHS services. They allocate funding and set priorities for health care providers that will influence the way that public health policy is applied.
- The **UK Health Security Agency** (UKHSA) monitors infectious diseases, environmental hazards and emergencies. This information is used to plan for these threats, and informs policies about the ways we can reduce the number of people who are at risk, or the level of danger.
- The **Faculty of Public Health** is a professional body that supports public health specialists. They do research, training and lobby people who are making policy, with the aim of promoting health and preventing avoidable disease.

Government and government agencies

The **Department of Health and Social Care** set overall priorities for health and social care. They provide funding for the NHS, the Office for Health Improvement and Disparities (OHID), the UKHSA and NICE. The Secretary of State for Health and Social Care has final responsibility for the health and social care system – to ensure it is effective, sustainable and ready to respond to public health challenges.

Pressure groups and campaigners

There are also charities, voluntary sector organisations and campaigning groups that influence public health policy. For example:

- **ASH** (Action on Smoking and Health) campaign for tougher control on the sale of cigarettes, banning smoking in more situations and stricter rules about advertising of tobacco products.
- **Age UK** advocate for the rights and wellbeing of older people.
- **Cancer Research UK** funds research, raises awareness and campaign to change policies and practices that relate to cancer.
- The **Equality and Human Rights Commission** (EHRC) do research to recognise the discrimination that different groups experience, and try to influence policy so that this is taken into account when policies are written, so that everyone should be treated fairly when dealing with health and social care services.

Charities and voluntary sector

- The **British Heart Foundation** funds research into heart related disease, and promotes things like improved diets, reducing smoking and improving treatments for heart disease.
- The **British Deaf Association** campaigns on behalf of deaf people, pushing for policies that improve access to healthcare for people with hearing impairments, increase access to sign language interpreters, and improve understanding of Deaf culture in healthcare settings.
- The **Alzheimer's Society** campaign for better care and support for people with dementia, and push for better funding for research into the disease.

International groups

International groups also influence public health policy in the UK.

- The **World Health Organisation** (WHO) set global health standards, and provides guidance on how to prevent and respond to outbreaks of specific diseases, such as HIV and the COVID-19 virus. They influence policies on the development of vaccines

> **Advocate** – To support or speak up on behalf of a group, to bring about changes in policy or practices.
>
> **Non-communicable diseases** – Diseases that cannot be spread from person to person, such as diabetes and asthma.

and best practices to reduce levels of non-communicable diseases.

- **Action for Global Health** is a network of organisations who advocate for global health equality. They push governments to increase funding for healthcare and to make sure that everyone has access to the health and social care services they need.
- The **United Nations** (UN) has a range of goals. They contribute funding to agencies such as the WHO. They also influence policies on issues such as disease prevention, maternal and child health, clean water and sanitation. The UN considers health to be a fundamental human right. They set long-term, international strategies through the UN Sustainable Development Goals (SDGs) which all member states agree to work towards.

Activity

Research the UN Sustainable Development Goals.

Choose one of the goals and use your research skills to identify a health policy that works towards that goal.

Recap questions

1. What is the role of the Faculty of Public Health?
2. What does a pressure group do? Give one example of a pressure group.
3. What is the UN's role when it comes to health?

End of Learning Aim Practice Activity

For this practice activity you should focus on public health policies around infectious diseases.

- Investigate how public health policies tried to reduce the spread of infectious diseases in the past.
    * How does this compare this to the way we try to control infectious diseases today?
    * What is the same and what is different between the approaches in the 20th and 21st centuries?
- What are the benefits to individuals of the current policies around infectious diseases.? What are good about them, and what prevents them from being fully effective?
- How have the current policies around infectious diseases been influenced by the Faculty of Public Health? What did it do with regard to infectious diseases?
- How might the public health policy on infectious disease have been different without the work of the Faculty of Public Health? Were there any recommendations that have been ignored or rejected? Why do you think this is?
- Are we now better at controlling and preventing the spread of infectious diseases compared to in the middle of the 20th century? How much of that progress do you think is due to changes in public health policy? How much is because of the work of the Faculty of Public Health? You must come to an overall conclusion that includes your own opinion.

This practice task will help you prepare for the following assessment criteria:

A.P1 Compare differences between the implementation of public health aims of the post-1948 public health policy and current practice.

A.P2 Discuss the influence of one national or one international group on current public health policy.

A.M1 Assess the benefits to individuals, of current ways of implementing one post-1948 public health aim.

A.M2 Analyse the influence of one national or international group on current public health policy.

A.D1 Evaluate the influence of post-1948 public health aims, and one national or international group, on current public health policy.

Learning Aim B: Examine the factors affecting public health policy and the impact of addressing these factors to improve public health

B1 Social policy development

Processes involved in social policy development

When developing a public health policy, there are a number of processes that must be completed.

The first is to identify the issue that this policy will address.

- For example, the policy may be related to some of the health issues that arise as a result of Britain having an ageing population. Life expectancy in the UK has increased a lot in the last hundred years, and people are also having fewer children. This means that a higher proportion of the population is elderly, whose health and social care needs are different from those in younger age groups.
- Another example would be a policy about preparations for potential public health emergencies, such as pandemics, natural or human-made disasters, or major accidents.

Evidence that supports policy development might come from data collected by UK bodies, such as the Office for National Statistics or the NHS.

Sometimes social policies are driven by political reasons – for example, something that a political party campaigned on during an election.

Evidence and research

Once an issue has been chosen, the next step is to conduct further research into the current situation, and explore evidence of how developments in policy could improve health outcomes. This may involve conducting research, or drawing on existing research from charities, special-interest groups, health and social care professionals and others.

- For example, when developing the increase in tax on sugary drinks, the UK government drew on the expertise of doctors, nurses, nutritionists and psychologists, as well as research from Cancer Research and diabetes charities, to decide the best approach to take.

Creating policy

A policy may be completely new or it may be a development or change to an existing policy. This can be a long and complicated process. If a policy requires new laws, or major changes to existing laws, then:

- The government sets out its plans in a **Green Paper**. This is a starting point for consultation and debate, and gives stakeholders a chance to feed into the policy detail. Stakeholders can include charities, pressure groups, and campaigners.
- Feedback from different organisations may be contradictory, so the government may need to conduct further research and collect more evidence.
- Eventually the Green Paper plans are turned into a **White Paper**, which is a firmer proposal for government legislation. It gives another chance for further debate and amendments.

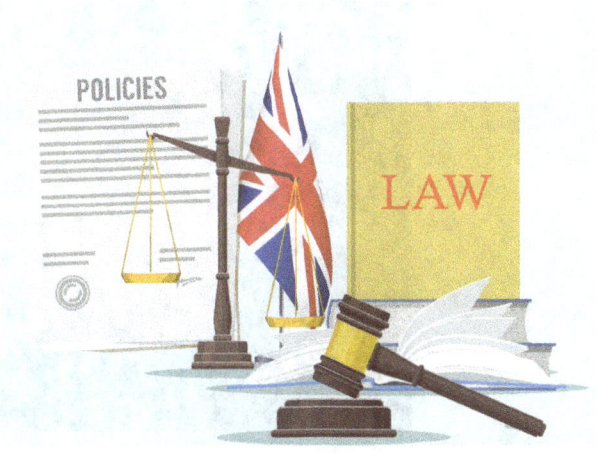

- It is then turned into a **Bill** which passes through Parliament. After further debate and passing through Parliament several times, a Bill becomes an **Act of Parliament**.

Implementing policy

Once a policy is finalised and written it must then be **implemented**. This means that the plan must be put into practice in the real world. This can also be a complicated process as it may require different government departments, local government, and a range of other organisations to work together.

For example, a policy may involve the Department of Health, the Department of Work and Pension, local authorities who have a budget for public health, and service providers such as hospitals, GPs, Integrated Care Boards, housing associations and voluntary sector organisations.

It is really important that this stage is done carefully, so that any consequences of the policy can be monitored and measured.

Impacts of policy reform

The data gathered from monitoring and measuring can then be used to analyse and evaluate the impact of the policy.

- Has it had the effect that was intended?
- If not, how should the policy be changed in the future to make it better?

Remember that the policy could be more or less effective in different contexts, so it's important to look at the changes it leads to locally, as well as at national or even international levels.

One example of a public health policy development process is the way that vaccines for COVID-19 were rolled out in the UK when they were first developed. Once a vaccine had been developed, and proven to reduce hospital admissions and deaths due to the COVID-19 virus, the Department of Health had to decide how to use it.

It was decided to target vaccinations at the elderly and those with underlying health conditions that made them particularly vulnerable. This was based on the available data about which groups were most at risk of serious illness from the virus.

Local NHS teams were then tasked with implementing the policy in their local area. As more vaccines were given to more people, the strategy was carefully monitored and the impact on the number of hospital admissions for COVID-19 in these groups was tracked. Gradually the vaccine was made available to younger and younger people. When potential side effects of one version of the vaccine were reported in younger age groups, the policy was adapted to give a different version to these groups, that caused fewer side effects.

As the NHS could gather all of this data efficiently, and compare results to people's existing medical conditions, it was able to generate very detailed and useful evidence of the way the vaccination policy worked. This information was used not only in the UK but shared with the World Health Organisation, to support effective vaccination programmes across many different countries.

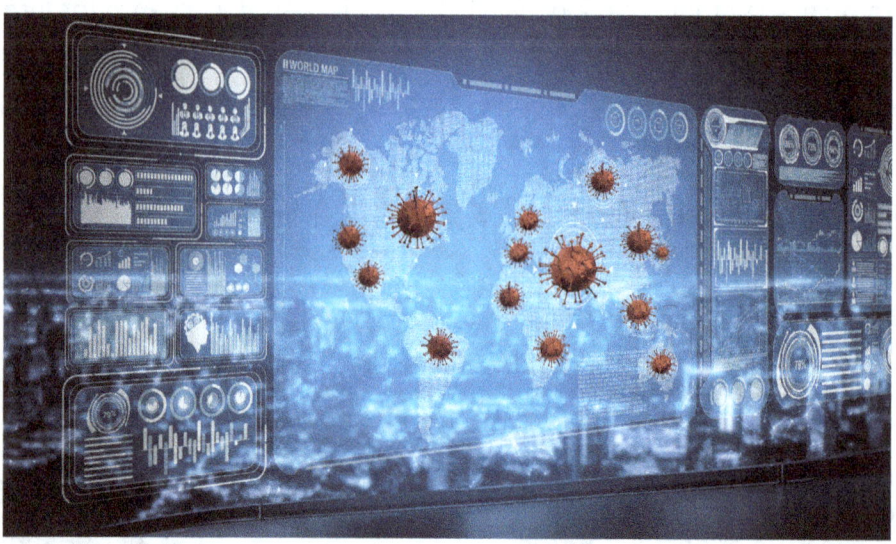

B2 Factors affecting the development and implementation of social policy

There are a number of factors that can affect the way that policies are developed and implemented.

Time taken to identify and highlight the issue

For example, evidence of the link between smoking and lung cancer was already clearly identified by the 1950s, but it took many decades for this information to translate into public health policy, such as the smoking ban in indoor public spaces that was only implemented in the UK in 2007.

Public opinion

The public's awareness, understanding and agreement with a public health policy has a big impact on the success of voluntary schemes such as screening and vaccination programmes.

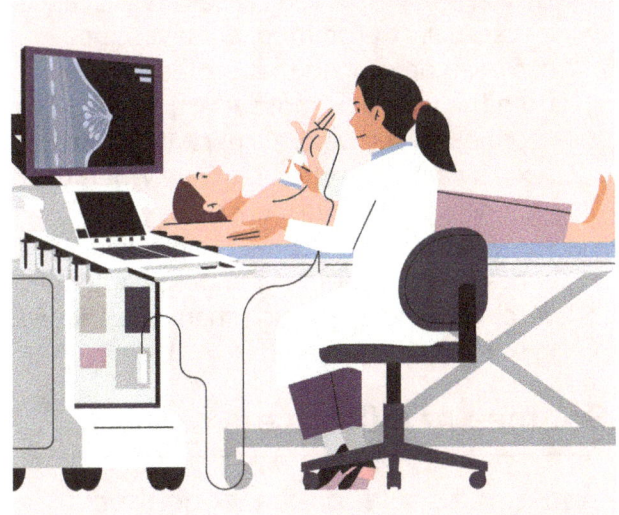

Breast cancer screening

Screening programmes

- Public awareness of the need for **breast cancer screening** has benefitted from sustained publicity, leading to many women attending scans to detect the early stages of breast cancer, before any symptoms appear. The proportion of eligible people in England who attended a scan in 2024 was 69.9%, according to The Department of Health and Social Care. This is less than before the COVID-19 pandemic, where the percentage was around 75%.

- Many people are uncomfortable talking about **bowel cancer** and historically were more hesitant to take part in screening. In 2015 57.3% of eligible adults in England attended screening. However, the number has been increasing since then, and according to the Department of Health stands at 71.8% in 2024. This is partly down to a new test that can be sent through the post, but is also due to increased awareness of the severity and frequency of the condition.

- The **National Chlamydia Screening Programme** (NCSP) is available for women aged 15-24. Department of Health data reports that just under 21% of eligible people took part in 2023. This low rate is likely to be because people do not know much about chlamydia, its effects, or the screening programme.

Vaccinations

There are a number of vaccination programmes in the UK.

- The **flu vaccine** is available for people aged over 65 (78% take-up in 2023/4) and other at-risk individuals (41% take-up in 2023/4). There has been a much better understanding in recent years that flu is not just a 'bad cold', but a serious disease that kills thousands of people each year.

- The **COVID-19** vaccine is still available for people aged over 65 and those who are at higher risk. Around 60% of over-65s took the part in the autumn 2024 booster programme, which is similar to the same period the year before. There is quite a difference between the flu vaccine take-up and the COVID-19 vaccine take-up for the same age range. Part of this is down to a difference in public opinion about the two diseases and the associated vaccines.

- **Measles** is a serious disease for which there has been a vaccine for many years. There is no question that the MMR vaccine, which covers measles, has saved many thousands of lives. However, the uptake of the vaccine in 2023/4 for one-year olds was 88.9%, which is less than in 2013/4, where 92.7% of children were vaccinated. The WHO recommends a 95% vaccination rate for measles to achieve herd immunity. The downward trend is almost certainly strongly influenced by public opinion on the topic. Unfortunately, there is a lot of misinformation about this particular vaccine, and vaccines in general. See the next section for more details about this.

- **HPV** is a virus that can cause cervical cancer. It is sexually transmitted, but a vaccine has been developed that protects people from the virus. It is most effective if the vaccine is given before a person becomes sexually active for the first time. When the vaccine was first introduced there was some resistance, as some people were concerned that giving younger people the vaccine would encourage them to engage in sexual activity earlier.

Sources of influence

Media and social media, conspiracy theorists and people with no expertise

Some public health programmes have been hampered by **conspiracy theories**, and misinformation, often available on social media channels and written by people who know very little about the subject in question.

- When the COVID-19 vaccines were developed, stories about potential side effects circulated on social media. These side effects were extremely rare, and the dangers of contracting COVID-19 are significantly worse, but the power of these stories in the media influenced many people to delay or avoid the vaccine altogether. At the same time, some people felt that they were being pressured into getting the vaccine, whether they wanted it or not.

- In another example, in 1998 a doctor incorrectly claimed a link between the MMR vaccine and autism. His study gained lots

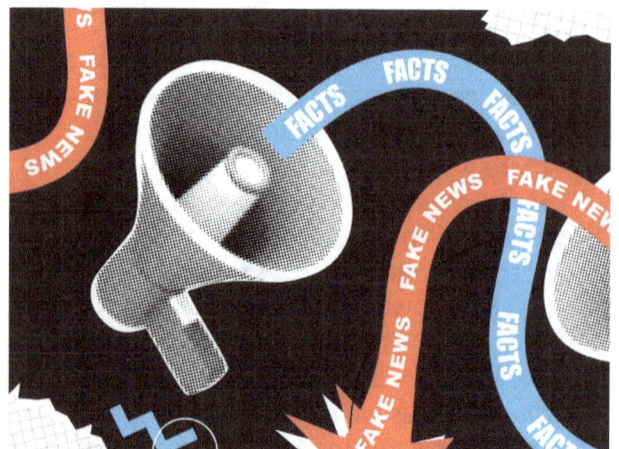

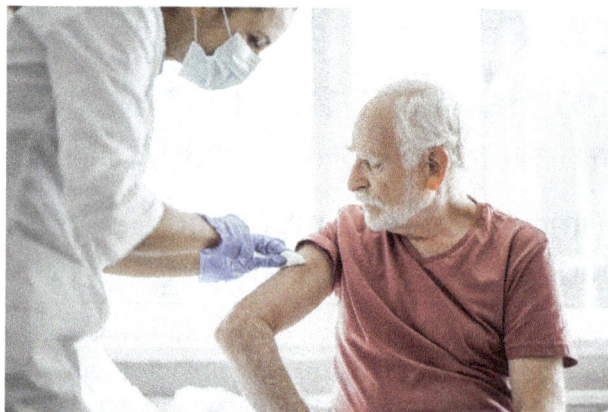

It is estimated that the COVID-19 vaccination programme saved 400,000 lives in England between December 2020 and March 2023

of publicity but was a fundamentally flawed piece of research. As a result, the study was later completely discredited and the lead author struck off the medical register. The mainstream media coverage, which was often uncritical of the original research, had a huge impact on public opinion. As a result, even today, a number of people remain hesitant to vaccinate their children with MMR. The MMR vaccine protects children from the dangerous diseases measles, mumps and rubella. There is no link between the MMR vaccine and autism.

Community leaders and family

Community leaders can have a big influence on how people engage with health and social care practitioners and institutions. If specific community groups are not engaging with a public health programme, winning over trusted community leaders can help get messages out much better. This is particularly true if a group have had negative experiences of institutions in the past.

Families can also have a significant impact on the way people engage with health and social care. For example, when someone dies, it is family members who will decide whether their organs can be donated.

Family members often have a big impact on the way we think about issues and how we approach things. This is particularly true for younger people. It is not a surprise, then, that members of the family can strongly influence people's engagement with public health policies.

International response

Different countries' approaches to the same health issues may also influence people's opinions.

For example, at the outset of the COVID-19 pandemic, different countries took very different approaches to managing the virus. For example:

- New Zealand quickly closed international borders.
- South Korea used intensive monitoring of the population through people's mobile phones.
- Sweden didn't use lockdowns or restrict people's movements, but attempted to achieve herd immunity by allowing many people to be exposed to the virus.

Public opinion in each country about the best way to deal with the pandemic was undoubtedly different, due to the difference strategies each government took.

Language

The language that is used around health issues can change the way that people respond to public health messages.

- **English is not everyone's first language**. Ensuring that policies and service descriptions are available in a number of different languages helps to ensure they are accessible.
- **Using simple language**, rather than complex jargon, to describe policies and services can help people to understand and feel more reassured.
- Official sources of information can **dispel myths and lies** that may be written and shared on social media.

Another example of the impact of language is regarding the HIV virus. When the virus first emerged it was not well understood and there were no effective treatments. People with HIV faced a lot of discrimination and were often described as 'victims'. As the scientific understanding of HIV has improved, we have developed treatments that mean that HIV is no longer a life-limiting condition. However, a lot of misinformation and myths persist. Changing the way we describe HIV patients to 'people living with HIV' rather than 'victims of HIV' completely changes the mindsets of both service users and the health and social care providers who interact with them.

> Herd immunity – When enough people in a community are immune to a disease it makes it harder for the disease to spread, protecting even those who are not immune.
>
> Side effects – Unintended reactions or symptoms caused by a medicine or treatment, such as headaches.
>
> Diagnosis – The process of identifying which illness or condition is causing symptoms in a patient.

Impact on practice

Implementing a new social policy can be complex. A new policy can change the way that organisations and services operate. For example, with regard to:

- hygiene procedures
- health and safety
- equality, diversity and inclusion
- meeting individual needs.

For example, the Health and Care Act (2022) was a major new piece of legislation designed to ensure that organisations in the sector work well together. There are many aspects to it, including the creation of new structures and organisations, such as Integrated Care Boards and Integrated Care Partnerships. It will take some time to see the impact of these structural changes on practice. It also set out the need for mandatory training on learning disabilities and autism for professionals. Implementing this means that, for example, organisations will need to ensure that new employees access this training, and that they can find training

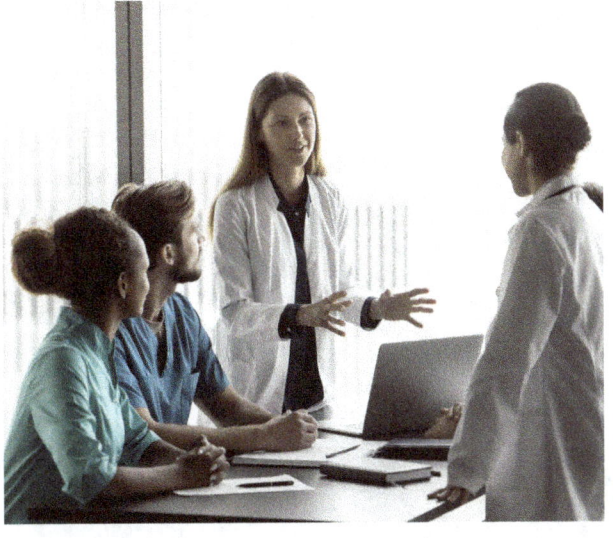

organisations who can deliver it.

Technology

Technology changes can have a big influence on the way social policy is developed and implemented. During the COVID-19 lockdowns, much health and social care provision shifted to being done over the phone and video calls. During the pandemic itself, people could report test results, and perform contact tracing, through an app. This would not have been possible without advances in technology.

Advances in artificial intelligence are being used to do tasks such as analysing scans and test results. The aim is that this should speed up diagnosis of, for example, cancers, so that people can get treatments quicker. These advances must be balanced with considerations around data privacy.

Economic conditions

Finally, the economic conditions in the country generally will have a significant impact on social policy. In the UK, health and social care provision is a public service, and is funded through taxation. This means that when the economy is doing well, and tax income increases, there is more funding for these services. On the other hand, when the economy is struggling, governments have less money to spend, and must make difficult choices about where to reduce funding.

The 2010s followed the 2008 financial crash, and marked a period of austerity in the UK. This impacted many public services and led to reduced funding for the NHS. NHS waiting lists increased from around 2.5 million to 4.5 million during this period.

> Recession – A period of time when the economy slows down. This means businesses may struggle to make profits, employers may lose their jobs and people have less money to spend.

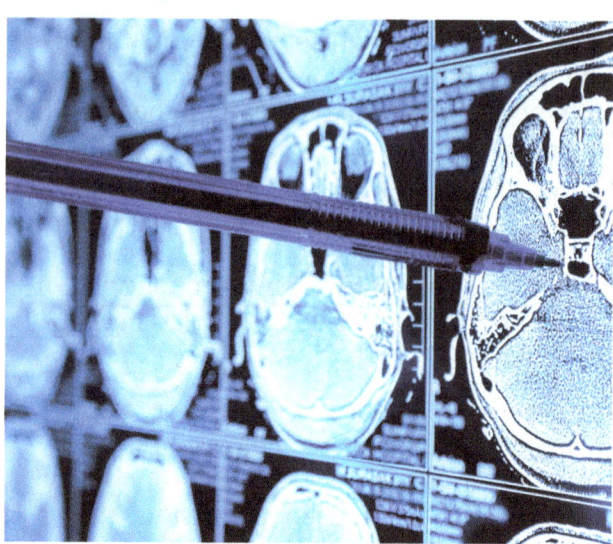

AI can now be used to detect abnormalities in scans

Find out more

www.eboru.com/BTEC-HSC-links

NHS waiting times.

Cancer screening rates.

Chlamydia screening rates:

An article in the Independent newspaper about the number of lives saved by the COVID-19 vaccine.

Recap questions

1. Which cancer does the HPV vaccine target?
2. Why were some parents hesitant to get their children vaccinated with the MMR vaccine after 1998?
3. Give one explanation of why the number of people on waiting lists for NHS treatment increased between 2010 and 2020.

B3 Social policy and its relevance to public health

Social policies relate directly to the health of the public in a range of ways.

Social factors

It has long been known that social factors have a large impact on public health. Some common social factors include:

- Socio-economic differences.
- Gender.
- Age.
- Employment.
- Disability.
- Education.
- Community services.
- New developments in medicine. These are not always rolled out on an equal basis, because of geographical funding differences. Some new treatments may not be available on the NHS and only used for private health care.
- The effects of climate change and natural disasters, such as flooding, tend to exaggerate other existing social factors. For example, crop failure due to climate change pushes up food prices, leading people with lower incomes to eat less healthily.

In 2010 the **Marmot Review** was published, analysing the state of health of the nation, and the causes of differences. It was called "Fair Society, Healthy Lives". It found strong and persistent links between **social**, **economic** and **environmental factors** and their influence on health outcomes and life expectancy. The report identified people living in poorer areas of the UK live shorter lives and spend more years in ill-health, compared to those in wealthier areas.

- For example, men in the poorest areas live up to 7 years less than those in affluent areas.
- The poorer someone is, the worse their health outcomes. This is referred to in the report as a social gradient.

The report also highlighted how early-life experiences have a lasting impact on health throughout a person's lifetime. People who have poor early-childhood experiences go on to struggle with education, employment and health.

> Social gradient – The link between socio-economic status and health, where poorer people tend to have worse health than wealthier people.

The Marmot Review recommended six objectives that should be implemented in all social policies:

1. Give every child the best start in life.
2. Enable all people to maximise their capabilities and control over their lives.
3. Create fair employment and good work for all.
4. Ensure a healthy standard of living for everyone.
5. Develop sustainable communities to promote health.
6. Strengthen the role of prevention in health services.

Policies designed to work towards these objectives include things like:

- free school meals for children living in families with a low income
- changes to welfare and benefits
- regulations about the quality of housing that is considered safe.

As well as economic differences, social policy is sometimes aimed at improving the wellbeing and health of other groups. For example:

- **Women's health policies** around providing free access to sanitary protections in schools and colleges, and better access to contraception and reducing maternal mortality rates.
- There are also policies aimed at **specific age groups**, such as free flu vaccinations for people over the age of 65, or school-age children.

Some policies aim to ensure equal access to health services for **people with disabilities**, for example by providing sign-language interpreters for people who are deaf.

Schools have a range of policies to support health and wellbeing, including sexual health, mental health and the importance of exercise.

In 2025 a cross-party inquiry will look into ways in which **young people who are not in education, employment or training (NEET)** can be reduced. In 2025 there were 900,000 people aged 16-24 who are NEET and it is well-established that they will have poorer health outcomes across their lives.

Health factors

Social policy can target specific health factors.

COVID-19

During the COVID-19 pandemic, many new policies were rolled out at speed. This included how to manage patients with COVID, social distancing, testing and tracking social contacts of people who had tested positive for the virus.

- The rollout of new technologies were accelerated. This included telemedicine, where many more appointments happened over a phone or video call.
- Extra funding for research into ways to tackle COVID was provided, which meant that vaccines were developed much faster than normal.

Obesity

Another health issue that is the target of specific health policies is obesity.

- In 2018 the UK government introduced a soft drinks industry levy (SIDL). This was commonly known as a 'sugar tax'. This was a tax that was added to soft drinks with added sugar. The aim was to reduce obesity by reducing the sugar intake of particularly children who consume a lot of soft drinks.
- In 2022 larger restaurants, cafes and takeaways were required to display calorie information on menus and food labels, with the aim that this will help people to make informed decisions when ordering food.

Smoking and substance abuse

Smoking cigarettes has a wide range of negative health consequences. According to the charity ASH, half of all smokers will die early, losing 10 years of life on average. There have been many social policy campaigns to help people to quit smoking:

> **Telemedicine** – The use of technology, like video calls, to provide remote healthcare.
>
> **Active travel** – Walking, cycling or other non-motorised transport, with benefits for individual health and the environment.

- Numerous media campaigns, including 'Smoking kills' and 'Stoptober'.
- A ban on smoking indoors in public places was put in place in 2006.
- Removal of logos and addition of disturbing graphic images of smoking-related diseases on cigarette packaging.
- Taxation on cigarettes to make them very expensive.

All of these methods have helped reduce levels of smoking to record lows.

In order to tackle drug abuse, the UK government introduced a **drug strategy** in 2021. The focus moved from criminal punishments for drug addicts to supporting people into treatment and recovery from their addiction. It aims to reduce drug-related deaths, and focuses police efforts more on drug traffickers, rather than on drug users.

Exercise

A social policy aimed at increasing the amount of **exercise** people do is the Cycling and Walking Investment Strategy. This policy promotes active travel such as cycling and walking. This has dual benefits of increased exercise and reduced air pollution from traffic. To comply with this policy, local authorities were encouraged to invest in cycle lanes and other changes to the way roads and paths are

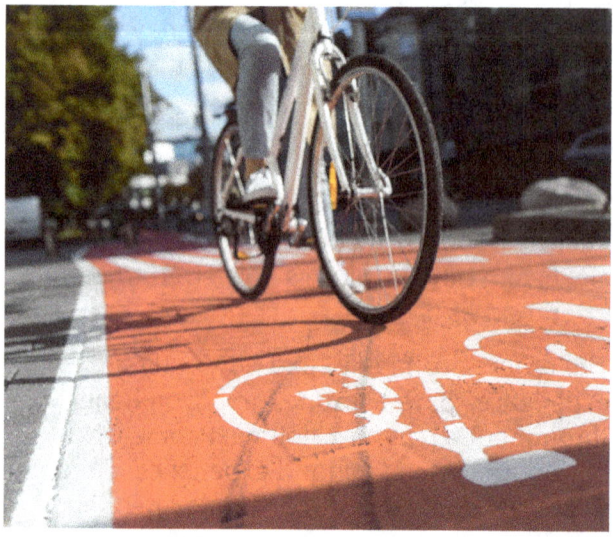

Dedicated cycle lanes encourage 'active travel'

laid out, to make it easier and safer for people to walk or cycle in their day-to-day lives. This policy should support the NHS recommendation that people should aim to do 150 minutes of exercise a week.

Emotional and mental health

Social policy not only focuses on physical health but also **emotional and mental health** factors. For example, the National Suicide Prevention Strategy (2023) sets out policies to target groups that are at higher risk of suicide. It suggests expanding mental health services, particularly for young people, so that people can access support early, before they become suicidal. It also recommends better counselling and practical help for families who have lost someone to suicide, and reducing stigma around mental health. As a result of this strategy, each local authority in England must have a suicide prevention plan that tackles the specific needs of the local community.

Recap questions

1. What is the link between health and income identified in the Marmot Review?
2. What products does the SDIL apply to?
3. How can a health service ensure that information is accessible to a deaf patient?

Access to public health services

Some groups of the population may find it more difficult to access health and social care services, so social policies should take these difficulties into account and try to minimise them.

- For example, the **NHS Accessible Information Standard** (**2016**) ensures that patients with hearing, sight, or communication impairments receive information in a format they can understand. This might include things like providing leaflets in large print, or having a British Sign Language interpreter for an appointment with a deaf patient.
- The **Learning Disabilities Mortality Review Programme** (**2015**) investigated health inequalities and premature deaths among people with learning disabilities. Based on the findings of the reviews, NHS providers can adapt and improve the way that they provide care to better meet the needs of people with learning disabilities.
- Similarly, the **Race Equality Framework for NHS England** (**2015**) investigated racial disparities in healthcare and aimed to tackle bias in treatment offered to patients by health and social care professionals.

There are also social policies that aim to support particular age groups.

- The **Healthy Child Programme** (**2009**) provided free health checks, vaccinations and support from pregnancy, through childhood up to the age of 19.
- NHS **Age Friendly Services** (**2018**) introduced a range of policies to make health care services more accessible to older people, for example by moving appointments from a clinic to be done in the person's own home.

B4 measuring the effectiveness of public health policy

Impact assessments and their role

An **impact assessment** is a tool that is used to evaluate how a policy, project or programme affects health outcomes and inequalities.

- Policy makers can also use them to try to predict the possible consequences of a new plan before it is put into practice.
- They can help to make sure that the policy achieves what it sets out to achieve, and doesn't have any unintended consequences.
- Gathering this evidence helps to decide which projects are worth funding, and which will not be such a good use of public money.
- They are also an important opportunity to include the voices of people that will be on the receiving end of the policy.

At a **local level**, impact assessments are used by local councils and by NHS bodies to assess health needs and include this information when developing strategies. For example, this could influence planning decisions about where to build key services such as health centres, and open spaces such as parks. This could help reduce levels of illnesses in areas where there is a high need.

At a **national level**, the government can use impact assessments to shape major policies, such as taxes on unhealthy foods or smoking regulations. For example, impact assessments helped the Scottish government to justify the introduction of minimum unit pricing for alcohol.

International organisations such as the World Health Organisation and the United Nations also use impact assessments to guide global policies. For example, policies about the best way to respond to emergencies such as outbreaks of disease, and the most effective ways to control these, or policies to tackle the impact of climate breakdown on people's health.

Types of impact assessments

Health Impact Assessment

A **Health Impact Assessment (HIA)** examines how the policy, plan or project in question will influence the physical, mental and social health and wellbeing of people.

For example, when planning a new housing development, a HIA will consider the additional need for access to healthcare services in the local area. It could mean that the plan should include increased capacity in local GP services, dentists and other services.

Environmental Health Impact Assessment

An **Environmental Health Impact Assessment (EHIA)** evaluates how environmental factors, such as pollution, climate change or housing conditions affect public health.

For example:

- Before expanding an airport, an EHIA will assess the impact of increased air pollution on people living in the flight path of the additional aeroplanes.
- Alternatively, to justify implementing a low-traffic policy in a city centre, an EHIA will assess the positive impacts this may have of the reduction of air pollution of people living and working in the city.

These impacts, and the associated costs to health care services for treating illness, should be weighed up against the economic benefits or drawbacks of the plan.

> Climate breakdown – The long-term, severe disruption of Earth's climate due to human activities, leading to extreme weather, rising temperatures and environmental damage.

Local impact assessments

A **Joint Strategic Needs Assessment (JSNA)** can be conducted by a local authority or the NHS to investigate the local health needs of the population.

If high levels of a particular need, such as rates of diabetes or mental health challenges, are identified in a specific area, this can influence how much of the budget of the organisation should be invested in services to address these needs.

Local councils and NHS bodies have targets for public health that they have to work towards.

> Infrastructure – The basic physical and organisational structures like roads, hospitals and power supplies, that support the normal functioning of society.

For example, a local NHS trust will have targets for how many vaccinations they give to local residents. Local health observatories will collect data and track this against policies that are in place, so that they can judge whether these policies are making a difference to the health and wellbeing of people in the local area.

Global and national impact assessments

World Health Organisation

The **World Health Organisation** conducts global impact assessments to make sure that any proposed interventions take into consideration health inequalities and social factors. For example, the WHO conducted an assessment of responses to the COVID-19 pandemic across different countries. This evidence will contribute to planning for future pandemics.

Centre for Disease Control

In the USA, the **Centre for Disease Control** conducts public health surveillance and impact assessments of changes to health regulations and policies. For example, they have reviewed different states' policies to tackle the crisis of addiction to opioid painkillers and reduce the number of deaths due to overdoses of this medication. The evidence can then be used to plan future policies that will have the best impact on this issue.

UK Health Security Agency

In the UK, the **UK Health Security Agency** (**UKHSA**) monitors threats to public health, and evaluates how effective policies are.

For example, in response to the COVID-19 pandemic, how effective were different lockdown phases. At times, there were different levels of lockdown in different parts of the country, in response to how many people in that area were being hospitalised with the virus.

Wales Health Impact Assessment Support Unit

The **Wales Health Impact Assessment Support Unit** (**WHIASU**) support public bodies in Wales to conduct Health Impact Assessments (HIAs) on a range of policies and projects. For example, in 2019 Public Health Wales, with support from WHIASU, conducted a HIA to evaluate the potential impacts of climate disruption on health and inequalities in Wales. It identified that air quality, extremes of temperature (both extreme heat and extreme cold) and flooding could have significant impacts on the Welsh economy, and could damage key infrastructure such as schools, hospitals, roads and the electricity grid. The assessment pointed out that specific communities in remote parts of Wales were particularly at risk and suggested that there is a need for specific plans to support these communities.

Legislation relevant to public health policy

There are a number of key pieces of legislation that are relevant to public health policy.

Health and Care Act (2022)

This law was passed with the aim of improving efficiency and patient outcomes from health and social care services.

- **Section 1.6** is about addressing health inequalities. It specifies that NHS bodies and local authorities are required to consider the impact of their work on reducing health inequalities, and to work to improve services for disadvantaged communities.

- **Section 1.8** encourages a greater focus on preventing people from getting ill in the first place, rather than waiting for illness and then treating it. In practice, this means an increase in screening programmes and health checks, because the early stages of many illnesses do not always have symptoms. Early treatment has better outcomes for the patient and is less expensive for the care provider.

- **Section 1.11** established **Integrated Care Systems (ICSs)** that brought together NHS services, local councils and community organisations to work together to tackle issues such as mental health and drug abuse.

Health and Social Care Act (2012)

This law created major reforms to the structure of the NHS in England. It moved responsibility for public health to Local Authorities. This means that local councils have responsibility for sexual health clinics, smoking cessation services and programmes to prevent obesity. It also increased the role of Health and Wellbeing Boards in planning local health strategies. It also allowed a greater involvement of private and third-sector organisations in public health services.

The Health Protection (Coronavirus Restrictions) (England) Regulations 2020

This legislation was rapidly passed at the beginning of the COVID-19 pandemic. It introduced legal restrictions and public health measures to prevent the spread of the virus. This included lockdowns and social distancing rules, business closures and limits on social gatherings. Later amendments to these regulations introduced mask-wearing guidance, protocols for testing, contact tracing, self-isolation and mass vaccination programmes.

Measuring effectiveness of public health policy

All of these social policies must prove their effectiveness. It requires **critical thinking** skills to make judgements about whether they are having the impact that they should. This includes:

- Selecting **reliable information** which has been **gathered from a range of sources**. This must include the people delivering the policy, and those who are on the receiving end.

- The evidence gathered must **be relevant**, **not be biased** and should have a high validity. This means that the way that the policy is being measured is reliable and genuinely measures how effective the policy is. This includes assessing if the right things are being measured. For example, if the policy being measured is a smoking ban, this should be assessed by how many people have stopped smoking, and not just how many people are aware of the policy.

- Once relevant and accurate data has been gathered, it must be analysed and synthesised.

- All of this allows for appropriate, reasonable and truthful conclusions to be drawn about how significant a policy has been in making a difference to the public health issue.

Validity – Whether a measurement truly measures what it claims to measure.

Analyse – Breaking down problems into separate parts, and identifying patterns and trends.

Synthesise – Piecing together different information to create new ideas, trends or insights.

Activity

The soft drinks industry levy (or sugar tax) was introduced in the UK in 2018. Which of the following options would be an accurate, valid and unbiased measure of the success of the policy?

- Tracking how much money was has been gathered in tax from the SDIL.
- Tracking levels of obesity in the target population.
- Asking soft drinks manufacturers how it has impacted their sales.

Find out more

www.eboru.com/BTEC-HSC-links

The Marmot Review.

Recap questions

1. Name two types of impact assessment.
2. What issues did the Welsh environmental health impact assessment find could compromise the Welsh economy and infrastructure?
3. Why is it important to assess the effectiveness of a public health policy.

End of Learning Aim Practice Activity

In this practice activity you will focus on public health policies that aimed to control the spread of the COVID-19 virus amongst elderly people.

- What were the main points of this public health policy?
- What influenced the way the policy was developed and implemented in order to protect elderly people?
- How was the effectiveness of this policy measured? What effect did this monitoring have on health of elderly?
- Can you assess the benefits of the policy for elderly people?
- Can you evaluate whether you believe these policies were effective in reducing the dangers of COVID-19 for elderly people? You need to offer a balanced argument, with both the positives and negatives of the policies, using evidence to back up your points. Make sure you consider how measurements that you discussed in B.P4 contribute to your evaluation of the policies. You must come to an overall conclusion.

This practice task will help you prepare for the following assessment criteria:

B.P3 Explain how two different factors affecting the development and implementation of public health policy, can impact a specific group.

B.P4 Discuss the effects of monitoring the effectiveness of public health policy, on the health and wellbeing of a specific group.

B.M3 Assess the benefits of public health policy to the same group, with reference to one method used to measure effectiveness of the policy.

B.D2 Evaluate the effectiveness of public health policy for the same group, with reference to one method of measurement used.

Learning Aim C: Examine the impact of social policy as a driver to improve outcomes in public health

C1 Impact of social policy on service provision

Social policies shape working practices for health and social care professionals in a range of ways.

Working practices

Policies like the **NHS Constitution** sets out the **values** that NHS workers should follow, and the expectations that service users can have of their healthcare providers. The NHS Constitution sets out the NHS's values as follows:

- Working together for patients
- Respect and dignity
- Commitment to quality of care
- Compassion
- Improving lives
- Everyone counts.

To make sure that the work of NHS staff aligns with these values, they are given training on these values at regular intervals. **Cultural competency training** helps practitioners provide inclusive care for all communities.

As part of the professionalism of NHS workers, they must all agree to follow the **6Cs of care**. These are: Care, Compassion, Competence, Communication, Courage and Commitment.

Continuous Professional Development (CPD) policies ensure that healthcare practitioners stay up to date with the latest guidelines.

National and global healthcare strategies

Social policies don't just influence individual health and social care professionals, they also impact on national and global healthcare initiatives, to tackle public health challenges.

National strategies in the UK include:

- The **Obesity Strategy** (**2020**). As part of this strategy calorie counts were added to menus, restrictions were placed on food advertising and the SDIL (sugar tax on soft drinks) was introduced.
- Another example is the **Mental Health Policy** that was part of the NHS Long Term Plan (2019) that increased funding for suicide prevention and mental health crisis services.

Global strategies operate across many countries. For example, the World Health Organisation's **Global Vaccine Strategies** aims to improve access to vaccines in parts of the world where there are high levels of disease. This involves coordination with countries where vaccinations are made, and countries where the need is greatest. Not only does this protect people in the parts of the world where levels of disease are high, but it also protects people in other parts of the world, if those diseases don't spread and mutate, becoming harder to treat and control.

Partnership working

Social policies increasingly try to integrate care, making sure that health care, social services and community organisations work together effectively. For example, the Health and Care Act (2022) established Integrated care Systems (ICSs). This means that the NHS and local authorities have to work together on things like mental health services and sexual health clinics. Joint Strategic Needs Assessments (JSNAs) mean that NHS, local councils and community services in a specific area work together to decide what the greatest needs are in their area, and then plan what services to pay for in order to meet these needs.

By working together, patients receive what is called joined-up care. They don't have to explain their situation over and over again. Different professionals from different agencies work together, focussing on the patient in the centre of each case. This leads to fewer hospital admissions and better care, particularly with long-term health conditions such as diabetes and dementia care.

Social prescribing is where GPs or other health and social care professionals recommend to patients that they join group or community activities such as exercise classes, gardening, craft or walking groups. These social activities have health benefits both in terms of physical and mental health.

Through the social policy encouraging joined-up care and social prescribing, this aims to reduce dependence on emergency hospital visits, help people who have been discharged from hospital, and increase the home-based care options for patients.

> Joined-up care – A coordinated approach to healthcare where different services and professionals work together to provide care for all aspects of a person's life.
>
> Social prescribing – When healthcare professionals refer their patients to non-medical services or activities such as community groups, exercise classes or other social activities that can support a person's mental and physical health.

Recap questions

1. What are the NHS 6Cs?
2. What three changes formed part of the Obesity Strategy (2020).

Apply your understanding

Mrs Patel is an 82-year-old widow living alone in a small flat. She has a number of health conditions including type 2 diabetes, arthritis which causes her a lot of pain and makes it difficult to walk and the early stages of dementia. This means that she is forgetful and sometimes gets confused about taking her medication. She is very lonely since her husband died. Her children live quite far away. She struggles to keep on top of the housework and sometimes misses medical appointments. She no longer drives and has to rely on getting the bus, which is not very frequent.

In a traditional care model, Mrs Patel might be seen completely separately by a diabetes specialist service, an arthritis specialist and a dementia specialist.

1. How could different health and social care professionals such as community nurses, pharmacists, social workers and community support work together to provide Mrs Patel with integrated care?
2. What would be the benefits to Mrs Patel of an integrated care approach?

C2 Partnership approaches towards promoting social policy development in public health

Key principles of collaborative working

There are key principles that should be followed when working collaboratively with different professionals from different organisations. These principles will make sure that partnerships will work well and that public health will improve.

Openness

This means that professionals are open about how they are making decisions and that everyone knows what their roles and responsibilities in working towards a social policy aim are. Where it is appropriate and doesn't compromise people's confidentiality, professionals can share relevant information, and their experiences of what works well.

Trust and honesty

Partners must trust each other to act in the best interests of the public, and not to put their own interests before the public good. By being honest about what is challenging or difficult, or what is not going to be possible, means that people are not let down.

Agreed shared goals and values

At the start of a partnership, it is important that everyone involved knows what the goal is, and why it's important. This way people are clearer on what they are trying to achieve. When organisations and professionals share the same core values, it is easier to collaborate because everyone is starting from the same understanding of what the problem is and how they are trying to tackle it.

Regular communication between partners

If a partnership is going to work well, it's essential that there is regular and clear communication between all organisations and professionals involved. This means that there is a shared understanding of what has been achieved at any time, which avoids unnecessary repetition of work, and helps to identify gaps and problems to be solved quickly before they get worse.

Global, national and local organisations

Global organisations

Partnerships can be local, national or international. The **World Health Organisation** is the largest global health body. This organisation coordinates responses to public health issues between countries. It conducts research and provides guidance and support to national health systems.

- For example, the **Global Polio Eradication Initiative** is a project that the World Health Organisation coordinates, in partnership with national and private organisations including UNICEF, Rotary International and the Bill & Melinda Gates Foundation. It aims to completely eradicate the polio virus. Through mass vaccinations and careful monitoring of outbreaks, polio cases have been reduced by over 99%.

- Another international partnership is the **European Health Alliance** (**EHA**), which brings together governments, research institutions such as universities, and other organisations across Europe. One of the EHA's projects is the EU Cancer Plan, which supports research into strategies to prevent cancer, detect it early and devise new treatments.

- The **International Initiative for Mental Health Leadership** is a global network to promote collaboration between people working in mental health. They support mental health training to improve the number of people trained to high standards and promote person-centred models of care for mental health patients.

National and local organisations

A key player in the development of national social policy is the government, including the Department for Health and Social Care, and the NHS. The Health and Social Care Act created 42 **Integrated Care Systems** (**ICS**) across England, to enable better partnership working between local authorities, different health and social care services, and other stakeholders to work together more effectively.

- Each ICS is run by an **Integrated Care Board**, which are NHS organisations that allocate NHS funding and services.

- Each ICS also has an **Integrated Care Partnership**, which is an organisation which works on longer-term plans to meet the health and social care needs for that area. Each ICS has an important role when it comes to developing new social policies with a partnership approach.

> Polio – A highly contagious virus that affects the nervous system and can lead to paralysis, long-term disabilities and even death.

Communication and collaborative working between different agencies

It is crucial that different organisations and people who are working to promote social policy change communicate and collaborate effectively. This is true whether we are considering a large multi-national organisation like the WHO, a national charity or business, a local community or even family groups. When groups work together, they can create a bigger impact than all working separately. Each person will bring a slightly different perspective to the table. For example, charities often understand the needs of vulnerable people, families can speak to the lived experiences of people with a specific health need, businesses can give information about the financial impact of policy changes or the most cost-effective ways to work.

Recap questions

1. What are the four principles that underpin collaborative working?
2. Give two examples of international partnerships towards public health.

Find out more

www.eboru.com/BTEC-HSC-links

The NHS constitution.

End of Learning Aim Practice Activity

In this practice activity you will focus on the obesity strategy.

- Which organisations are relevant to the obesity strategy?
- How do two of them work together to achieve this strategy? What impact does it have on service users when these different organisations work together effectively?
- How can partnership working between these two organisations help to develop a model of integrated care?
- Can you assess the importance of collaborative working in order to reduce obesity?
- What would be missed or less efficient if they were not working in an integrated way?
- Can you analyse partnership working between these organisations? What are the advantages and disadvantages of the ways that these organisations work together, and how do they relate to the obesity strategy? Include your opinion about the barriers to collaboration, and what you think would improve these ways of working. Make sure you come to an overall conclusion.

This practice task will help you prepare for the following assessment criteria:

C.P5 Explain the potential impact on users of services, when health and social care organisations work as partners to provide care.

C.P6 Explain the significance of partnership approaches to developing an integrated care model in health and social care organisations.

C.M4 Assess the importance of collaborative working between different agencies in promoting social policy change

C.D4 Analyse the ways in which health and social care organisations work collaboratively to promote social policy change.

Unit 5 Promoting health education

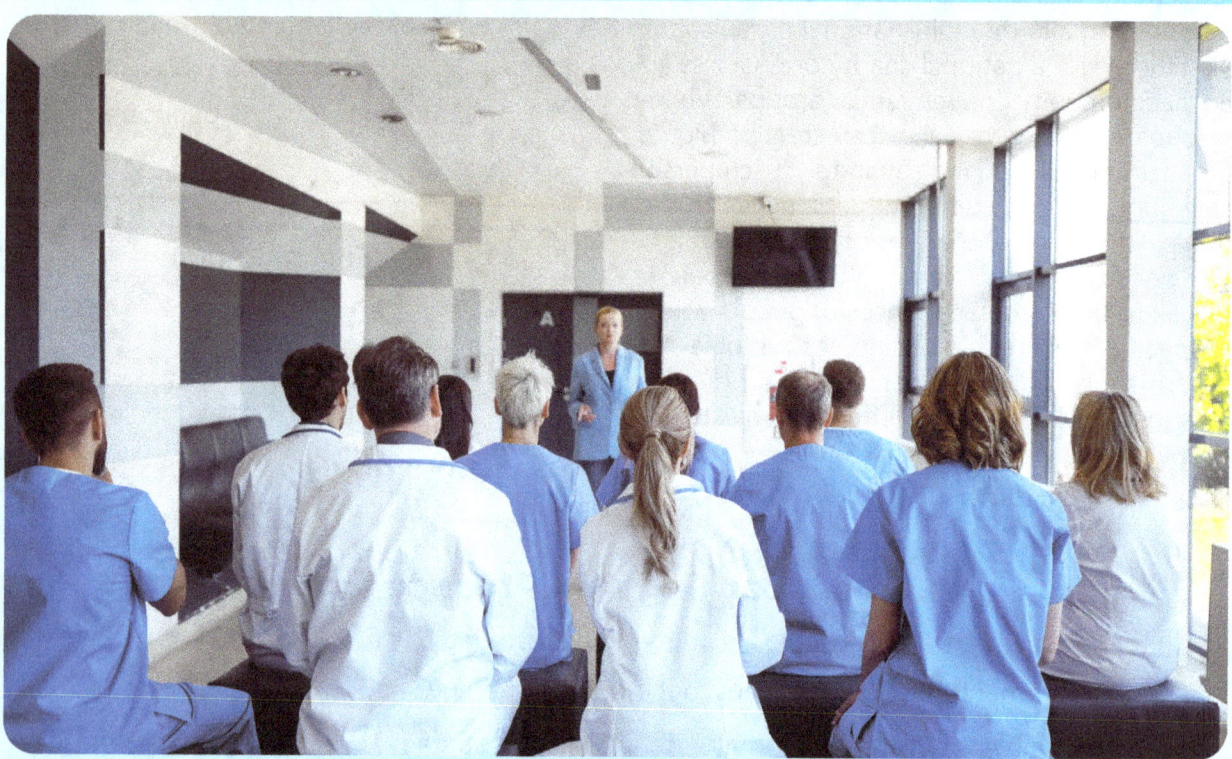

By the end of this unit, you will learn about the role of health education and how it can impact key health outcomes.

You will learn about:

- The purpose and role of health education.
- The organisations involved in health education.
- Legislation and regulations that impact health education.
- Health issues.
- Factors that affect health and wellbeing.
- Models and approaches to promote health and wellbeing.
- Planning health education events.

How you will be assessed?

In this unit you will be assessed through an internal assessment consisting of a series of tasks, covering Learning Aims A, B and C. The assignment is set by the awarding body and marked by your tutor.

Learning Aim A: Understand the purpose of health education

Learning Aim B: Explore key issues and priorities for health and the factors that affect health and wellbeing

Learning Aim C: Examine approaches to health education campaigns and their impact on health and wellbeing

Learning Aim A: Understand the purpose of health education

A1 Purpose of health education

Health education is a critical component of health promotion. It aims to improve the health outcomes of the population. Before action can be taken to improve the health of the general public, awareness needs to be raised about health risks, prevention methods and healthy lifestyle choices.

Health education also applies to professionals, to aid their understanding of health conditions and who is most at risk.

The main purposes of health education are as follows.

Develop an understanding of health risks and risk-taking behaviour

Health education helps to raise awareness of the causes and consequences of health risks.

- Health risks can include choices such as smoking, alcohol and drug abuse, an unhealthy diet and lack of physical activity.
- Health education also seeks to explain the factors that contribute towards risky behaviours, including peer pressure and stress.

Raising awareness about the risks associated with lifestyle choices and behaviour allows individuals to make informed decisions.

Reduce the cause and incidence of ill health

Giving people all the facts allows them to make informed decisions. This will lead to a good number of individuals deciding to change their lifestyle or behaviour to reduce their chances of developing ill health in the future. Examples include:

- Smokers quitting cigarettes as they understand the high risk of lung cancer and other diseases in the future.
- People who live a sedentary lifestyle deciding to add 120 minutes of exercise each week, reducing their chances of a whole range of diseases and health conditions.
- Parents fully appreciating the risks of measles and how safe and effective the vaccination is for their children.

As well as awareness of risks and healthy behaviour, education can also include resources or programmes that support the reduction of ill health.

Understanding the cause of illness, and how conditions can be spread, means the incidence of ill health can be promoted through education. This means the prevalence of new cases of illness is monitored and promoted through vaccinations, hygiene practices and regular health check-ups.

Control the occurrence of infectious diseases

This can be done by raising awareness of the causes of infectious diseases and how they spread. This might include:

- Preventative measures against infectious diseases, such as vaccinations or good hygiene.
- What to do if you or a loved one develop symptoms of a disease.

Protect against environmental hazards

Education strategies also cover environmental hazards that can affect health. For example:

- An understanding of the impact of **air pollution** can change people's behaviours, such as turning off a car engine while stationary, or avoiding a busy road when walking with children.
- **Mould and damp** are bad for people's health, particularly children and older people.
- **Water safety**. Most rivers in the UK are polluted, which means it is not safe to swim in them.
- The risks of **skin cancer** from sunshine and how to protect from it.

Promote equity and empowerment for the nation

Providing information and education helps to address health inequalities between different groups. It also empowers people to make positive choices about their health and their future.

Education programmes can be specifically tailored to different groups, tackling specific inequalities and promoting equity and empowerment for all. This helps to create a more equitable society.

> Equity – Fairness
>
> Prevalence – The total number of cases of a disease or condition compared to the overall population.
>
> Demographic data – Facts and figures about the number of people and their different characteristics. This could include, for example: age, sex, ethnic group, earning, education, and health status.

A2 The role of health education

Identify health priorities at a national and local level

In order to change health outcomes, we need to know what the problems are in the first place. So, the first step in health education is to understand the **prevalence of risky behaviours and diseases.** This means understanding:

- The geographical spread.
- How common they are in different groups within the overall population.
- The risks they pose for different groups and for the whole population.

This helps to establish the **overall need for health education,** both nationally and locally. This determines what this will focus on and who it needs to be pitched at.

Use demographic data

Demographic data collected by government organisations can be used to help to identify health priorities and intervene with the needs of a population. This means:

- Regular reviews of health data to highlight the current health risks and diseases.
- Determining a plan to further educate individuals on the most pressing issues.

Address health challenges and reduce exposure or risk

After identifying health challenges, health education programmes ultimately aim to address these challenges and reduce people's risk of developing ill health.

They do this by providing the correct level and type of information on current health challenges. For example, COVID-19 posed a critical threat to the nation's health. Health education programmes covered things such as encouraging people to wear face masks, to practise social distancing and to avoid gathering indoors with larger groups. Advertisements and other information sources aimed to educate individuals about all this and more, in order to reduce the risks of contracting or passing on the virus. For some people, contracting COVID-19 led to serious illness and death.

Recap questions

1. Identify two purposes of health education.
2. Outline one of these purposes.
3. Which purpose of health education is linked to pollution?
4. Which purpose of health education is linked to lifestyle choices?
5. Give an example of a risky behaviour that poses health risks.
6. Give an example of a health challenge.
7. Give an example of a preventative measure that can help reduce exposure or risk of disease.

Activity

Consider and answer the following questions:

1. Why is health education important?
2. What are the possible implications of not having health education?
3. Discuss the importance of reducing exposure to illness and disease and consider ways this can be implemented.
4. How do these roles impact the level of health education provided?

Apply your understanding

A small coastal town has recently seen a rise in unexplained respiratory problems and residents have also reported that they have experienced nausea and skin rashes in the last two months. The town has been recently suffering with a bout of heavy rainfall and floods which has caused issues with the town's main water supply. The local council have occasionally shut the water off due to reports of the water having an odour. Residents have been quick to blame a new factory that has recently opened, but officials believe that algae and other debris may have entered the water system.

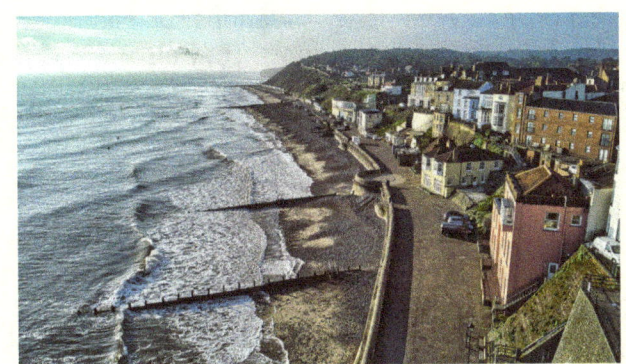

1. What do you think are the health priorities for this local area?
2. What health education do you think this local population needs?

A3 Organisations influencing health education

An important aspect of health education is the support and influence of global, national and local organisations.

The **World Health Organisation (WHO)** is a global organisation that was founded in 1948 to connect 'nations, partners and people to promote health'. The WHO has a responsibility to respond to health challenges and emergencies as well as promoting a healthier life for all individuals. The WHO is involved in a number of health education initiatives, including:

- A range of guides, factsheets and information on a range of health issues.
- The establishment of a Health-Promoting Schools framework, to help schools integrate health education with the school curriculum.
- The WHO also supports members to develop health literacy in their own countries, including advising about training for health professionals.

NHS England is in charge of the training and education of the NHS workforce. Historically, it has also been responsible for identifying and setting priorities and strategies to promote public health, including:

- Campaigns and partnerships to address key health risks, including obesity and mental health issues.
- Partnering with wider services such as schools and local authorities, in order to educate about health issues and actions people can take to prevent ill health.

However, it was announced in early 2025 that NHS England is being abolished. Its role as an administrative body that runs the NHS will be absorbed into the Department for Health and Social Care.

Local Education and Training Boards (LETBs) were introduced in 2013. There were 13 local education and training boards that represent all the areas of England. These local organisations assessed priorities in their local area and implemented relevant health education, with a focus on addressing the health challenges faced by their communities. LETB's responsibilities have now been assumed by NHS England.

The **UK Health Security Agency** (UKHSA) is an executive agency of the Department of Health and Social Care. They are responsible for protecting the nation from environmental hazards and infectious diseases. They lead the response to emergency situations such as heatwaves or radiation incidents. They also provide health education for at-risk groups, the general population and for health professionals

The **Department of Health and Social Care** (DHSC) is a government department responsible for implementing government decisions about health and social care policy. Its remit is to enable people to live more independent, healthy lives for longer. With the abolition of NHS England, it will have direct control of the NHS in England.

- The DHSC is ultimately in charge of national health policy and funds associated health education campaigns.
- It defines and supports health education campaigns and health outcomes for local authorities.
- It co-ordinates health campaigns with other government departments, such as the Department for Education.

Integrated Care Systems (ICS) are responsible for ensuring health care services, social care services and any other relevant organisations form partnerships and work together. England is split up into 42 ICSs, which can then target and respond to local issues. There are two main parts to each ICS:

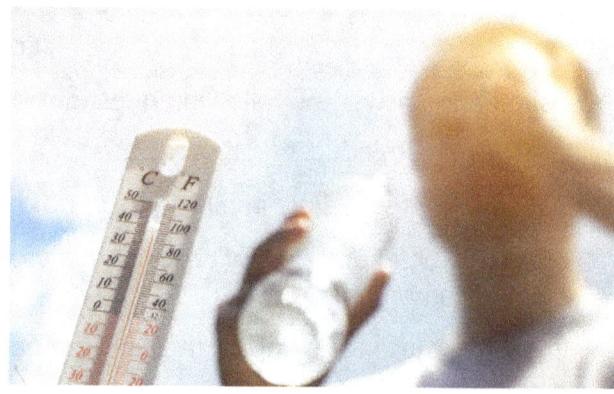

The UKHSA provides advice and leads the response to emergencies such as heatwaves

- **Integrated Care Partnerships** (ICP) create long-term strategic plans for the health needs of the local area. They are made up of representatives from a number of different sectors, such as education and housing, as well as health and social care. They try to prevent ill health, so health education is important.

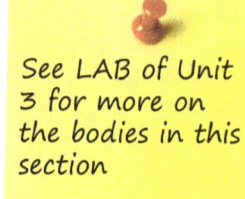

See LA3 of Unit 3 for more on the bodies in this section

- **Integrated Care Boards** (ICB) plan, commission and fund NHS services for the local area. They are responsible for the day-to-day running of services, and try to implement the ICP's plans.

Integrated systems are influential over health education as they consider the needs of local populations to implement health education and practices to support health outcomes.

Local authorities are branches of government in charge of a local area such as a city or region. They are responsible for many services that affect day-to-day lives and are run by elected councillors. They are legally responsible for delivering public health services. They also have a responsibility to improve the health of people in their area, which includes health education programmes such as 'stop smoking' clinics and providing information about healthy eating. These initiatives are based on the specific needs of the local community.

The **Faculty of Public Health** is a national membership organisation that sets the standards for public health practice across the UK. They provide training, courses and learning material for new professionals to become qualified, and continuous professional development (CPD) material for existing professionals. They also campaign and advocate for public health issues.

Activity

1. Explain why you think it might be important for global, national and local organisations to work together to deliver health education.

2. Describe three consequences of these organisations failing to communicate with their partnering organisations.

Find out more

www.eboru.com/BTEC-HSC-links

The WHO.

Local education and training boards:

The UKHSA.

The Faculty of Public Health.

Recap questions

1. Identify a global organisation with influence in health education.
2. Identify a national organisation with influence in health education.
3. Outline how local organisations influence health education.
4. Using an example, explain how a national organisation can influence local authorities in their health education.

A4 Legislation and regulations impacting on health education

Sustainable development goals

The member states of the United Nations adopted the 2030 Agenda for Sustainable Development in 2015. This included 17 **sustainable development goals** that aim for a world free of 'poverty, hunger, disease and want'.

Whilst all the goals have a direct or indirect impact on health, **Goal 3** is **Good health and wellbeing**. The target for goal 3 is **to ensure healthy lives and promote wellbeing for all at all ages**. The targets within this goal cover much of the work of the WHO that relates to health education. These targets include things such as:

- Reducing **maternal mortality** – the number of women who die in childbirth.
- Provide universal access to sexual health services.
- Halve the number of global deaths and injuries from road traffic accidents.

There are many other targets too. Educational programmes play a part to help address them, enabling people to make healthier informed decisions.

Health and Care Act (2022)

The **Health and Care Act (2022)** is a piece of government legislation that aims to support collaboration and partnership across the NHS and social care services. Part of the Act included the establishment of Integrated Care Services – see Section A3.

Other parts of the Act include:

- Extra powers for the government to direct other public bodies, such as the NHS or an ICS, to carry out public health measures.
- Restricting advertising to children of unhealthy foods.
- Better data sharing between health and social care bodies, to enable better public health planning and response.

Health and Social Care Act (2012)

The **Health and Social Care Act (2012)** is another piece of government legislation that included major reforms to the NHS and public health services.

Section 12 of this Act gave local authorities a legal responsibility to improve public health in their local area. This meant that local authorities became responsible for programmes on things such as:

- smoking cessation
- sexual health

> Cessation – Stopping doing something.
>
> Maternal mortality – Death of a woman linked to pregnancy or childbirth.
>
> Multi-disciplinary teams – A group of professionals that work together to meet the needs of a specific individual.

- substance misuse
- healthy eating.

Local authorities each appointed their own Director of Public Health to lead on community-focused public health issues.

Care Act (2014)

The **Care Act (2014)** regulates the delivery of social care in the UK.

Part three of this Act says that local authorities must:

- Promote the integration of care and support with health services.
- Promote the well-being of both adults being cared for and their carers.
- Prevent or delay the onset of development needs.
- Improve the overall quality of care and support for adults and carers.

This means there is a focus on creating partnerships between local services through multi-disciplinary teams. Health education also plays a part in ensuring that:

- Service users can make appropriate informed decisions about their care.
- Conditions are prevented or delayed by recognising symptoms and by making healthy lifestyle choices.

Activity

Discuss how important you think legislation is as part of health education. Consider the possible implications of legislation not being involved in health education. Do you think health education would still be as impactful?

Recap questions

1. Identify the WHO's sustainable development goal.
2. Give an example of a change the Health and Care Act (2022) has promoted.
3. Which piece of legislation considers the carers in their health education campaigns?
4. Which piece of legislation was developed in 2012?

Find out more

www.eboru.com/BTEC-HSC-links

WHO Sustainable Development Goal 3.

The Health and Care Act (2022).

The Care Act (2014).

The Health and Social Care Act (2012).

A5 Monitoring the health of the nation

You need to understand where sources of information can come from when determining patterns of health and ill health, as well as how this data is then used to monitor and address health issues.

Sources of information are a vital mechanism when monitoring the health of the nation. Methods such as health surveys, medical records and public health data play an important role in identifying health and ill health patterns and monitoring the rate of decrease or increase.

World Health Organisation

The **World Health Organisation** (WHO) outlines **key priorities for monitoring health and wellbeing** through indicators such as life expectancy and maternal and child mortality. They also consider the social determinants of health inequalities, such as education, socio-economic status and environmental factors.

By monitoring key indicators and possible causes, it allows an evidence-based approach to tracking global health outcomes and implementing measures to combat issues.

Government methods

The UK government also set out their own methods for monitoring patterns and trends in health and wellbeing at a local and national level.

- **Epidemiology** is the study of the distribution and causes of health and disease. The data and insights from these studies are used to identify problems and direct future prevention strategies. For example, the UK's Health Security Agency (UKHSA) oversees the National Cancer Registration and Analysis Service, which monitors cancer trends and registrations. This then allows the shaping of public health interventions, such as education about risk factors, with the aim of improving the health of the nation.

- **Regional and local reports** can be used to monitor patterns and trends of health and ill health within specific communities, to provide more localised data. Data such as hospital admissions, community health surveys and general practice records can all be used to identify health needs and target services and improvements.

- **Demographic data** provides insight into how factors such as gender, ethnicity and age impact on the health status of individuals and groups. This can help tailor interventions and health education strategies. For example, areas with an ageing population may need to prioritise services for age-related health conditions, such as high blood pressure and type 2 diabetes.

The government publishes a wide range of data on the 'Fingertips' website: fingertips.phe.org.uk

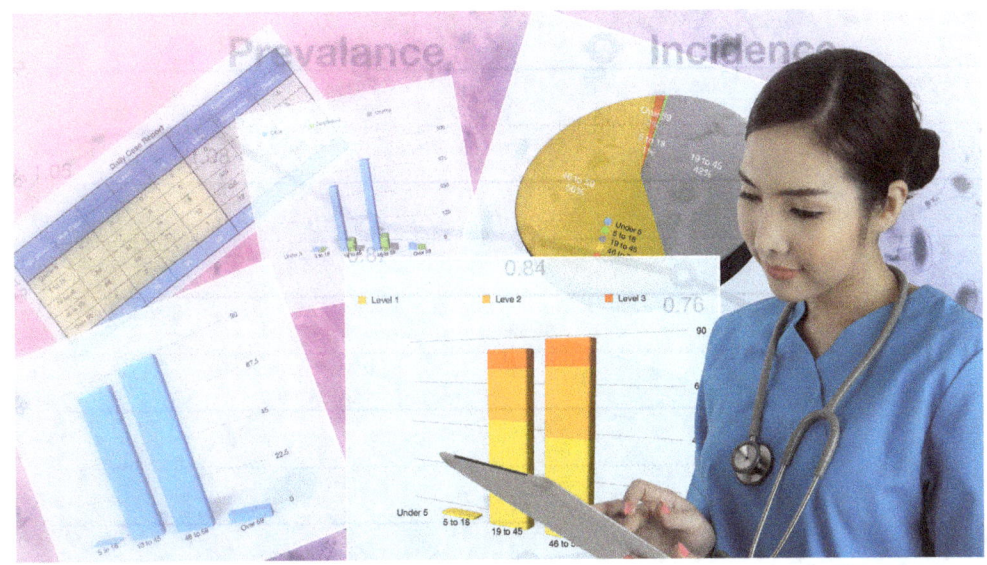

Public health practitioners

Public health practitioners use all the data sources above to **monitor and respond to public health issues** by identifying patterns and trends and then targeting interventions and education.

For example, during the COVID-19 pandemic, data was regularly reviewed and analysed to determine how vaccines were impacting hospital admissions, and how hospitals were coping with the demand of inpatients, based on admission data.

Social determinants – Non-medical things that affect how healthy people are – For example, where they live, how much they earn, their employment status.

Inpatients – A term to describe when a patient is admitted into hospital for a period of time.

Activity

1. Discuss the impact of not using data on the health of the nation.
2. Which government method is the most effective for monitoring patterns and trends of health and wellbeing?

Recap questions

1. Identify two ways data can be collected to monitor health and ill health.
2. Describe epidemiological as a government method.
3. Give an example of demographic data.
4. Using an example, explain how data can support public health practitioners in making changes.

Learning Aim B: Explore key issues and priorities for health and the factors that affect health and wellbeing

B1 Health issues and priorities

See Learning Aim C of unit 1 for more information on key health issues.

Smoking

According to the NHS report **Statistics on Public Health, England 2021**, 74,600 deaths were attributed to smoking in 2019. Smoking is the biggest cause of preventable illness and death in the UK, causing numerous cancers, chronic obstructive pulmonary disease (COPD) and cardiovascular disease. Around 500,000 people over 35 are in hospital because of smoking-related conditions. This places a large financial strain on the NHS.

It is a public health priority to reduce smoking rates to prevent illness and death. In 2024 the UK government introduced the first reading of the Tobacco and Vapes Bill, which would phase out tobacco sales from 2027, meaning that anyone born after 2009 in the UK would never be able to buy cigarettes.

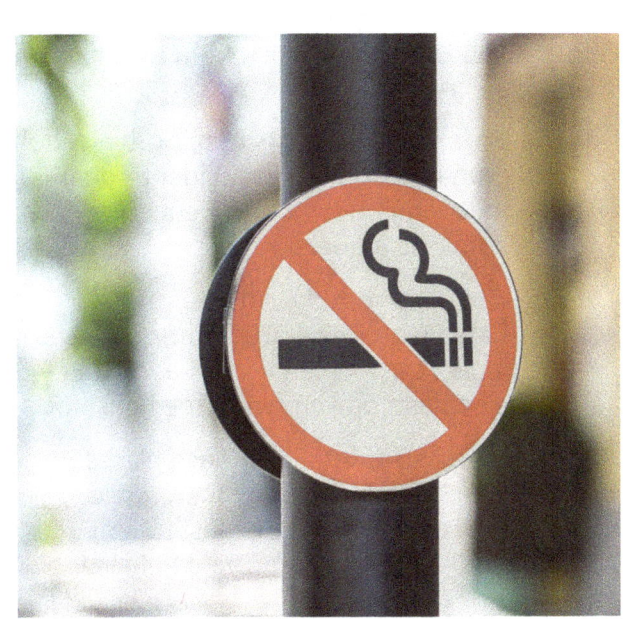

Diet and nutrition

In 2022, the World Health Organisation (WHO) reported that 2.5 billion adults worldwide were overweight, with 890 million being obese and 390 million underweight.

Obesity can pose significant health risks such as cardiovascular diseases, type 2 diabetes, and mobility problems, as well as minor symptoms such as fatigue and lethargy.

Diet and nutrition are heavily influenced by socio-economic status. For example, convenience foods, which are higher in fat and salt and with fewer nutrients, are often cheaper than fresh food. This means that people on lower incomes are at higher risk of obesity and the associated health risks.

A public health priority is to encourage healthy eating through balanced diets and the availability of affordable, nutritious foods.

Health education in schools helps to promote healthy eating habits, through health campaigns such as Change4Life. These strategies also help address health inequalities, so that disadvantaged groups experience reduced rates of diet-related illness.

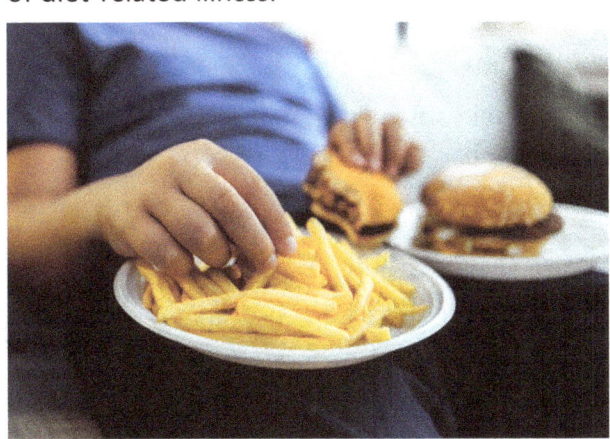

Alcohol, drug and substance misuse

Long-term excessive alcohol consumption can lead to many health conditions, such as cirrhosis, liver disease, liver cancer, high blood pressure, strokes and mental health issues such as depression.

Drug and substance misuse also poses health risks. While different drugs pose different risks, they often include death from overdose, cardiovascular risks (heart attacks and high blood pressure), lung damage, serious mental health problems, organ failure and infectious diseases like HIV and hepatitis from needle sharing.

- There are also other risks from both alcohol and drug misuse, such as accidents, deaths due to driving under the influence, violence and domestic abuse.
- Social impacts include violence, crime associated with illegal drug trafficking, and the impact on people's lives of addiction – homelessness, broken family relationships

Alcohol, drug and substance misuse places a huge strain on the NHS and other public services such as the police. The Institute of Alcohol Studies estimated in 2024 that alcohol

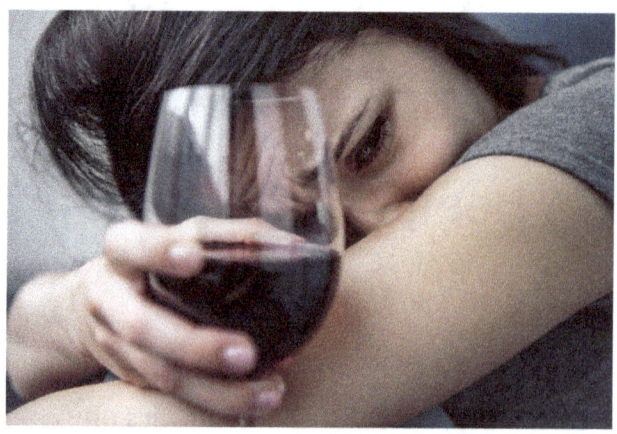

abuse alone costs England £27 billion per year.

Reducing alcohol and drug use is another priority for the health of the nation. This can be done through:

- Increased taxation on alcohol products.
- Education campaigns, such as Drinkaware.
- Implementation of addiction services such as Alcoholics Anonymous
- Rehabilitation services, such as therapy and medication-assisted treatments for drug users.

Pollution

Air pollution has a negative impact on people's health. The government guidance 'Air pollution: applying All Our Health' estimates that between 28,000-36,000 people die each year in the UK due to human-made air pollution, with a cost to the NHS of at least £1.6 billion.

Health issues associated with air pollution include:

- Asthma.
- Chronic obstructive pulmonary disease (COPD).
- Lung cancer.
- Pregnancy complications.

It has a larger impact on children, the elderly, and people with existing respiratory conditions.

Air pollution comes from cars and transport, fossil-fuel power stations, industry, agriculture and residential sources (such as wood-burner heaters).

Water pollution has less of an impact in the UK as drinking water is amongst the safest in the world. However, pollution in rivers and the sea can cause health issues for swimmers and other recreational users.

Public health policies that try to tackle air pollution include the implementation of stricter emissions regulations, clean air zones in cities (e.g. Ultra Low Emission Zone in London), renewable energy investments and public transport enhancements, to reduce car use.

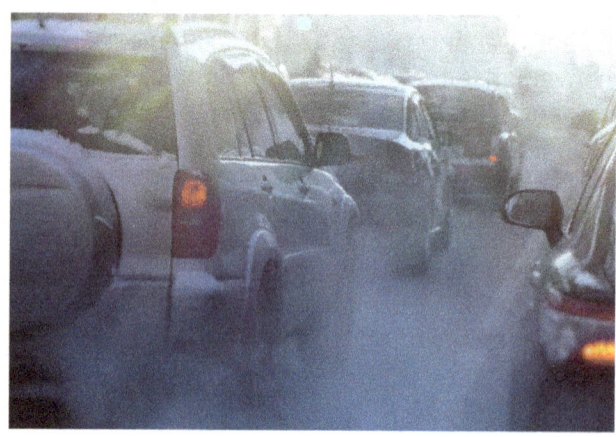

Mental health

Mental health conditions are a growing public health concern.

- According to the mental health charity Mind, 1 in 6 people suffer from common mental health conditions, such as depression and anxiety, each week.
- There are over half a million people in England with a more severe mental health condition, such as schizophrenia or bipolar.

Mental health issues affect overall wellbeing. They can also lead to feelings of loneliness and isolation, panic attacks, self-harm, suicidal thoughts, hallucinations and delusions. They can also affect people's ability to work and lead to substance misuse. People with severe mental health issues have a life expectancy 20 years less than expected.

The stigma around mental health has shifted in more recent years. Society is more open and responsive to mental health issues now because of a rise in health education.

- National campaigns such as 'Time to Change' have seen this stigma reduce by encouraging conversations about mental health.
- Media coverage, such as ITV's 'Britain Get Talking' campaign, has also helped raise awareness.

Increased awareness makes it more likely that people with mental health issues will choose to seek appropriate and effective support.

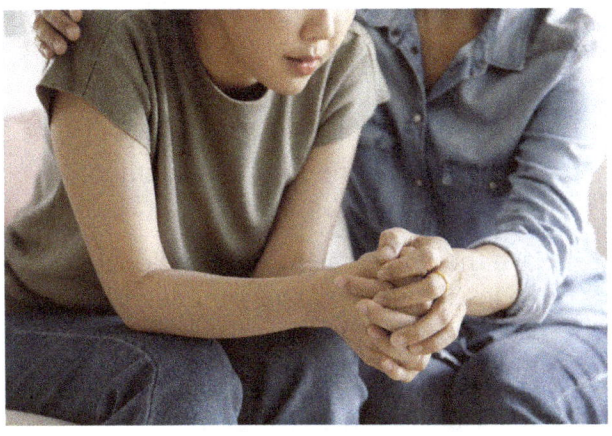

Cirrhosis – A condition that causes scar tissue to replace healthy liver cells which can then lead to liver damage.

Determinant – The cause of something.

Recap questions

1. Identify a health risk associated with air pollution.
2. Describe the priority for reducing the amount of people smoking.
3. Give an example of an education campaign designed to reduce alcohol misuse.

Better start in life

A **better start in life** refers to a growing understanding that the environment and experiences of babies and young children impact them for the rest of their life. This includes their future health, behaviour, opportunities and mental wellbeing. According to the government report 'The Best start in life', the first 1000 days of a child's existence, including in the womb after conception, are recognised as being critical for brain development, impacting on intellectual, emotional and social development.

Factors such as poverty or neglect are determinants of future health issues, such as developmental delays and increased risk of future health problems such as asthma. Better start programmes aim to minimise these

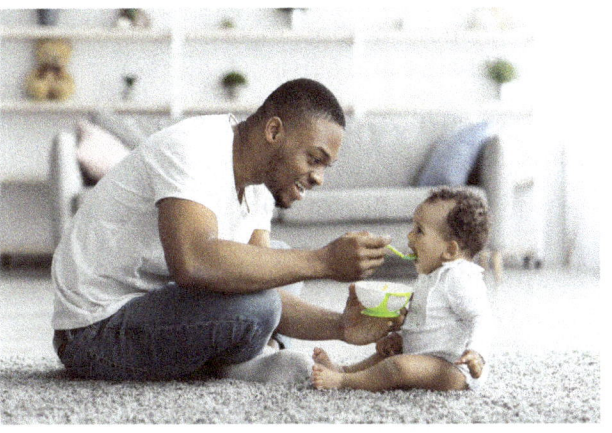

factors, so that babies and young children:

- Are kept safe from harm, neglect and abuse.

- Are raised in clean and safe environments.
- Have a strong, nurturing and loving bond with at least one main caregiver, to meet their emotional development needs.
- Have a healthy diet, to promote good physical development and encourage healthy eating habits.
- Have their physical, social, emotional and intellectual development needs met through stimulation, interactions, play, movement and relationships.
- Are included, regardless of their background.

Ultimately, each child should have the opportunity to reach their full potential.

For all these reasons, public health programmes are put in place to support babies, children and parents, and educate people about lifestyle choices that might disadvantage children, or put them at risk.

- The **Healthy Child Programme** is a UK national initiative to provide services and support for children aged 0-19. For children aged 0-5, health visitors play a leading role in assessing needs and involving other services as required. For children aged 5-19, school nurses play a similar role.
- The **Healthy Start scheme** entitles some pregnant women and new parents/carers to receive healthy foods such as milk and fruit, and vitamins to support the foetus or child's growth and development. This intervention is targeted towards low-income families who may struggle to afford good nutrition to support child development.
- **Child-health clinics** are run by health visitors and GPs. They provide **childhood vaccination** in order to protect young children from preventable diseases such as mumps and rubella. They also run health and development reviews to identify any problems at an early stage.

These public health schemes aim to eliminate health inequalities, so that all children have the best start in life.

Sexual and reproductive health

- **Sexual health** refers to the prevention of **sexually transmitted infections (STIs)** and disease, and the forming of healthy sexual relationships as adults. The UKHSA reports that in 2023 there were 4.6 million consultations delivered by sexual health services in England.
- **Reproductive health** covers the health of the male and female reproductive systems, including fertility, contraception, conception, pregnancy, abortion, menstruation, menopause and gynaecology.

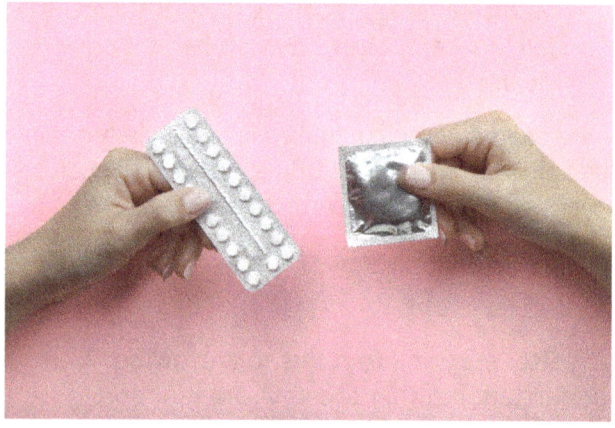

The consequences of poor sexual or reproductive health include:

- The transmission of STIs such as chlamydia, gonorrhoea and HIV. Each STI has its own symptoms and impacts upon health, some of which are very serious.
- Unplanned pregnancies and abortions.
- Cervical cancer.
- Poor maternal and child health.
- Under-18s pregnancies.
- Psychological harm from sexual abuse.

Health education is very important to promote safe sexual health practices, such as the use of contraception to prevent unplanned pregnancies, barrier methods such as condoms to prevent infection and disease, and the increased risks of multiple sexual partners.

- **Education** on sexual and reproductive health typically begins for adolescents in schools as part of the curriculum.
- **Sexual health clinics** are part of the NHS and provide free testing and treatments for STIs, advice about safe sex and access to contraception methods.

- **Online sexual health services** can send free testing kits and contraception through the post, and include advice and information.
- **Women's health hubs** support women's and girls' reproductive and sexual health. These are a new initiative set up by Integrated Care Boards in each local area.

By providing these services for free it ensures barriers to accessing care are reduced and individuals are encouraged to seek support.

Fertility – When the reproductive systems are able to produce and support healthy eggs and sperm.

Gynaecology – The area of medicine that specialises in the female reproductive system.

Activity

1. Discuss the societal impacts of alcohol misuse.
2. Choose one health issue covered in this section. Explain how it can impact the holistic health of an individual.

Recap questions

1. Identify a public health priority for the health issue of mental health.
2. Which health issue is associated with the campaign Healthy Start?
3. Identify an effect of poor sexual health.
4. Which health issue can lead to issues such as malnutrition?

Find out more

www.eboru.com/BTEC-HSC-links

Deaths caused by smoking

Health data linked to malnutrition

Air pollution: applying All Our Health

Mental health conditions

The healthy child programme

NHS support for parents and children

Sexual health statistics

Women's health hubs

B2 Factors affecting health and wellbeing

Social factors

Social relationships can have significant positive and negative effects upon an individual's health and wellbeing. These relationships include:

- family members
- friends
- work colleagues
- other social groups.

Positive social relationships are based upon mutual trust and respect, providing emotional support and a safe and encouraging environment. These relationships provide a good platform for positive overall health and wellbeing.

Negative social relationships, which harbour conflict, peer pressure, aggression, abuse or neglect, are detrimental to health and wellbeing. They are more likely to lead to an increase in stress, cause other mental health issues and result in poor lifestyle choices such as substance abuse. They are also more likely to lead to future negative relationships.

As well as the direct effect of relationships on health and wellbeing, social relationships influence people's behaviour regarding health and wellbeing. What is considered 'normal' behaviour is often defined by friends and family. For example:

- If parents give their children healthy food choices, and discuss the impact of poor food choices on health, then children are more likely to adopt a healthy diet as they grow up.
- If someone's friends do not drink alcohol or smoke, and enjoy sports and exercise, then it is more likely that they will do the same. However, if someone's friends all smoke, then it is more likely they will be tempted to try smoking in order to fit in.

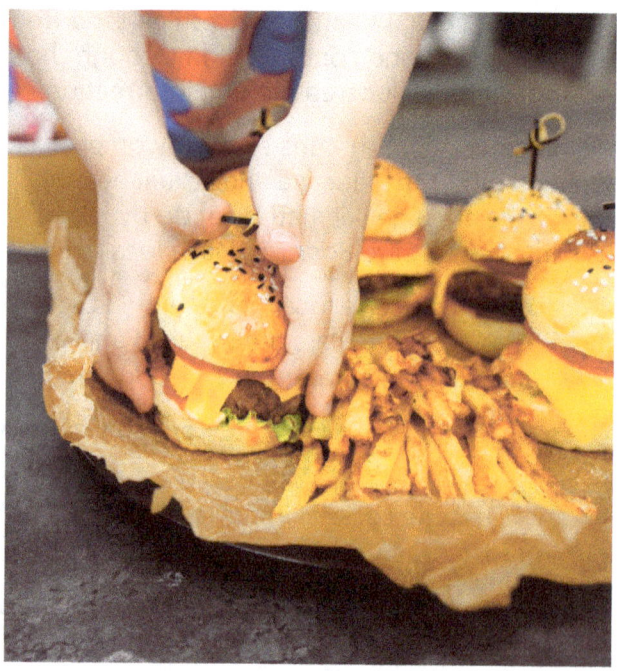

A child's diet impacts their future health and behaviour

Economic factors

Economic factors are those which relate to money. There are a few related economic factors:

People with more **income,** often because of a well-paid job, can afford a lifestyle and resources that can **prevent ill health.** For example:

- They are more able to afford fresh fruits and vegetables and higher-quality ingredients to maintain a healthy balanced diet.
- They may be able to afford things such as gym memberships and fitness classes.
- Their job may provide extra benefits, such as private health care, allowing them to see a doctor immediately if they have any concerns.

However, those with a low income, those who are not in employment, or those in poverty may struggle to afford services that can prevent ill health. For example, a lack of money can mean:

- People cannot afford transport to attend appointment

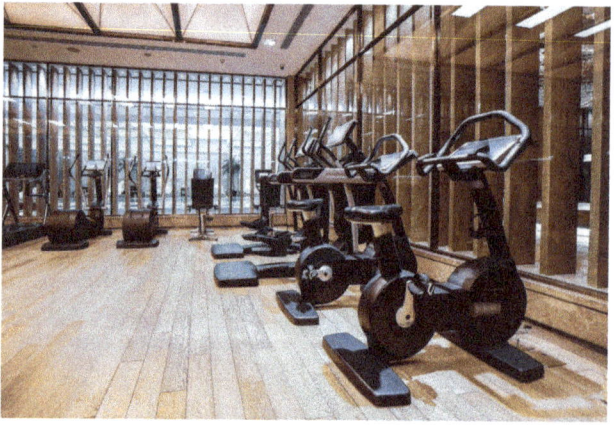

Gym memberships can be expensive

- People cannot afford prescription costs
- People are unable to afford an active social life, leading to loneliness and mental health issues.

There are clear links between people's economic situation and their health outcomes.

Environmental factors

Environmental factors are linked to:

- Geography.
- The availability and quality of health services in the local area.
- The availability and quality of other services in the local area, such as housing and leisure.

Where an individual lives can determine the number of services available. This is known as the **postcode lottery**. For example:

- Some areas of the country have more or less demand placed upon services. For example, the number of patients per GP differs across the country.
- The quality of health and social are services can be different in different locations.
- Those living in urban areas are more likely to have access to a wide range of leisure activities compared to those in rural areas, which can encourage a more active, healthy lifestyle.
- The types of **housing** a person lives in is also determined by the area in which they inhabit. For example, people in more deprived areas may have access to poorer housing. Poorer housing might be too small, too cold in winter, and contain damp and mould. All of these can lead to poorer health outcomes. Damp and mould can seriously affect the respiratory system.
- The **types of referral services available** differ in different parts of the country. A **referral system** is when individuals are sent to other services and professionals for further support or treatment, for example when a GP refers a patient to a specialist. If these specialist services are not available locally, then individuals may need to wait longer and struggle to attend appointment further away.

> **Marginalised** – When a person or group are pushed out of society because of a specific characteristic they possess.

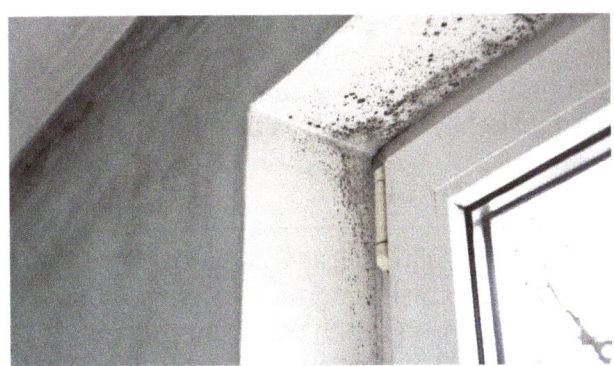

Mould and damp are very bad for people's health

Behavioural factors

Behavioural factors are very important for health and wellbeing. These include habits, attitudes and actions. The reasons for people's behaviour can be complex.

Discrimination

Some people's behaviour and decisions about health, and the services that can help them, can be informed by negative experiences they have had with health and social care services in the past, particularly stereotyping, prejudice and discrimination.

- **Stereotypes** occur when individuals or groups of people have an assumption about other characteristics, behaviours or attributes.
- Stereotypes typically stem from **prejudices**, which are preconceived ideas about other people without necessarily knowing that person or group.
- Prejudices and stereotypes can then lead to **discrimination**, which is the unfair treatment of an individual or group based on a particular characteristic such as gender, age, sexual orientation and religion.

These experiences can negatively impact health and wellbeing. For example:

- Increased stress levels.
- Biases in health care impact the quality of care given, which then negatively affects health outcomes.
- Marginalised groups can be left isolated.

The **Equality Act 2010** makes it illegal to discriminate against anyone on the basis of nine protected characteristics.

217

Compliant behaviour

Compliant behaviour is when individuals or groups choose to adhere to rules and norms of society, to avoid conflict or to gain approval of others.

In health and social care compliant behaviour can mean:

- People choosing to follow treatment recommendations leading to increased recovery rates.
- People voluntarily following guidance to reduce the risk of infection or spread of disease, for example through maintaining personal hygiene.
- People vaccinate their children against common childhood diseases, to protect them and others.

However, being over-compliant can open people up to being misled, for example succumbing to peer pressure and carrying out harmful behaviours such as binge drinking.

Empowerment

The aim of health education is to **empower** individuals to make informed decisions about their lifestyle and health conditions, so they understand what support is available, how they might access it and why they might need it. In order to do this, individuals need to be provided with clear information about why certain behaviours and actions are recommended. This can be a challenge as the issues can be complex and technical.

Individual personalities

Each person has their own unique **personality**

> Norms – The expected ways of behaving in society, for example lining up in a queue and not pushing in.
>
> Conscientious – Performing a task well and with care.
>
> Negative disposition – Having a negative attitude or view of something which can impact the way individuals adapt to challenges that arise.

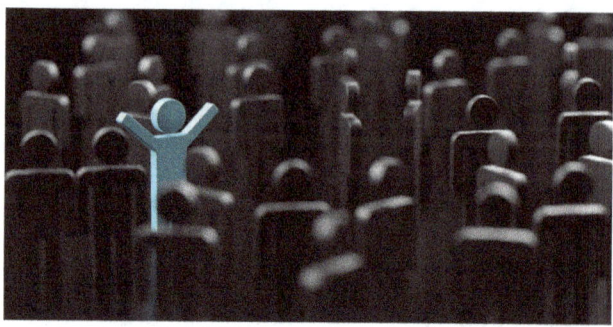

Everyone has their own individual personality

made up of traits, behaviours, quirks and patterns of thinking, which gives us our sense of who we are. Our personality influences decisions about health and wellbeing. For example:

- Personality traits such as resilience can support individuals who are recovering from health conditions.
- Someone who is open to ideas is more likely to listen to and comply with medical advice if it is fully explained.
- Conscientious people are more likely to be organised and keep up good health habits, such as consistently exercising.
- People who worry a lot, or who have a negative disposition, may lead more stressful lives, with more anxiety and illness.

Education

On average, a person's level of **education** is linked to health outcomes.

- A higher level of education can lead to a higher-paid job, which leads to the economic factors discussed earlier.
- Greater financial stability leads to better housing conditions and less financial stress.
- A higher level of education can lead people to fulfilling work and a sense of purpose, which is particularly important for mental health. A higher level of education also tends to give people more options when it comes to work, which leads to a greater feeling of control – again, this is important for mental health.
- Someone with a higher level of education may be more likely to **access and engage with continued learning**. This means they more likely to be aware of different health issues, health services available, symptoms, and how best to reduce lifestyle risks.

- They may be better equipped to understand more complicated advice and navigate more complicated medical systems.
- A lower level of education often leads to lower-paid jobs, which leads to the economic factors discussed earlier.
- Financial insecurity, such as finding it difficult to pay bills, can cause stress and illness.
- A lack of education can cause individuals to make unhealthy and risky decisions, as they may be less aware of the consequences of certain behaviours.

Overall, education has a direct impact on people's health, and also an indirect impact due to people's awareness of illness and how it might be prevented.

Media influences

Media refers to sources of information about any given topic. Common sources of media include the news, television, newspapers and magazines, social media platforms, and websites.

The media has a big impact and can shape the behaviours and choices of individuals and groups.

- Media campaigns can help raise awareness of health conditions such as mental health or cancer.
- Websites of well-known and respected sources such as the NHS, or charities who campaign on an issue, contain lots of very useful and trusted information. This is a good place to start when trying to understand heath conditions and health policies.
- Ideas and viral trends can swiftly gain traction on social media. Sometimes these can have positive benefits, such as healthy eating, exercise or giving up alcohol.

However, the media can also misinform people. For example:

- It can create unrealistic expectations about appearance or behaviours.

> **Recap questions**
>
> 1. Give three examples of geographical factors that can lead to poor health.
> 2. How might economic factors affect health and wellbeing?
> 3. How can compliant behaviour improve health?
> 4. Describe how access to education can impact an individual's physical health and wellbeing.

- Social media and website can contain information that is completely wrong.
- Unlike mainstream media (TV, newspapers, magazines) most social media accounts do not have any editorial checks. This means that no-one objectively checks whether statements are true or not. People who post on social media may know little, or nothing, about a subject but still present opinions as 'facts'. This can be very dangerous, particularly when it comes to health.

It is important that individuals are aware of both the benefits and risks of the media and take precautions when viewing or reading content. It is always good practice to check any give facts against a separate trustworthy source such as the NHS.

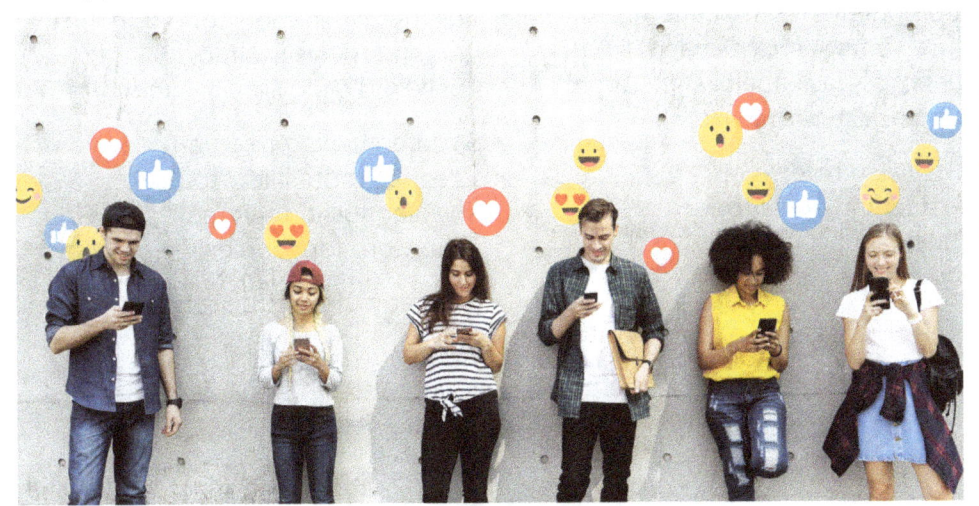

Health inequalities

Health inequalities are caused by a range of determinants.

This table outlines some of them and their possible health effects.

Social determinant	Health inequality	Health outcomes
Social class	Middle or upper-class people tend to have: - Better access to health and social care services. - Better diets. - Healthier lifestyles. - Better living conditions.	Upper and middle-class people tend to: - Live longer lives - Are healthier for longer. (See Find Out More for source.)
Race and ethnic or national origin	People may face discrimination on the basis of race, ethnic group or nationality. This can include: - Language barriers, so people do not understand the available options and services. - Concerns being taken less seriously by professionals. - Unequal treatment by services. - Care may not be culturally appropriate. All of this can lead to mistrust in services and professionals. Discrimination in wider society means that some groups are more likely to be affected by the other determinants in this table, for example, lower income, living in more deprived areas, working in more hazardous jobs.	Some groups have: - Higher infant mortality rates - Higher maternal mortality rates - Higher rates of diabetes. - Poorer outcomes across a range of infectious diseases. (See Find Out More for source.)
Sex	Inequalities occur between men and women. - Women can receive less attention for reproductive health conditions because some services and professionals lack abilities to support and empathise with women. - Men can also receive less understanding and support for mental health.	- Women live longer but spend more time in ill health. - The average diagnosis time for the debilitating condition endometriosis is almost 9 years (See Find Out More for source.) - Women having heart attacks are 50% more likely to be misdiagnosed than men. (See Find Out More for source.) - Higher male suicide rates.

Social determinant	Health inequality	Health outcomes
Disability	Inequalities occur based upon individuals' ability to access services physically and financially. For example, a disabling environment causes issues with individuals attending services due to inappropriate physical barriers such as no ramps for wheelchair users.	• Mortality rates for disabled people are double that of the general population. (See Find Out More for source.) • Poorer access to health services • Poorer mental health • More likely to feel isolated or lonely
Age	Older adults can experience ageism and be limited in the opportunities presented to them, due to them being viewed as vulnerable and incapable of remaining independent.	• Barriers in affording health care • Greater risks of isolation and withdrawal from society • Mental health conditions are under-diagnosed and under-treated in over 65s (See Find Out More for source.) • Many older people experience worse access to key services, including cancer care and end-of-life services (See Find Out More for source.)
Sexual orientation	Inequalities occur from a long history of systemic discrimination against individuals amongst the LGBTQIA+ society. This has resulted in stigma leading to issues with health and social care treatments.	• Poorer mental health • Double the risk of suicide and self-harm (See Find Out More for source.) • More likely to face direct discrimination.
Geographical location/ region	Urban locations typically have higher levels of services than rural locations. Areas of higher deprivation have worse health outcomes. There are clear regional differences between health outcomes across the UK.	• Housing issues • Pollution effects • Hospital admission rates for infectious diseases are twice as high for people in deprived areas. (See Find Out More for source.)

Activity

1. Discuss the impact that one health inequality can have upon mental health.
2. Discuss how health education can reduce the impact of discrimination on health.

Recap questions

1. Which factor considers prejudices and discrimination?
2. Identify two social determinants that can lead to health inequalities.
3. Explain how social factors can impact the health issue of substance misuse.
4. Explain how economic factors can influence the 'better start in life' health issue.

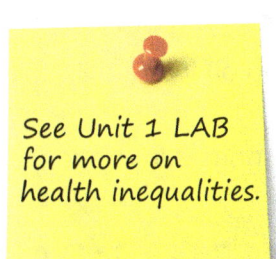

See Unit 1 LAB for more on health inequalities.

Find out more

www.eboru.com/BTEC-HSC-links

Find out more about the data behind the following health inequalities:

Social class.

Race, ethnic or national origin.

Sex.

Disability

Age

Sexual orientation

Geographical location.

End of Topic Practice Activity

In this practice activity you will look health education around alcohol misuse.

Write down your ideas about the following:

- What do you think is the role and purpose of health education in relation to alcohol misuse?
- Can you explain which organisations are involved in education about alcohol misuse?
- Can you explain which legislation is involved in education about alcohol misuse?
- What sources of data are there about alcohol misuse? What methods are used to gather this data?.
- How is data about alcohol misuse used by public health practitioner?
- What factors, and health inequalities contribute to alcohol misuse?
- Can you discuss how this all impacts individuals' holistic health, and wider society?
- Can you justify the need for health education about alcohol misuse, and for monitoring and responding to it? You should back up your arguments with evidence.

This practice task will help you prepare for the following assessment criteria:

A.P1 Explain the purpose and role of health education.

A.P2 Explain organisations and legislation involved in health education.

B.P3 Explain one health and wellbeing issue affecting the health and wellbeing of individuals at a local and national level.

B.P4 Explain factors affecting the health and wellbeing of individuals and wider society in relation to the chosen health issue.

A.M1 Discuss how the health of the nation is monitored through organisations and legislation.

B.M2 Discuss the impact of factors affecting health and wellbeing on individuals, their holistic health and wider society.

AB.D1 Justify the need for health education, monitoring, and responses in relation to factors that affect health and wellbeing at a local and national level.

Learning Aim C: Examine approaches to health education campaigns and their impact on health and wellbeing

In this section you will investigating health education campaigns at an international, national and local level. You will need to understand how models and approaches in health education campaigns support behavioural changes.

C1 Current and ongoing health education

International campaigns

Some examples of international campaigns organised by the **World Health Organisation (WHO)** include:

- **World Health Day** – 7th April. This is a general health education campaign that is reactive to health concerns that affect people all over the world each year. For example, World Health Day 2024 focused on educating people about their right to access good quality health care services, education and information.
- **World Immunisation Day** – 24-30 April.
- **World AIDS Day** – 1st December.

National campaigns

The UK has a wide range of health education campaigns, implemented by various organisations.

Department of Health and Social Care and NHS

The **Department of Health and Social Care** and the **NHS** have run many campaigns to educate the public about a range of health issues. These include:

- **Act FAST** – to educate the public on the signs of a stroke, so that individuals can get the necessary health care support quickly.
- **Help Us Help You** – A campaign to urge people to seek medical care for their health needs, after evidence had suggested that 1 in 10 people choose not to ask for support due to believing they are burdening the NHS.
- They have run campaigns to encourage people to get medical attention for:
    * Cancer
    * Vaccinations
    * Heart attacks, stroke and hypertension

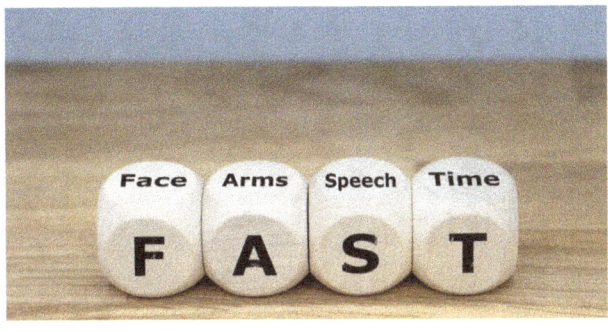

They also provide education on NHS 11 and primary care services so that the public understand where to go for medical support for issues that less serious.

Charities

Charities support government and NHS campaigns with their own. For example:

- **Cancer Research UK** have run various Be Clear on Cancer campaigns to teach the public about identifying early signs of cancer.
- The **British Heart Foundation** run an ongoing campaign to deliver training to perform CPR.

Local campaigns

A **local** health education campaign target the health needs of the local population. For example:

- The **local authority** in Cardiff identified issues with obesity rates based on national health data and launched the 'Move More Eat Well' campaign to promote a healthier lifestyle. It promoted a better diet more exercise, to help reduce obesity and the associated health risks.

- **NHS organisations** in Liverpool have embedded the 'Know your numbers' campaign about high blood pressure after statistics showed that 31,000 people in Liverpool were not aware they had high blood pressure. High blood pressure (**hypertension**) is 'responsible for half of all heart attacks and stroke in the UK', The campaign was set up by the charity Blood Pressure UK, and explains what the numbers mean in a blood pressure reading, where people can get their blood pressure checked and what to do if they think they have high blood pressure.

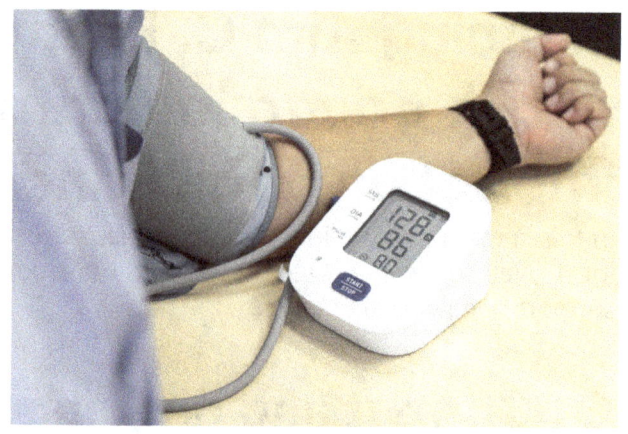

Recap questions

1. Describe the function of international health education campaigns.
2. Identify an example of a national campaign.
3. Identify an example of a local campaign.

Activity

1. Research your local area to find a health education campaign. Explain the purpose of this campaign.
2. Discuss the importance of health education campaigns being evidence informed.

Find out more

www.eboru.com/BTEC-HSC-links

WHO's international health education campaigns.

The FAST campaign.

The Help Us Help You campaign.

The British Heart Foundation CPR resources.

The Cardiff local authority campaign.

The Know Your Numbers campaign in Liverpool.

C2 Models and approaches used in health education to promote health and wellbeing

The health campaigns identified in C1 will need to be considered in relation to the following models and approaches.

Models of behaviour change used in health education

Health Belief Model

The **Health Belief Model** considers how an individual makes decisions regarding their lifestyle choices and health behaviours. This model believes individuals make decisions by weighing up the costs and benefits of engaging with healthy behaviours. Rosenstock and Becker argued that individuals make choices regarding their health by weighing up:

- **Perceived susceptibility** – do they believe are susceptible to an illness or condition?
- **Perceived severity** – how much do they believe their life will be affected by the illness?
- **Perceived benefit of recommended behaviour** – do they believe the recommended behaviour will reduce their risk of illness?
- **Perceived barriers to recommended behaviour** – do they believe the recommended behaviour is possible, achievable and will work?

Health education campaigns consider this model by breaking key health behaviours down so that individual can process their belief. For example, for a smoker:

- **Perceived susceptibility** – A campaign might clearly state how many people get smoking-related illnesses.
- **Perceived severity** – A campaign could make it clear that these illnesses are serious and often fatal or life-changing.
- **Perceived benefit of recommended behaviour** – A campaign could state how giving up smoking extends life expectancy.
- **Perceived barriers to recommended behaviour** – Examples could be given of how there are methods to help quit smoking, such as nicotine patches or e-cigarettes.

In addition, the model considers:

Self-efficacy – which means how much control they have over the recommended behaviour, such as where to get nicotine patches from.

Cues to action – things that might prompt people to think about the change, such as warning signs on cigarette packaging.

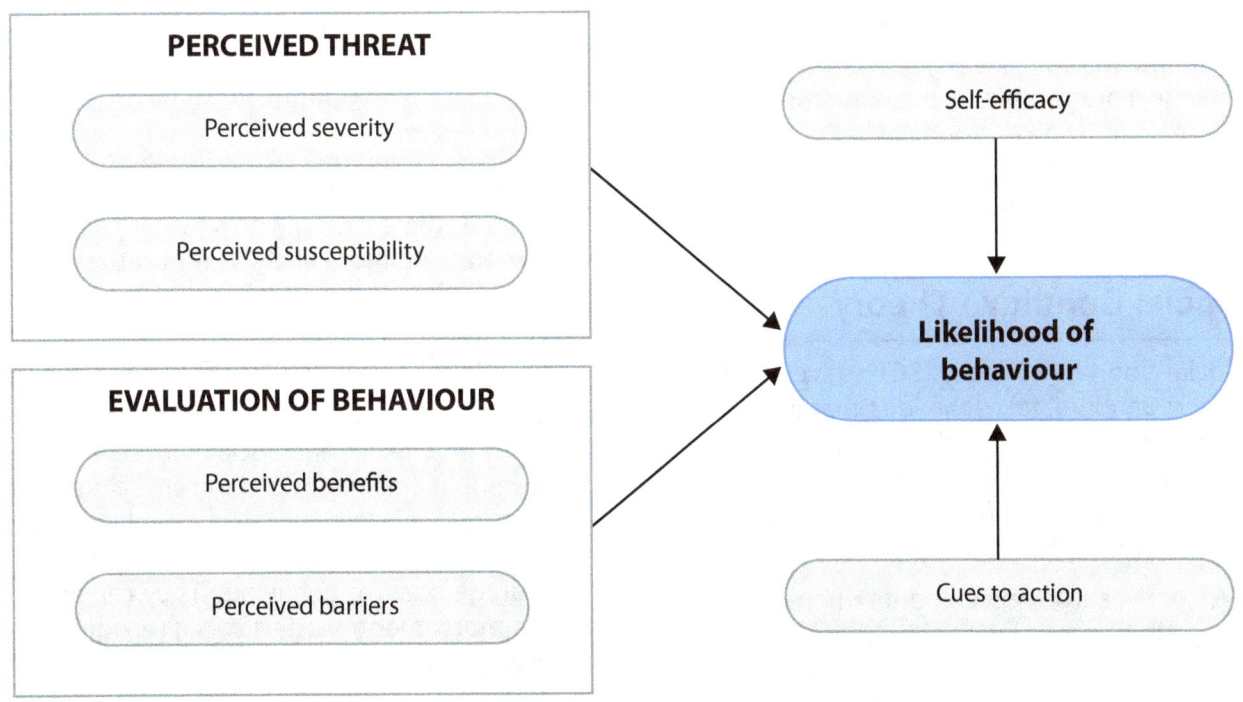

Transtheoretical Model (Stages of Change Model)

The **transtheoretical model** consists of six stages that an individual experiences before they ultimately change their health behaviour.

Table outlining the stages of the transtheoretical model

Stage	Description
1. Precontemplation	Individuals have no awareness of a problem or have no intention of making a change in their health behaviours.
2. Contemplation	The individual has started to think about a change in behaviour.
3. Preparation	Individuals begin to plan how they will change their behaviour and when they want to have achieved this by.
4. Action	Individuals work towards changing their behaviour.
5. Maintenance	Individuals continue to work at the desired behaviour, so they don't revert to old behaviours.
6. Termination	Individuals maintain their new behaviour and have removed the old behaviour.

Health education campaigns need an awareness of these stages, so they target people at different stages to help guide behavioural change. For example, at the contemplation stage an individual may have been given news about their health by a professional that provides them with the motivation and desire to change.

Social Cognitive Theory

Social Cognitive Theory (**SCT**), developed by Albert Bandura, takes the idea that individuals' thoughts, behaviour and environment are interlinked, so that each of them influences each other. A key insight from SCT is that individuals' behaviour is influenced by other people.

SCT derives from experiments where children saw adults interact with a 'bobo doll' in

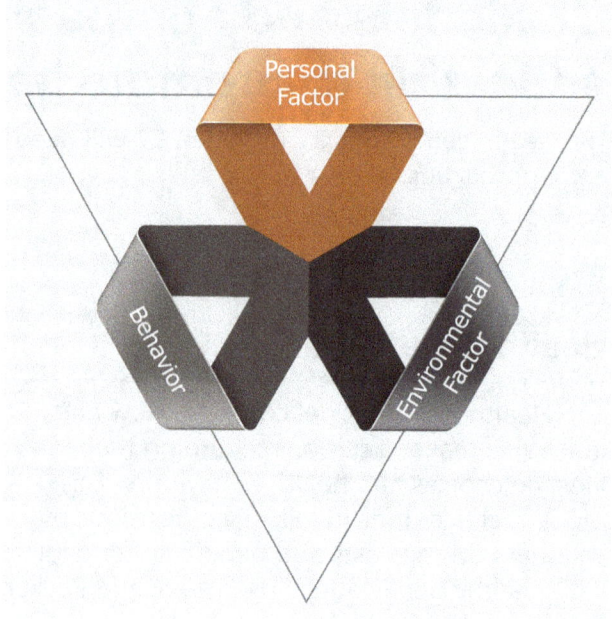

There are three aspects to SCT

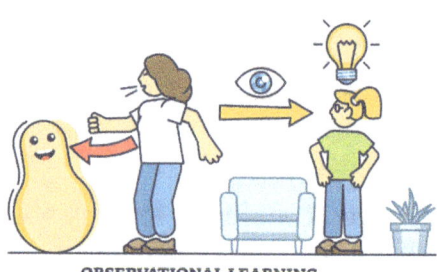

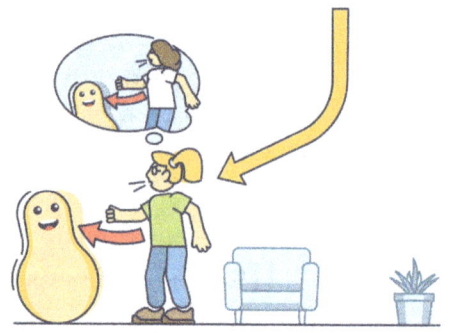

Bandura's bobo doll experiment

an aggressive manner. Some adults were 'rewarded' and some were 'punished'. Bandura found that the children who saw adults being rewarded were more likely to replicate the aggressive behaviour. This highlights how social influences – other people – and the environment contribute to people's behaviour.

This theory can then be applied to behaviour changes in a health and social care context. For example, health education campaigns can use role models, such as relatable people or celebrities in their advertisements, to encourage positive behaviour. They can also use reinforcement, such as social recognition, to encourage change.

Theory of Reasoned Action

The Theory of Reasoned Action focuses on a person's intention to behave in a specific way. It believes that individual actions are a product of people's own free will. This theory says that **intention** is the best predictor of behaviour change, and intentions are shaped by social norms and the person's attitudes. If behaviour change does not happen, then work must be done to change the perception of social norms and/or the person's attitude to the change. Once that happens, behaviour change is likely.

> **Holistically** – Considering the whole of something, not individual parts.
>
> **Autonomy** – To be independent and make your own decisions.

In practice this might mean educating people about health issues, and changing attitudes and norms about healthy behaviours. Together, this model says this is enough to lead to intent, which will lead to behaviour change.

Joint health and social care approach

It is important for health and social care to take a **joint approach** to health education of individuals and populations. **Partnerships between organisations**, such as the NHS and local authorities, are crucial to:

- Co-ordinate the approach so there are no unnecessary duplicates.
- Agree on priorities across topics or services.
- Ensure that education messages are consistent and do not contradict each other.
- Ensure that there are no or gaps in coverage.

A joint approach is a more efficient way to work, as it ensures that work is not duplicated unnecessarily. This reduces pressures on NHS and social care services budgets.

Promoting healthy behaviours

Prevention is better than cure. For this reason, health and social care professionals have a responsibility to **promote positive health behaviours** as part of their day-to-day practice. Educating and providing accurate information empowers people to make informed decisions.

The **Making Every Contact Count** (**MECC**) programme encourages health and social care professionals to use every interaction with service users to discuss improvements they could make to their health and wellbeing. Typically these improvements are around smoking, drinking alcohol, exercise and diet.

> **Find out more**
>
> www.eboru.com/BTEC-HSC-links
>
> Making Every Contact Count.

Holistic health and wellbeing

Professionals need to consider health and wellbeing holistically when promoting health behaviours and running education campaigns. They should consider the potential barriers a person or group may face when accessing services or changing behaviour.

For example, a health campaign aimed at encouraging older adults to exercise would need to consider that high-impact activities such as running is unlikely to be suitable for lots of people in this age group.

> **Recap questions**
>
> 1. Which model of behaviour change conducted a study on role models with children?
> 2. Which model of behaviour change places on focus on intentions?
> 3. Which model of behaviour change can be divided into six stages?

Person-centred approach

Health education should take a **person-centred approach** so that people can make **informed choices** and have autonomy over their care. This supports them in making their own choices, based upon evidence provided by a health education campaign.

In practice, this might mean:

- Tailoring one-to-one advice or discussions to the individual in question.
- Running education campaigns that target specific groups or demographics, because each may have quite different circumstances, barriers and motivations.
- Working with local communities to get feedback on how education campaigns or sessions might work best for them.
- Providing facts and information in a balanced and reasonable way, rather than lecturing or instructing people.

Addressing health inequalities

Effective health education campaigns need to consider health inequalities to ensure that they are truly effective.

Health inequalities mean that not everyone is at the same starting point. Campaigns should recognise this and consider which factors lead to inequalities in the groups that are being targeted.

- For example, advice about healthy eating for people living in a deprived area might need to consider some of the underlying factors, such as a lack of nearby shops that sell cheap or healthy food. Perhaps this group have less experience of cooking meals with fresh ingredients.

Campaigns should also very carefully consider **equality and diversity**.

- Is the language fully inclusive and sensitive?
- Do the images represent a cross section of the target audience?
- Are there specific needs of a group that are not covered in the campaign?
- What other barriers do people face?

Government and societal approaches

Government and societal approaches to changing the **physical, economic** and **social environment** also have a big impact on healthy behaviour.

- Approaches to adapting the physical environment include improving housing, more access to green spaces and reducing air pollution.
- Approaches to adapting the economic environment include the minimum wage, help to return to work, providing free services (such as computer skills training), and investing in more deprived areas.
- Approaches to adapting the social environment include community centres, setting up community groups, supporting families and eliminating discrimination by training staff.

All of these have an impact on overall health outcomes. Education campaigns need to understand the barriers and opportunities that impact an individual's decisions and behaviour.

Impact of health education

Successful health education campaigns can have a very positive impact for the following:

- **Families**. Effective campaigns can help foster a healthier home environment. Healthy behaviour can be worked into daily routines, and older family members act as role models to younger members. This can have a large impact because children that grow up with healthy behaviours are more likely to be healthy as adults, and also pass this behaviour on to future generations too.
- **Communities**. Effective campaigns can ensure that peer-pressure and community expectations act in positive ways, to benefit everyone's health. When communities are actively engaged in campaigns, they are more likely to succeed, and even campaign

themselves for further improvements, such as better community exercise spaces. Successful community campaigns can also help to reduce health inequalities across different groups.

- **Individuals.** Effective campaigns enable self-efficacy, where people take control of their own health to support positive outcomes. This means that people are more aware of conditions, when to seek health, which lifestyle factors pose risks for them, and which behaviours they should adopt

> **Self-efficacy** – When individuals believe in themselves to conduct behaviours to produce a desirable outcome.
>
> **Qualitative** – Written information that usually provides an explanation for something.
>
> **Quantitative** – Numerical data that measures the amount of something.

as a result. Health education campaigns support this approach by empowering people to make their own decisions.

Measuring the effectiveness of health education

It is very important to measure how effective a campaign has been. There are a number of categories against which the effectiveness can be measured.

- **Benefits to individuals of early intervention and lifestyle changes.** These can be measured through reductions in hospital admissions, recorded conditions, healthcare costs or community services. Alternatively, they could be measured through questionnaires where people assess the benefits to themselves. For example, someone who has completed the 'Couch to 5k' programme may report that they feel fitter, stronger, have less anxiety and sleep better. Those benefits would be hard to track through official statistics.

- **Lifelong health outcomes** are tracked through the overall rates of ill health issues. For example, health statistics about obesity or diabetes can show whether these health issues are declining or increasing.

- The **effect on holistic health** is more difficult to track. However, questionnaires covering intellectual, emotional and social impacts on people can help to link education campaign to overall health. It might also be demonstrated through reductions in mental health services or diagnoses.

- A **reduction in the use of specialist services for medical interventions** is another way to track the impact of a campaign. Specialist services include things such as kidney dialysis or chemotherapy. A reduction in use of these services implies that fewer people have contracted the disease or condition, which might be linked to the education campaign.

- A final way of measuring the effectiveness of health education is by monitoring the **what behavioural changes have taken place** as a result of the campaign. For example, a rise in the use of preventative services such as vaccine centres or sexual health clinics can demonstrate a shift in individual responsibility for their own health outcomes. Similarly, questionnaire data about behaviour might indicate changes in behaviour, such as reducing alcohol consumption, whose effect will not be seen in hospital admissions data for many years to come.

The data collected can be qualitative or quantitative.

> **Recap questions**
>
> 1. Identify a responsibility of health and social care professionals when promoting positive health behaviours.
>
> 2. Define the term **autonomy**.
>
> 3. Identify two ways of measuring the effectiveness of health education.

> **Activity**
>
> 1. Discuss the impact that the Health Belief Model of behaviour change has upon the effectiveness of health education.
>
> 2. Discuss why it is important to aim health education campaigns at families and communities as well as individuals.

C3 Planning a health education event

Task 2 of your set assignment (PSA) requires you to plan a small-scale health education event.

Your plan for a health education event must include the following.

- **Aims and objectives of the event**. An **aim** is a testable statement of what someone sets out to achieve in the long term. **Objectives** are the steps you need to take to achieve the aim.
- The aims and objectives must be:
    * **Specific** to the health and wellbeing issue. This means they are clearly defined and are relevant to the issue outlined in the aim.
    * **Measurable** – this means they can be tracked, so that you can see the effect of the campaign. A timeframe must also be provided for when each objective and the aim needs to be met.
    * **Realistic** – this means they are achievable and relevant to the health and wellbeing issue, as well as for the demographic the campaign is aimed at.
    * They must also show that you understand the **starting point** for the intended audience. This means that the event will not be too advanced or too simplistic for your target audience, and use language and approaches that they will be able to access and understand.
- As this is a health education event you must choose a **model of behaviour change** to support you in your event. You must be able to justify your decision.
- Your work should be present information **clearly and accurately,** and the plan should show how information will be **presented and communicated appropriately** for the target audience.
- Your plan will need to explain of how you will **challenge and correct misinformation, prejudice, stereotypes** and **discrimination.**
- **Target groups** – who will your event be targeted at and how might this impact different groups in society? A consideration of equality and diversity should be demonstrated.
- Your plan should discuss the options for an **integrated approach** – this includes consulting with and explaining which agencies, organisation and people your event will include.
- **Demographic data** – you should include researched demographic data to inform your health event. This data should show that the health and wellbeing issue covered by your event is an area of concern.
- **Ethical considerations** – you should consider the rights of individuals, others and how confidentiality can be maintained for people when delivering your health education event.
- **Educational resources** – you need to plan and create resources that could be used in the event. For example, this could include:
    * a visual display
    * poster
    * leaflet
    * in-person activities
    * digital resources.
- **Measuring impact** – you must create a plan for how you will measure the effectiveness of the event through. You can do this through different data collection methods such as:
    * questionnaires
    * focus groups
    * observations
    * interviews.

Throughout your planning of your health education event, you must provide reasonable justifications for your decisions. Finally, it must only be a plan – you do not need to carry out the event.

End of Topic Practice Activity

Read through the extract taken from a health education event and answer the questions. These questions are linked to the knowledge and skills needed for M3, M4 and D2.

Tackling Lifestyle Choices and Obesity in Adolescence

Obesity in adolescents is a growing public health concern with data showing a significant increase in obesity-related illness in the past few years. According to the World Health Organisation (WHO) the prevalence of obesity amongst adolescents aged 12-19 years has more than tripled over the last two decades. In the UK, 24% of adolescents are classified as obese with 80% of them continuing to be obese into adulthood. This means health issues associated with obesity, such as type 2 diabetes, cardiovascular issues and depression, are also on the rise.

This health education event will begin with a presentation of the causes and risk factors associated with obesity to adolescents within a local school. In this presentation, adolescents will be provided with evidence from national and global statistics to highlight the prevalence of obesity in the UK. The goals of this event will be shared, and they will then be presented with healthy alternatives to lead a healthier lifestyle, encouraging healthy weight or weight loss.

After the presentation, adolescents will be involved in an interactive workshop where they will complete peer-led activities to demonstrate healthy behaviours, such as meal preparation or exercises and exercise routines. These workshops will include providing adolescents with case studies of individuals with obesity, so they can analyse and discuss possible interventions.

By the end of this event, 85% of participants reported a better understanding of the health risks associated with obesity, and 70% said they understood the importance of leading a healthy lifestyle.

Consider and answer the following questions:

1. What percentage of adolescents are classified as obese according to the extract?
2. What is the aim of this health education event?
3. How has the data been used to determine the focus of the health education event?
4. How effective do you think this health education event been for the aim?
5. Which model or approach has been demonstrated in this event? How do you know this?
6. What do you think about using this model for this event?
7. What is good about the health education event and what could be improved?

This practice task will help you prepare for the following assessment criteria:

C.P5 Explain models and approaches used in health education campaigns.

C.P6 Plan a small-scale health education event for one health and wellbeing issue.

C.M3 Assess the effectiveness of models and approaches used in health education campaigns, with reference to data.

C.M4 Assess the effectiveness of planning a small-scale health education event with reference to one health and wellbeing issue.

C.D2 Justify the proposed plan for health education event with reference to the health and wellbeing issue, models and approaches used.

Unit 6 Safe environments in health and social care

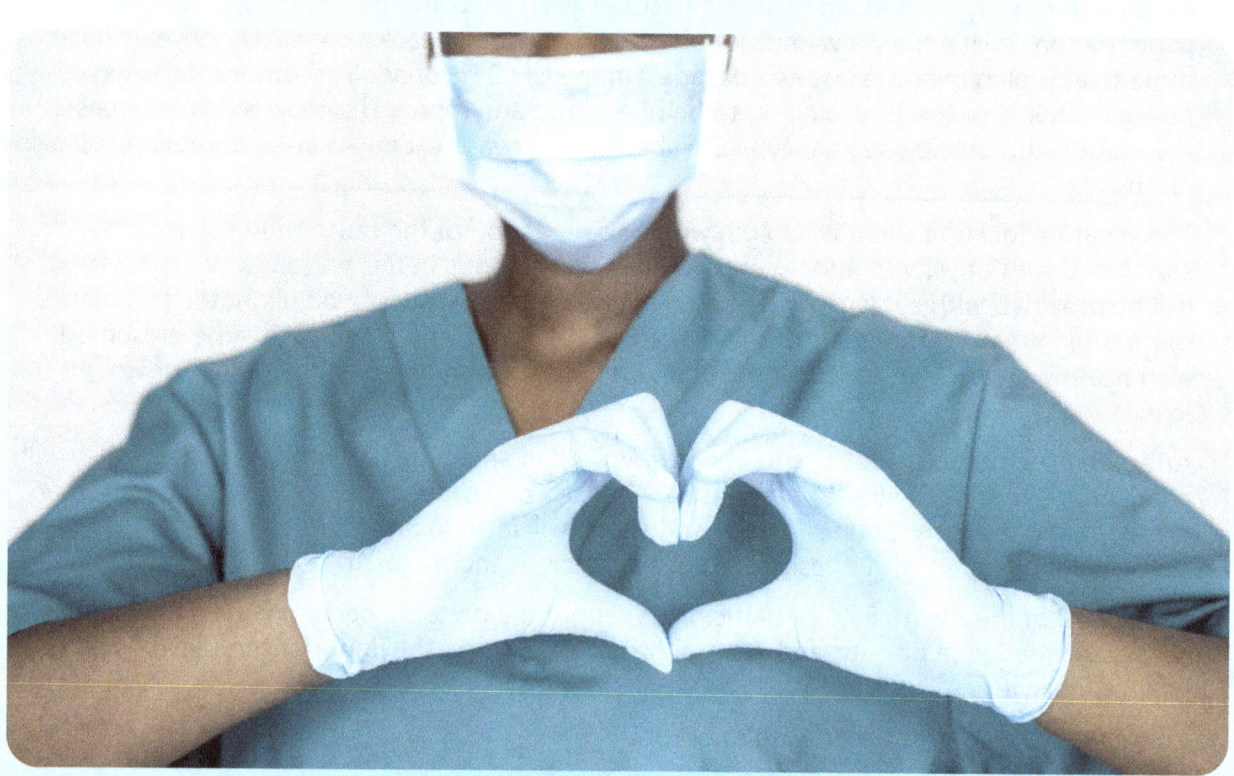

In this unit students will learn about safe working practices and professional responsibilities in health and social care services.

You will learn about:

- Local health and social care services and the challenges they face.
- Health and safety legislation and regulations, and how they are important for safe working practices.
- How a duty of care is important to maintain the safety and wellbeing of vulnerable individuals.
- The responsibilities and statutory requirements for effective record keeping and maintaining confidentiality.

How will I be assessed?

In this unit you will be assessed through an internal assessment consisting of a series of tasks, covering Learning Aims A, B and C. The assignment is set by the awarding body and marked by your tutor.

Learning Aim A: Explore appropriate care environments for individuals at different life stages

Learning Aim B: Explore aspects of legislation, policies and regulations that support safe environments in health and social care settings

Learning Aim C: Examine aspects of monitoring and maintaining safe practice in health and social care environments

Learning Aim A: Explore appropriate care environments for individuals at different life stages

A1 Meeting individual's needs in health and social care settings

There are many different health and social care services that provide care for individuals across many sectors, including physical health, mental health, learning disabilities and rehabilitation.

These can be arranged in different environments to meet the unique needs of individuals.

Local services

One of the ways to meet the needs of individuals is to offer support locally. These are services that are based in communities that serve the needs of local residents. They are generally easier to attend and make use of.

Local services can include the following.

Acute care

Acute care services offer short-term treatment for injury or illness. These offer care for sudden symptoms for brief periods of illness. These include:

- Emergency care
- Urgent care
- Trauma care
- Surgery recovery
- Critical care

These can be based locally to ensure they can be used by individuals when they are needed to help to meet the needs in an appropriate time, particularly for physical health.

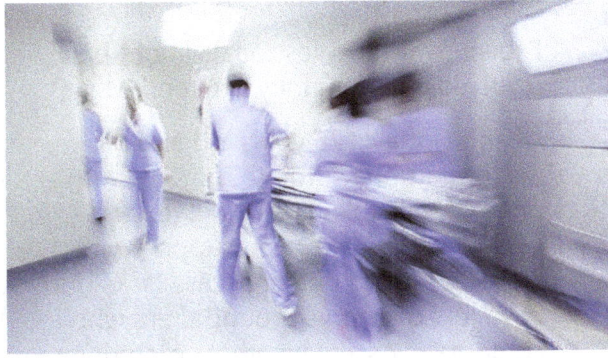

A common example of an acute care service is an Accident and Emergency department in a hospital

> Cessation – The process of ending something.
> Primary care services – Services that individuals can access directly.

Community health services

There are many different types of **community health services**. They are usually primary care services. They can include:

- Sexual health and smoking cessation clinics
- GP surgeries
- Pharmacies

There are often many different community health services in a local area, to ensure there are enough to serve the needs of all the people living in the area. They can each offer their own support but can also make referrals to secondary support if needed.

These services can be particularly useful to support physical and mental health.

Residential social care

There are different types of residential homes to cater for a variety of needs. These include residential care for:

- Individuals who need nursing support.
- Elderly individuals with poor physical health.
- Individuals of any age with severe learning disabilities.

Residential social care services are often based in local communities, so that individuals can stay in an area they are familiar with, where family and friends can visit frequently. This helps people maintain relationships with others outside of the residential care home.

The different types of residential homes can meet the needs of different types of individuals, as the focus of care will be widely understood. This can be particularly useful to support individuals with poor physical or mental health, or those with learning disabilities.

Community social care

Community social care is mainly provided by domiciliary care. This is when care services are given in the individual's own home, and is carried out by trained professionals such as care assistants. The type of activities they may help with include:

- Getting dressed
- Taking care of personal hygiene
- Taking medication
- Completing household chores
- Cooking meals and making drinks
- Changing dressings on wounds

This care allows an individual to continue to live at home and allows them to maintain their independence for as long as possible. This can give them confidence in their own abilities and allow them to maintain their dignity. This can help individuals with poor physical or mental health, those with learning disabilities and people undertaking rehabilitation.

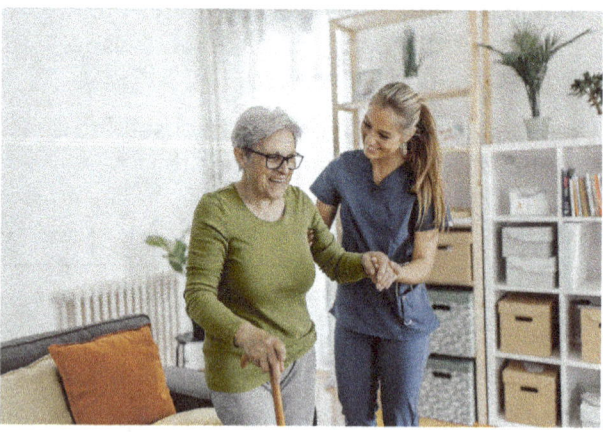

Domicilliary social care

> Domiciliary care – Services put in place to support an individual in their own home.
>
> Dignity – Being treated as worthy, and with respect.

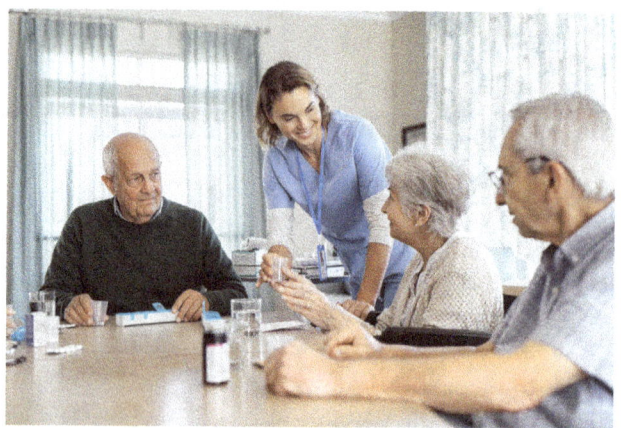

Residential social care

Recap questions

1. What is the difference between residential care and domiciliary care?
2. What do community health services include?
3. Why are community care (health and social care) services important?

Activity

Look again at the information regarding community care and residential care. Consider the following questions. Try to justify your answers.

1. What are the positives of community care for an individual needing support?
2. What are the positives of residential care for an individual needing support?
3. Explain which professionals might be involved in residential care and why.
4. Explain which professionals might be involved in community care and why.
5. An individual is 26 years old and has just undergone surgery. They live with one of their siblings and will recover in 4-6 weeks. They need support with medication and personal care tasks but have lots of people around them who could help. Assess whether community care or residential care services would be best for them, justifying your reasons.

Dental services

Dental services are used by all individuals in a community, regardless of age. These services meet individual needs through providing:

- Routine check-up appointments to reduce the risk of more serious issues
- Emergency appointments if urgent care is required
- Private dental work if required

Dental services are set out across communities to ensure local people can easily access them. This can help to reduce the risk of longer-term problems and the need for further services later.

Hospice services

Hospice care is offered to individuals who have a terminal illness. It is offered from the moment they are made aware their diagnosis is terminal until the end of their life.

- Palliative care is offered once the terminal diagnosis is made. It offers guidance and support regarding medication and treatment to ease pain or improve mental wellbeing.
- This may then turn into end-of-life care, where pain management, spiritual guidance and emotional support are given not only to the individual but to their whole family.

Hospice care is based in local areas, to ensure family and friends can visit as much as possible so the individual can get as much time with them as they can. Family members can make the room personal to the individual, with furnishings, pictures and plants that make them happy, which helps to meet the needs of individuals.

> **Terminal illness** – An illness predicted to lead to death.
>
> **Palliative care** – Care for the terminally ill and their families.
>
> **End-of-life care** – Health care provided in the lead up to an individual's death.
>
> **Multi-disciplinary team** – When professionals from the same service but with different roles work together to meet the needs of an individual.

Virtual wards/hospitals

A **virtual ward** or **virtual hospital** is when a ward-like room is set up in an individual's own home. This ensures that individuals get the care they need in familiar surroundings. This can be extremely important if they would otherwise struggle to access care. It can also be really beneficial for emotional and mental health to stay at home with loved ones.

Multi-disciplinary teams are used to ensure each of the individual's needs are met in a virtual ward. For example, they might need to be prescribed intravenous medication and have clinical teams visit regularly to check on their progress. In this situation, a multi-disciplinary team could consist of professionals from the community nursing team and general practitioners or specialist medical professionals as needed.

Recap questions

1. Explain what a virtual ward is.
2. Assess some benefits of using hospice care for an individual and their family.

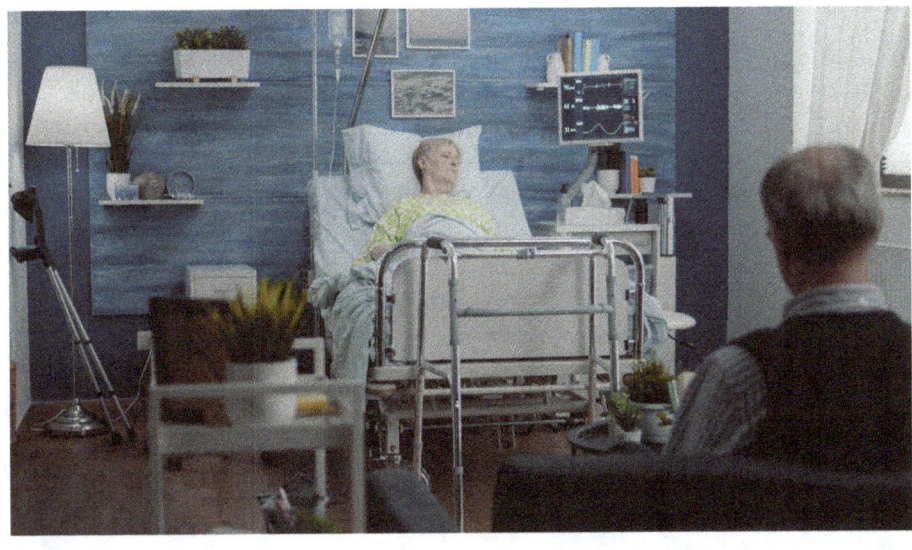

A hospice

Apply your understanding

Leo is in his 60s and has suffered from ill health for a while. He has had multiple strokes as well as a bleed on the brain. He has also had heart disease for many years. Despite this, he has not suffered mentally except for some brief periods of confusion. He has been married to his wife for 40 years and they have never spent more than one night apart. Leo struggles to go to the toilet by himself and he cannot get upstairs well. He has four grown-up children, two of whom live close by, but they work full time and have small children, so can only offer limited support. His wife has been dealing with an arthritis diagnosis.

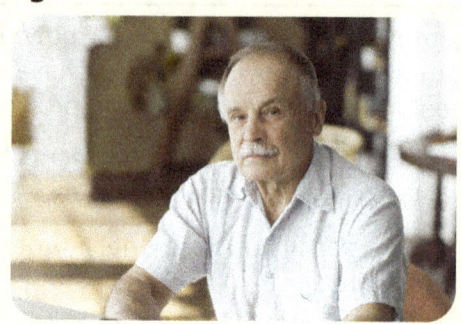

1. Make an argument for Leo to stay at home with the use of a virtual ward, where he can access adapted toileting facilities, as well as a hospital bed and medication when needed. Consider the wellbeing of himself and his family.

2. Make an argument for Leo to be moved to a residential home. Consider the wellbeing of himself and his family.

3. Assess the possible outcomes for each choice.

Meeting individuals' needs in health and social care environments

There are many things that can be done to meet the needs of individuals safely and with positive outcomes. Some of these strategies are discussed below.

Recognising what service users can contribute

Service users need to be involved in as much of their care as they are able. They are the ones who are living through the care journey and will have to work with the professionals tasked to help them, so it is important they are fully on board and committed to the care being given.

Recognising the journey they have been on, and will continue on in the future, can ensure they feel ready for the next steps.

It is important for professionals to understand the lived experience of service users, which is the knowledge individuals have gained from first-hand experience. Because they are the ones experiencing care, they may have understanding and insight that is different to the care team. By understanding lived experience:

- Agreements about further care can be made more easily
- Individuals feel their experience, good or bad, has been taken into account

> **Lived experience** – Knowledge gained through first-hand involvement in something
>
> **Advocate** – Someone who speaks regarding a person's case on their behalf.
>
> **Holistic approach** – This is when support is provided for the whole person, including all parts of their development.

- Changes to care can be made as appropriate.

Using a person-centred approach

Using a **person-centred approach** means that an individual's wants, needs and wishes are taken into consideration, and the individual is at the centre of all decision making. This includes making sure they are present in all meetings and that they agree with all decisions. It may involve the use of an advocate to ensure individuals can express their thoughts and feelings. It can ensure that a holistic approach is taken, including all aspects of their physical, intellectual, emotional and social health and development.

Using a person-centred approach can help to meet an individual's needs by:

- Ensuring they feel heard in discussions and meetings

Apply your understanding

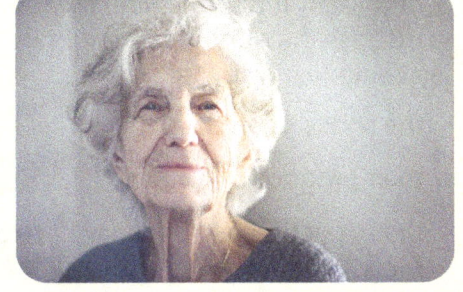

Betty is 78 years old and has recently had a hip replacement. She has led a very active life – she was a dental nurse in the army and has lived in a variety of different countries. She needs the hip replacement because she was recently hit by a car. This has led to her being in need of support and care at home.

A meeting was arranged with various care professionals to discuss her care needs. The professionals included a social worker, a home carer, a GP, the surgeon who completed the surgery and Betty. Due to her age, the professionals in the meeting were rather dismissive of Betty's contribution. They made assumptions about what Betty did and didn't understand, regardless of her medical background, and they didn't ask her opinions.

1. How do you think Betty would feel in this meeting?
2. How much would Betty want to work with these professionals in the future?
3. Assess how professionals could use a person-centred approach in this situation.
4. Explain why 'lived experience' could be helpful here.

- Ensuring they will take the decisions and care given seriously
- Reducing time being wasted by professionals, ensuring the most appropriate care can be given.

Using integrated care

Integrated care means that different types of care, and different parts of the care plan, work together to support the individual. This helps to focus on the specific needs of the individual, as well as the needs of their friends, family and carers. It helps ensure that everyone can get along with each other, supporting the outcomes of care, leading to it being more productive and beneficial for all.

This will help to meet their needs as:

- They will feel confident that everyone is working together
- They will know where to go for help if needed
- Everyone will have a good understanding of the role of others.

An example of an integrated care system could be within a residential care home. A care manager would take responsibility for the care plan and share this information with other professionals. They would ensure that these professionals work with residents when needed and that local authority professionals,

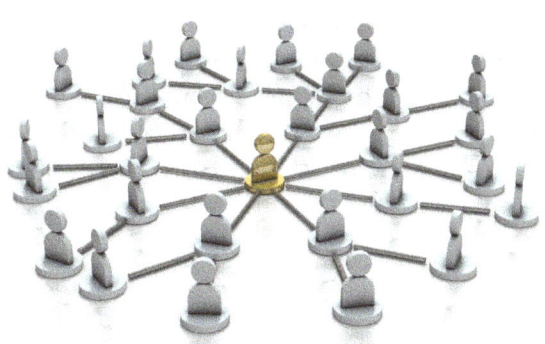

Care should be person-centred

Integrated care – When different parts of the given care are coordinated and work well together.

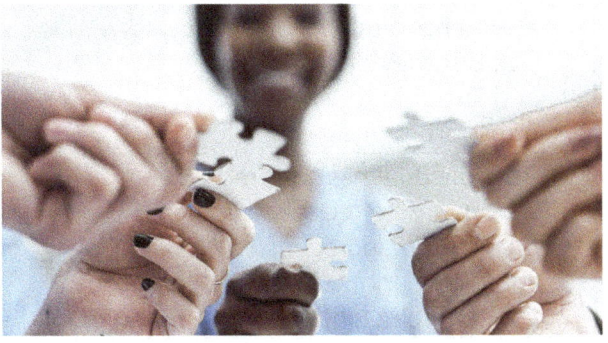

such as social workers, have access to residents as required. The manager would ensure that regular meetings are held amongst all professionals, to understand each other's roles and the preferences of individuals and their families.

Reducing distress

It is important that professionals work to reduce any **distress** that individuals might be feeling. They could feel distressed due to:

- the shock of an accident
- their prognosis
- the impact their needs may have on their friends or family.

Distress can be reduced by using person-centred care, and including friends and family in decisions. This can enable them to focus on what is important to them to improve their health.

Managing risk and supporting risk taking

Risk is the possibility that something bad will happen. Risks need to be managed so that the potential for harm is reduced as much as possible, but in a positive way. Risks could be due to an individual's physical needs, their mental health needs, or their environment. In order to manage risks, an individual's holistic health needs must be considered, alongside the potential hazards they may face. The barriers they may face in managing these risks, such as financial barriers or a lack of understanding, must also be considered.

Some risks may need to be taken to make positive changes to an individual's life. For example, this could include taking new medication, moving into a residential home or taking up new hobbies. Managing risks, and positive risk-taking, consider the specific circumstances of the individual, helping to meet their needs. They can help ensure positive changes are made to the individual's life.

Recap questions

1. What is 'lived experience'?
2. Explain what may be needed when using a person-centred approach.
3. Assess why some individuals might struggle with managing risks.
4. Analyse what might be a cause of distress for individuals.

Activity

Consider the following examples of risks that may be experienced by individuals. Complete the table to show what barriers may prevent the risk being managed and how these can be overcome.

Risk	Barriers	Overcome
An individual has lost the support of their informal carer		
An individual needs to attend hospital in a different city, but they do not drive and struggle to use public transport		
An individual has suffered serious side effects from medication and needs to change to another type, but they are reluctant to do so		
An individual has made the decision that they want to stay in their own home and not move to a residential home after suffering a stroke		

The impact of health conditions

The health conditions that individuals are suffering from can have a profound effect on whether their individual needs can be met, and how this can be done. The health conditions can impact not only themselves, but others around them too.

The impact of health conditions on the individual and others

When an individual has a health condition, it can impact on everyone around them in many different ways. These can include:

- **The individual themselves** – this could be due to the distress or upset from a diagnosis, they could be worried about their future, or they could physically ill from the condition itself.

- **Family and friends** – this could be due to the extra worry or burden placed on family members or friends, such as giving them extra caring responsibilities. This could also lead to them feeling worry or concern for their family member, as well as the possibility of them also suffering from a genetic disorder.

- **Professionals** – this could be due to the extra demands placed on professionals, such as nurses or care workers, if an individual has a life limiting health condition. This could lead to numerous providers being involved in caring for an individual and increase the level of support needed.

> Profound – Very great or intense.
>
> Institutionalisation – Being placed in a residential institution, usually for their own safety.

The effect of long-term health conditions

Long-term health conditions can affect many areas of an individual's life.

- One of these could be the **physical impact of the condition,** such as their ability to continue to do the physical activities they have previously enjoyed and their ability to do things such as shopping for themselves.

- Another impact could be the fact that they may become **dependent on others.** This could be for personal care or daily household activities, such as cleaning or laundry. This could lead to them feeling worthless, and as though their ability to make choices has been taken away from them. This could also lead to a loss of personal space, as they may need others to care for them, which could make an individual feel uncomfortable in the long term.

- Institutionalisation may also be needed for specific long-term health conditions. This could drastically change the daily lives of an individual, meaning they will lose their freedom and ability to make many decisions for themselves, but it would ensure their needs are met 24 hours a day.

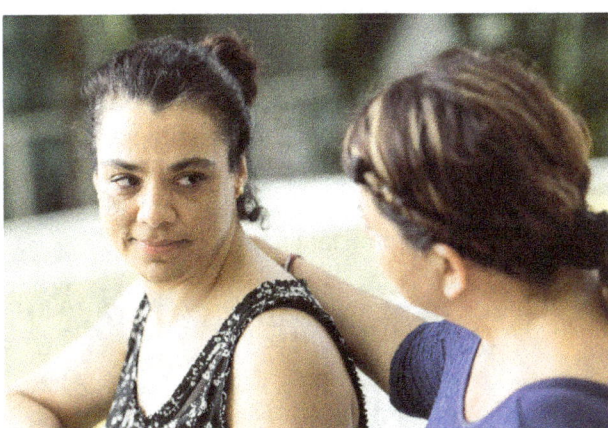

Family and friends are also impacted by health conditions

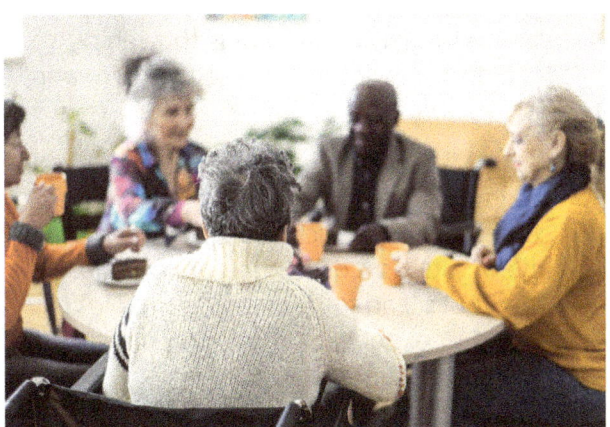

There is a risk of institutionalisation in a residential care home

The impact of health conditions on emotional and mental wellbeing

When an individual is suffering from a health condition, it can have a deep impact on their emotional and mental wellbeing. This is because it can lead to upset, trauma and concern for their welfare. The mental and emotional impact could include:

- **Fear** – This could be due to diagnosis itself, the fear of treatment or the long-term outcomes of the condition itself.

- **Learned helplessness** – This can occur due to individuals giving up on trying to do things for themselves and can lead to them being unable to in the long run, leading to poor mental health and a lack of confidence.

- **Frustration** – This can occur due to timescales of treatment or appointments or frustration due to the side effects of medication. This can lead to them feeling unable to get along with others and find it hard to see anything in a positive light.

- **Anger** – This can occur due to individuals feeling angry at the diagnosis of their health condition or angry at themselves, perhaps for their lifestyle choices. Individuals may also be angry at professionals if they feel they are not being offered the care they deserve.

- **Depression** – This can occur when individuals realise how their lives will change due to their health condition and they feel unable to change the outcome. They may feel that their future has been taken out of their hands and that they can no longer do the things they enjoy, leading to feelings of low self-esteem and depression.

- **Anxiety** – This can occur due to individuals feeling worried and nervous when it comes to things such as appointments or investigations regarding their condition. This could lead to them being unable to attend or experiencing poor mental health prior to appointments.

- **Confusion** – This can occur if professionals have been unable to explain an individual's condition effectively, perhaps due to a learning disability or due to professionals not understanding their needs effectively.

> **Apply your understanding**
>
> Blake is 22 years old and has just been diagnosed with a long-term health condition. He is at university and enjoys taking part in sports such as football and likes going out with his friends. His university course is also very physically and mentally demanding, as is his part-time job.
>
> Describe three emotional and mental impacts that he may be experiencing, why he may have to deal with these, and how this will affect his life overall.

The social impact of health conditions

The social health of an individual is very important, as it can impact their holistic health and development. For example, it can affect their emotional and physical health through the activities they are invited to take part in and how these affect their self-esteem.

Suffering with a long-term health condition can lead to:

- **Social exclusion** – This is when individuals are excluded from specific activities due to their condition, such as sports or leisure activities. This can lead to a lack of confidence and self-esteem, as well as boredom and resentment for those who have excluded them.

- **Discrimination** – This is when individuals are treated negatively or unjustly based on their long-term condition, such as not being given a job role they have applied for, or amendments not being made to enable them to take part in activities.

- **Isolation** – This is when an individual is isolated from others, perhaps on purpose if they have been negatively subject to discrimination, or due to specific circumstances, such as geographical location or financial circumstances.

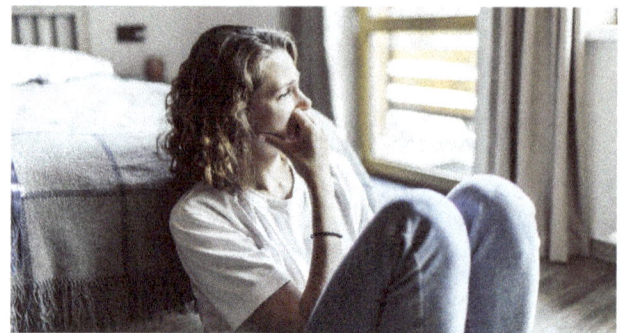

The organisational impact of health conditions

When an individual suffers from a long-term health condition, there are often many things that professionals need to keep control of and organise.

One of these is the **management of staff** who are working with the individual. Depending on the health condition, there may be many different types of staff supporting the individual in many different ways, such as carers, nurses, GPs and occupational therapists, for example. These need to be managed effectively to avoid professionals repeating work done by others, as well as to ensure the individual knows who they can turn to and when.

The wellbeing of staff is also important when they are working with individuals with long-term health conditions. This could be due to the time spent with the individual, which could be extremely time-consuming and stressful, affecting a professional's physical and mental health. Therefore, it is vitally important that managers are aware of their staff's wellbeing and offer guidance and support whenever possible.

Another organisational role of professionals includes day-to-day planning and the allocation of resources needed to support individuals. This can be important if an individual is in a residential home or in need of specialist resources. If resources are organised effectively, it can help to reduce stress on professionals and the individual themselves, as well as lead to better long-term outcomes. Any issues with limited resources can impact service users but also increase the stress on professionals, who know what service users need but are unable to provide it. This could then negatively affect the care and outcomes for individuals.

Occupational therapists – Professionals who help individuals to maintain their standard of living following an accident, injury or illness.

Diversity – The practice of involving all people, perhaps due to race, gender and ethnic background, for example.

Equality – Being and feeling equal in status, rights and opportunities.

Inclusion – Providing equal access to opportunities and resources for all.

Recap questions

1. Can you recall what social exclusion is?
2. Name one organisational role professionals may need to take on.
3. Name two emotional impacts of having a long-term health condition.

Activity

Explain why each of the following may be an issue for individuals with long-term health conditions and how they can be overcome with help from professionals.

	Why it may be an issue	How it could be overcome?
Isolation		
Discrimination		
Social exclusion		

The importance of diversity, equality and inclusion in health and social care environments

In order to ensure the needs of individuals with health conditions can be met, it is important that diversity and equality are respected to promote inclusion within health and social care environments.

Cultural competence of staff

It is important that the professionals working to help to meet the needs of individuals can work effectively to support all individuals, regardless of their cultural background. Not only this, but professionals also need to include the individual's culture into the support they give to ensure they feel included and are not discriminated against. This should include their culture, ethnic origin, nationality, gender, age, religion, beliefs, sexual orientation and ability.

Cultural competence means professionals understand the culture and background of the individuals they support. This leads to positive working relationships, allowing them to depend on each other and agreeing on the support needed and how to manage needs. This will lead to inclusion and equality being possible across different settings used by individuals.

Promotion of individual rights, choice and opportunity

In order to meet the needs of individuals, it is important that professionals promote individual's rights. These can include their right to independence, their right to be protected from abuse and their right to be treated equally. By ensuring individuals' rights are upheld, it can help to meet their needs, as they will feel safe, secure and understood.

Promoting an individual's independent choices also helps to meet their needs, as it will create opportunities for them to be able to improve their own health and wellbeing and be happy with the care and choices they are given. This helps uphold their dignity and promotes autonomy.

The types of choices that could be promoted by professionals include:

- Financial decisions.
- Decisions about the professionals involved in their care.
- Where they want to live.
- The medication and treatment they want.

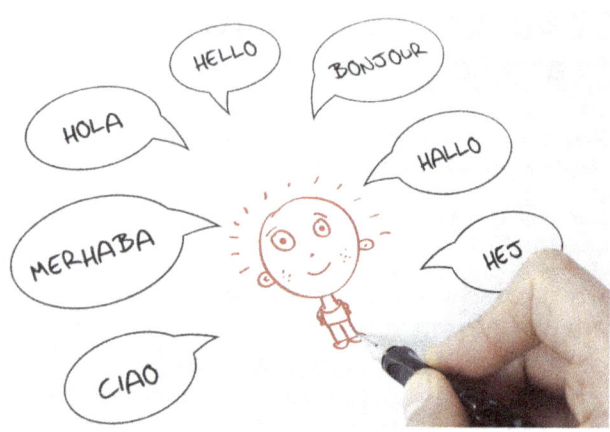

Respect for the cultural context of an individual's life

We have already discussed the importance of professionals understanding the lived experiences of individuals needing care and support for their needs, but it is also important for professionals to take into consideration how an individual's culture and background may also impact how they receive care, as well as their wants, needs and wishes regarding care.

Respecting an individual's cultural context will help professionals to make positive and workable suggestions to individuals and their families, ensuring positive decisions can be made and good relationships can be built.

An individual's culture may impact their experience of health and social care in the following ways:

- They may have felt discrimination previously and be reluctant to accept help again.
- They may have a language barrier.
- They may not be confident when communicating with professionals.
- They may need and/or want the support of their extended family.

Apply your understanding

Abigail is 69 years old. She has recently been moved into a residential home due to being diagnosed with dementia four years ago. Her symptoms have been declining over the last year and she agrees with her family that she should move into a residential home. Abigail was a nurse in her working years and is a devout catholic, praying daily and attending regular church services. She isn't as old as some of the other residents but needs to move due to the progression of her illness.

Make a list of the things professionals can do to show Abigail and their family they are culturally competent, taking into account the information you have about her.

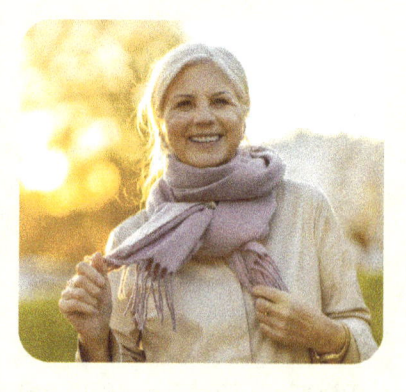

- They may be restricted regarding the treatments available to them, which needs to be respected.

If professionals working with individuals can understand these, and offer support to overcome them where necessary, it will lead to professionals feeling more fulfilled in their role and reduce the chances of conflict occurring.

Policies and procedures in the environment

There are many policies and procedures which are essential in all health and social care environments to **promote inclusivity, challenge discrimination, empower individuals, improve participation** and **promote dignity and respect**.

These include the following policies:

- **Safeguarding** – To ensure all concerns about the safety of an individual are reported effectively so action can be taken where necessary. This will ensure all professionals know who to make reports to and how to do this.

- **Equal opportunities** – To ensure that everyone has the same opportunities of care, activities and a private life, and that all professionals are aware of how to do this.

- **Record keeping** – To ensure appropriate records are kept regarding personal details, medication taken and concerns raised, to support future care and protect individuals.

- **Confidentiality** – To ensure no documents or records are able to be handled by people not authorised to do so. This also applies to verbal information, to protect the wellbeing of individuals.

- **First aid** –To ensure professionals know their roles and responsibilities should an incident arise, or who to turn to if first aid is needed.

- **Complaints/whistleblowing** To ensure all staff, individuals and their families are aware of how to raise a complaint and how it will be dealt with. For professionals, this will include giving them protections regarding their employment should they whistle blow after raising concerns.

- **Administration of medicines** – To ensure medicines are stored and managed correctly, including making sure dosages are correct and the correct medication is given to specific individuals.

- **Health and safety** – It is the responsibility of all staff to ensure the safety of all who visit the service. This can include what to do in the case of emergency as well as who to report issues to across buildings.

> Autonomy – The ability to make their own informed decisions.
> Dignity – Feeling worthy and being proud of oneself.

Recap questions

1. What decisions should be made by individuals needing support to meet their needs?
2. What are two examples of policies used in health and social care services?
3. Give one reason why an individual's culture may affect them accepting help and care.
4. What does it mean for professionals to show cultural competence?

Activity

For each of the policies listed below, explain how they can promote inclusivity and promote dignity for individuals needing care and support.

Policy	Promote inclusivity	Promote dignity
Safeguarding		
Equal opportunities		
Record keeping		
Confidentiality		
First aid		
Complaints / whistleblowing		
Administration of medicine		
Health and safety		

A2 The impact of environmental factors and the care experience

In order for individuals to feel able to access the services they need, buildings and environments need to be appropriate. Individuals may have specific needs regarding their accessibility to services due to sensory impairments, physical disabilities, or cultural barriers, for example.

> Sensory impairments – When one or more of the senses is not working as well as it should, such as hearing or sight.
>
> Proximity – How close or far away something is.

Geographical location

The **geographical location** of a service includes:

- where it is located
- how easy it is to access
- the distance to the individuals needing to use the service, which could be positive or negative.

There are often many 'local' services, such as GP and dental services, for example. These are often easy to access due to being in close proximity to the community they serve, reducing the need for transport as these can often be reached on foot. However, even these services can be difficult to reach in a rural area. These may also be difficult to reach if individuals are dealing with a physical disability, for example, making even the smallest journeys more difficult.

Secondary and tertiary services, such as hospitals, hospices and specialist care units, tend to be in more central locations. They need to meet the needs of many people and so are usually in the centre of bigger towns and cities. This can create a geographical barrier because users need transport to get there, requiring extra time, effort and cost.

For example:

- If an individual is suffering from a long-term disabling condition, they may not be able to make longer journeys because they interrupt their medication and care routine.
- Individuals may also be dealing with poverty and be unable to afford the cost of public transport, limiting their ability to attend appointments and access care.
- The geographical location could impact on family members' ability to offer support, such as accompanying people to appointments.

Apply your understanding

Finn is 30 years old. He has just been to see his GP regarding a skin condition he has developed. He called to make an appointment and was able to go after work as they stay open until 6:30pm. The GP surgery is also a 10-minute walk from where he lives and his workplace.

His GP refers him to the dermatology clinic at the hospital. Finn doesn't drive, and to make the hospital appointment he would need to take two buses, taking around two hours to get there and two hours to get back.

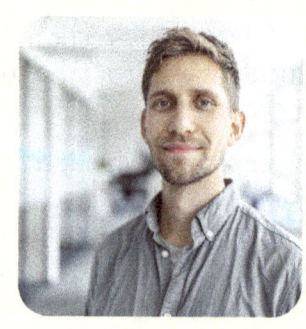

The hospital appointment is scheduled for 11:30am on a weekday. Finn will need to take the day off work as he would need to leave around 9:30am and, depending on the length of his appointment, he would return around 2pm. He doesn't get paid for being off work and would also need to pay for the bus journeys.

Consider the following questions:

1. Describe three reasons why Finn might be less likely to attend the hospital appointment.
2. What could be the long-term consequences?
3. Evaluate how the services could help to overcome the geographical barriers Finn is facing.

Design and accessibility of buildings

The design and accessibility of a building is vitally important to ensure that those who need to access the service can do so. The design of the building needs to take the following into consideration.

Use of ramps and lifts

These are important both inside and outside to ensure individuals can get into the building and navigate around once inside. This will help to support an individual's independence and dignity as they will feel able to go wherever is needed without help. These are particularly important for individuals with physical impairments or disabilities.

Use of signs

This is important to ensure individuals know where they are going when attending services. This can reduce confusion and anxiety for individuals. It also reduces the workload of professionals, as individuals don't have to ask for directions.

The use of signs is important inside and outside the building, and will need to take into account sensory or language barriers.

Cost of access

The location of the service might incur additional costs for individuals. This includes:

- public transport costs
- parking costs.

It is essential that these costs do not make it more difficult for individuals to access the services they need, and that concessions are made when possible.

Parking availability

Poor parking facilities can make people feel more anxious or worried about accessing services.

- They could feel anxious about finding a space to use
- They might worry about how they will be able to walk from the parking space to the building if they suffer from a physical disability.

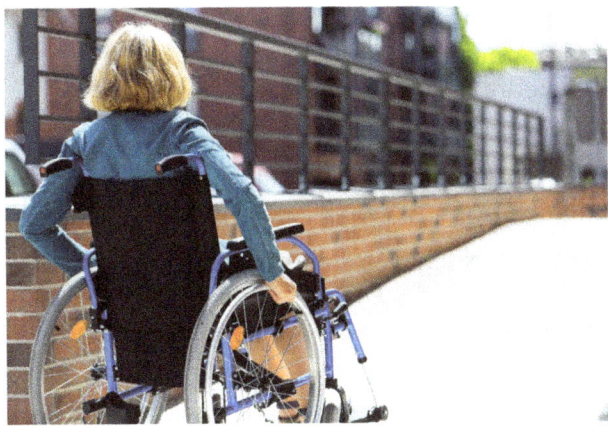

An accessible ramp

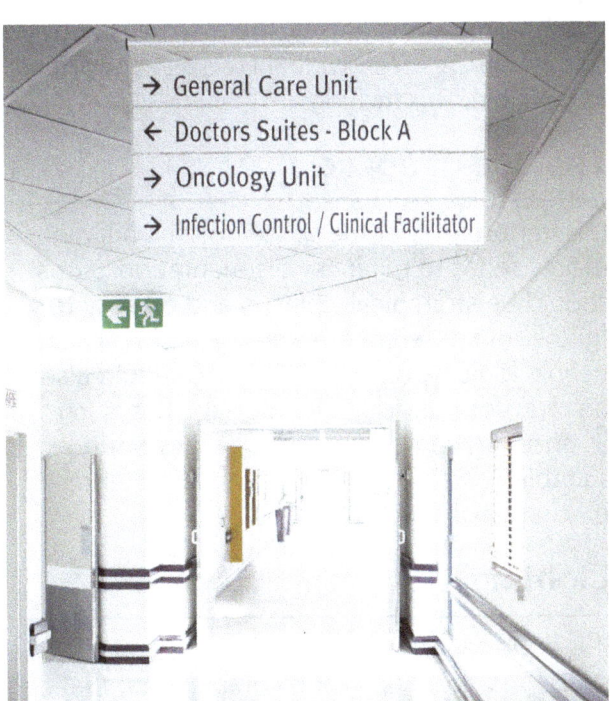

Availability of private space

There are some services where access to private space is important, such as when attending an appointment with a professional, or in services such as residential homes.

Access to private space is important to maintain an individual's dignity and to give them the opportunity to seek the support they need. This could include:

- rooms with doors that close
- curtains
- Places they can access independently..

Access to outside areas

Being able to spend time outside, in gardens and seating areas, can make a big difference to the mental wellbeing of individuals.

Mental wellbeing can also be improved through the use of windows, especially if an individual is unable to get outside.

In services such as residential homes, nursing homes, hospital wards, and hospices, being able to access outside space can be vitally important.

Recap questions

1. Name one adaptation that could be helpful to improve accessibility to buildings for people with a physical disability.
2. Explain one cost that individuals might face when accessing services.
3. How can mental wellbeing be improved around buildings?

Layout of buildings

The layout of the inside of the building is also important to alleviate any stress or panic, but also to ensure an individual feels as comfortable as possible. This includes:

The use of space

It is important that the space inside a building makes sense to minimise disorientation. Signs should be strategically placed and be easy to follow, and different areas in the building should be in a logical position. The space should also be clear for individuals with disabilities, such as ensuring corridors are clear, that flooring is suitable and that there are minimal potential blockages of space.

Lighting

It is important the lighting is suitable for the space and the tasks being completed in that space. For example, bright lighting should be used in areas where physical examinations are being conducted to ensure clear vision for the professionals. This would also be needed for corridors to reduce the risk of trips or falls. However, in places where individuals may need to rest or sleep, softer lighting may be more useful, such as lamps or dimmable switches.

Aesthetics

Depending on the service being used, there may be more requirements to promote a comfortable environment. For example, at a dentist surgery, a calming colour on the wall and some nice pictures may be all that is needed to ensure individuals feel comfortable. However, in a residential home, long-term care ward or hospice, for example, more will be needed. This could include decor that gives a 'homely' feel, such as curtains, carpets, cushions, bedding, sofas and ornaments. These will help individuals to feel more comfortable and help it to feel less clinical, especially when they are there long term.

Engaging service users in designs

In places such as a residential home or hospice, it is positive if the individual is included in the design of their environment, such as choosing colours and materials to use and by bringing personal objects of their own, such as pictures or bedding.

Activity

Imagine that you are moving into a residential home and consider the following:

1. What colour options would you choose and why?
2. What five things would you insist on taking from home to help you to feel more comfortable?
3. How and why would these help you to feel settled?
4. How would you feel if you couldn't take these?

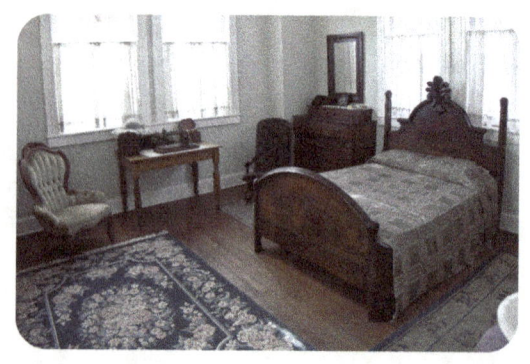

The scheduling of activities

When activities are scheduled in health and social care services, it is important that these are appropriate for the individuals taking part and that they are held at an appropriate time and in an appropriate place. If activities are too strenuous for the individuals, it could lead to injury or a reluctance to take part, leading to poor mental and physical health for individuals.

Also, if the space used is not appropriate, it could lead to overcrowding as well as stress and anxiety for individuals if the space used is too small or doesn't have the right equipment to complete the activity, such as inappropriate flooring, for example. Timing is equally important to consider, especially for individuals who require routine. If the activity is inappropriately timed, such as near the time when medication is given or before mealtimes, it could lead to frustration, upset or worsening physical health if medication is delayed.

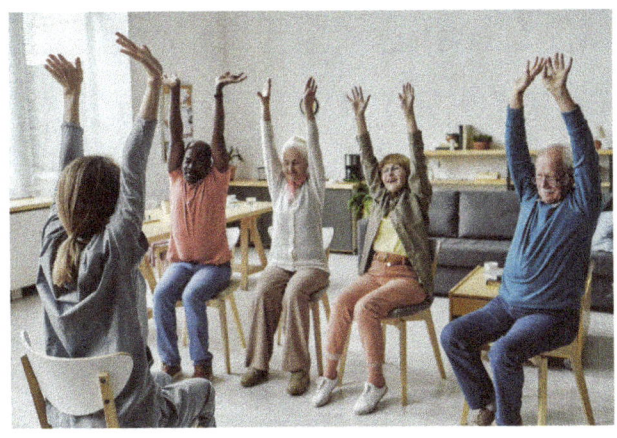

However, if activities are appropriate and offered in an accessible way at a time that suits the individuals, it can enhance their care experience and improve their chances of socialising with others. This can improve their self-esteem and confidence and open up new possibilities for them intellectually, therefore improving holistic health.

The impact of noise

The level of noise from things like traffic or other external sources can have a big impact on an individual's care experience. External sources could be permanent or temporary, which can affect their impact on individuals in the long term.

Activity

Consider what the impact could be on individuals experiencing the following noise complaints. Think about how this would impact their daily life, thinking about their physical, intellectual, emotional and social health and how this could be supported or overcome.

Noise complaint	How it affects daily life	How it could be overcome
A residential home is on a busy road where there is constant traffic noise.		
A hospital is undergoing building works. There is constant noise from diggers and machinery from 6am to 6pm right next to the children's ward.		

Recap questions

1. Why is the use of signs important in health and social care buildings?
2. Explain how the geographical location of a service might affect an individual's ability to access it.
3. Why would it be positive to include a service user in making decisions about their own environment?
4. What do professionals need to consider when scheduling activities?

A3 Challenges to providing appropriate care environments

Unfortunately, there may be many reasons why it is a challenge to meet the care needs of an individual, perhaps due to the services available to help or due to the needs of the individual being complex and difficult to manage. These can all affect the care and support offered and the chances of having their needs met.

Needs of individuals

The needs of individuals may be complex due to their age and stage of development. The difficulties due to each life stage could be:

- **Infancy (0-2 years)** - Challenges could arise due to the small size of individuals and their underdeveloped immune system. This could lead to an increased risk of complications when making decisions about their care and their vulnerability means they need constant 24-hour care.

- **Childhood (3-8 years)** - Challenges may arise with this age group due to their inability to understand the care decisions being made on their behalf. They should be included in decisions they can make, with the support of an advocate, making things like meetings perhaps a little more difficult.

- **Adolescence (9-18 years)** - Challenges may arise with this age group due to an advocate being needed whenever meetings are held to ensure these individuals can understand and be involved in decision making, ensuring person-centred care is given. There are also many potential obstacles with this age group to consider, such as education, social needs and the changes and developments from puberty.

- **Early adulthood (19-45 years)** - Challenges may arise due to the independence required by individuals in this age group, such as within higher education and to uphold their rights to a private family life. Professionals may find it difficult to get adults in this stage to make any long-term decisions, as the immediate future is often their priority. There are also minimal long-term care environments for individuals of this age group.

- **Middle adulthood (45-65 years)** - Challenges may arise within this age group as individuals may find it more difficult to make changes to their lifestyle, even if it has created a health condition such as obesity or cancers. Professionals can give help and support, but it is down to individuals themselves to make changes, which at this age may be met with resistance. There are, again, minimal long-term care environments to support individuals of this age.

- **Later adulthood (65+ years)** - Challenges to meeting care needs at this age may be down to mobility and their ability to access the services offered. They may live in a residential home or may be unable to get to appointments, affecting their health. Also, they may be suffering from age-related illnesses, such as dementia, making decisions and person-centred care more difficult.

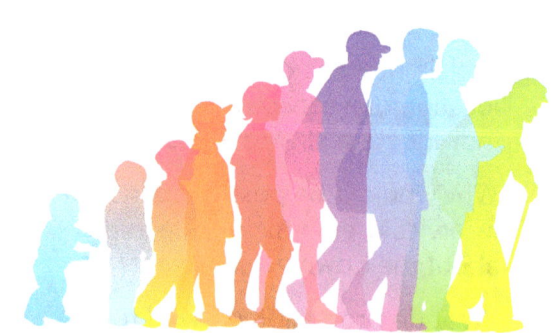

> **Apply your understanding**
>
> John is 55 and is suffering from heart failure. He is a teacher and has been extremely independent since his diagnosis. He has two children who live far away, and he is married. John and his wife have recently retired, but his condition has deteriorated, and he is needing more care due to suffering a number of small strokes, so residential care is likely.
>
> 1. Assess the possible difficulties in finding John an appropriate environment to receive his residential care in the long term. Think about his age and people around him.
>
> Noah is 15 years old. He is suffering from a degenerative medical condition. His parents both need to work and his needs are increasing on a daily basis. His family are adamant that he continues at school to give him the childhood he deserves, but they are now struggling to meet his needs as well as the needs of his 2 siblings. It has been agreed that he should be moved into alternative care.
>
> 2. Assess the possible difficulties in finding Noah an appropriate environment to receive his care. Consider his age and the things happening in his life.

Meeting individual's expectations

In order for care to be effective, individuals themselves need to be on board. The best way to ensure this happens is to promote **person-centred care**. This is so:

- the individual has been involved in the decision making
- they have had the opportunity to voice their own preferences, so these can be taken into consideration before any decisions have been made.

This is more likely to result in the individual accepting the care they are offered, as it will meet their expectations and make them more likely to cooperate with the professionals supporting them.

> Degenerative – A disease that will get worse over time.

Another potential challenge could be due to the outpatient and inpatient services available. It may be that an individual has spent time at an inpatient service and is now able to return home with outpatient services. However, if the outpatient services available at that time cannot meet the needs of the individual, they may then need to remain an inpatient until this can be resolved. This can lead to individuals staying in places like hospitals for longer, even though it is not the most appropriate for them at that time. This can lead to individuals feeling let down and struggle to accept help in the long term.

Length of time requiring care

The **length of time** an individual requires care may affect professionals' ability to find an appropriate service for them.

- Some services only offer short-term care, such as specific hospital wards or mental health facilities, which often have a set number of weeks to allocate to an individual. This can lead to individuals not using that service, or using it but feeling let down once the support has ended.
- Equally, an individual may only need short-term care, but there are only longer-term care facilities in their area. This can lead to individuals feeling let down by the services around them and lead to professionals feeling like their hands are tied and are unable to help those who are most in need.

Once an assessment of an individual has been completed, it is the role of professionals to seek out the most appropriate service to support them and discuss this with the individuals themselves. Discussions should be had in relation to what an individual wants and whether particular services can match these, such as the time needed to be allocated to them and the facilities they have available. If an individual is to be in a care environment, such as a residential home, for a long time, it is important they have facilities such as outside space and communal areas to enable them to meet the holistic needs of individuals.

Integrated care system approach

The **Integrated Care System** (**ICS**) approach was created in 2022 to support communication between professionals and partners across health and social care services. The aim of the integrated care system approach was to focus on prevention, improve outcomes for individuals and reduce long-term health inequalities. (NHS England, 2022). These will help to increase the opportunity individuals have to access good quality healthcare in their times of need, and as people are living longer with health conditions, the demand for services will only continue to increase.

There are **42 Integrated Care Systems** in England, made up of NHS organisations, local councils, the voluntary sector and social care in each area.

- Each ICS runs a committee called an **Integrated Care Partnership** (**ICP**) who work with local providers in sectors such as housing, education and employment with the aim to improve health and wellbeing in local areas. All ICPs have a role to develop a long-term strategy to support this and work alongside other services to enable this strategy to be implemented.

- Each ICS area also has an **Integrated Care Board** (**ICB**) who implement and oversee a five-year plan, including the budget, to ensure the NHS can contribute to the ICP long-term strategy effectively.

Resources

Each ICS ensures they have the resources necessary to implement their strategy through partnerships working with local services. This ensures that specialists are working in their area of expertise and that individuals are receiving all-round support to improve their lives. This could include support from the NHS with a health condition, support from social care regarding housing and financial support as well as support from employment services to improve their prospects.

In order to increase their pool of resources, two trusts can bring together their resources to work in multiple places, therefore increasing the range of professionals available for individuals in those areas. This happens particularly with acute health care and mental health support.

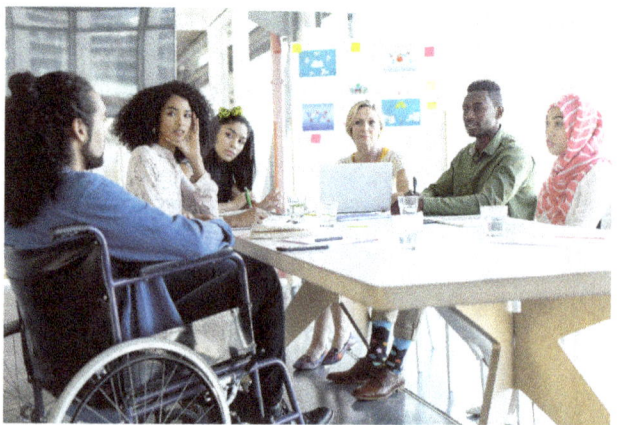

Sharing information

As with all partnerships of professionals working together, information sharing is vitally important. By sharing information effectively, ICSs can:

- Reduce variation in the services provided, ensuring equality for all,
- Provide mutual aid,
- Ensure consolidation of services to prevent replication, providing better outcomes for all.

(NHS England, 2022)

There may be difficulties when sharing information across these teams. This could be due to:

- Time available and working hours,
- The variation of job roles and responsibilities across the team,
- The variation in priorities among members of the team.

These could make it difficult for decisions to be made across the teams and lead to disagreements and animosity. It would be the role of the ICP to ensure all those involved are working towards achieving the long-term strategy to support the needs of the local community.

If working together in these partnerships is ineffective, it could lead to:

- Poor relationships between professionals,
- A lack of collaborative working,
- Individuals not having their needs met,
- Individuals losing confidence in professionals, therefor affecting their ability to work together.

Local availability

There are 42 integrated care systems across England.

Activity

Use the following link to see where your local Integrated Care System and Integrated Care Board is.

https://www.england.nhs.uk/integratedcare/integrated-care-in-your-area/

Now find out the following information:

1. Who is the chair of your local ICS?
2. Who is the CEO of your local ICS?
3. Who is the ICP chair?

Click on the link for the most local ICB and make a note of:

- The local areas they cover.
- At least 5 areas from their long-term plan.

Click on the link for the most local ICS and make a note of:

- At least one key priority they focussed on.
- When the next ICP meeting is and when the last one was held. What was one key priority from the last meeting?

Working with others

When supporting individuals in care environments, including their own home, it is vital for professionals to work with others who may support an individual. This could include:

- Family members
- Friends
- Advocates
- Legal representatives

It is important for professionals to recognise the contribution of other people in the lives of an individual they are working with to ensure they are working together for the good of all.

Developing good working relationships with others can help to reduce stress and anxiety on the individual and could result in a decrease in the replication of work, such as personal care responsibilities for example. It could also ensure the professionals receive important pieces of information that can lead to more effective support being given. For example a friend or family member may relay information about:

- a fall the night before

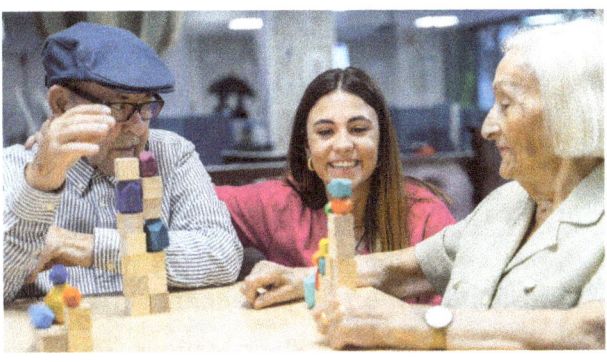

- how a particular medication is causing side effects, which the individual themselves may not communicate,

This can lead to the care environment being adapted to suit as much as possible.

Recap questions

1. What does ICS stand for?
2. What is the role of the Integrated Care Partnerships?
3. Why might it be difficult to find an appropriate care environment for a very young child?

End of Topic Practice Activity

Carol is 30 years old and has a genetic heart condition which will get progressively worse. She is married and has one child but lives far away from any other family members, after moving away for work. She needs to attend regular check-ups at the hospital with specialist cardiologists and also attends regular GP appointments. She cannot drive and her husband is often busy with work. She has visited Accident and Emergency department of the hospital a number of times in the last few years, due to issues being brought on by stress.

Choose **one** of the following local services that could support Carol:

- Acute care
- General practice clinic
- Pharmacy

Then complete the following:

- Explain the purpose of your chosen service and the roles of the professionals within them to meet Carol's needs.
- Describe what factors may impact on Carol's ability to access the chosen service. These factors must relate specifically to Carol.
- Assess what impact each of these factors have on providing services to Carol, and the challenges of giving care that meets her specific needs. Remember to think carefully about Carol's circumstances.
- Evaluate the challenges the service may face when trying to give care to Carol in appropriate, safe and well-maintained environments, and how these could be overcome.

This practice task will help you prepare for the following assessment criteria:

A.P1 Explain the purpose of health and social care services and how they meet the needs of two individuals.

A.P2 Describe the factors that may contribute to service provision and influence the care received by two individuals.

A.M1 Assess the impact of factors on service provision and the potential challenges to providing appropriate care to meet the needs of two individuals.

A.D1 Evaluate the challenges of providing an appropriate care environment for two individuals.

Learning Aim B: Explore aspects of legislation, regulations and policies that support safe environments in health and social care settings

B1 The influence of legislation and policies on safe practice

It is important that all current legislation is followed to ensure safe practice in all health and social care settings. For this to happen, it is essential that all professionals are up to date with current legislation and that they are supported by those in charge to fulfil their roles.

Core legislation

The Care Act 2014

The **Care Act 2014** helps to ensure that local authorities maintain the independence and wellbeing of individuals. The Act ensures that local authorities uphold their responsibilities to provide and arrange services for individuals needing care and support.

In order for local authorities to fulfil their responsibilities to the Care Act 2014, they need to:

- Understand what services and facilities are available in the area,
- Identify people in the area who might have needs that aren't being met,
- Identify carers in the area who might have needs that aren't being met. (Gov.UK, 2019)

There are six principles of safeguarding embedded within the Care Act 2014:

Empowerment – To support and encourage individuals to make decisions for themselves.

Prevention – To take action before harm occurs.

Proportionality – To take the least intrusive response to risks presented.

Protection – To support and protect individuals in greatest need.

Partnership – To promote local solutions and encourage partnerships within communities.

Accountability – To promote transparency to hold all professionals accountable.

(Social Care Institute for Excellence, 2024)

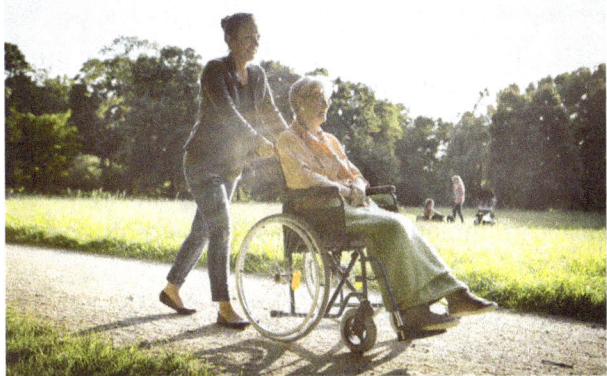

Candour – Being honest and telling the truth.

Health and Social Care Act 2008

The main role of the **Health and Social Care Act 2008** was to create a central regulator which could inspect health and adult social care services, to hold them to account and ensure a minimum standard of care is met. This role was given to the Care Quality Commission (CQC) who aim to uphold 14 fundamental standards across health and social care (Care Quality Commission, 2024). These are:

- Person-centred care
- Visiting and accompanying
- Dignity and respect
- Consent
- Safety
- Safeguarding from abuse
- Food and drink
- Premises and equipment
- Complaints
- Good governance
- Staffing
- Fit and proper staff
- Duty of candour
- Display ratings

When the CQC inspects a health and social care service, these are the areas where judgements are made. This helps to ensure that all services and professionals are held to the same high standards and that meaningful judgements can be made regarding the effectiveness of a service. The reports and judgements made by the CQC are made available to the public to enable individuals to make positive choices when choosing where to receive care.

Children and Families Act 2014

The **Children and Families Act 2014** was introduced to protect and safeguard the rights of children under the age of 18 years, as well as their families. It is particularly important to protect the rights of vulnerable children, such as those with special educational needs and disabilities. This helps to ensure those who are more vulnerable have the support they need to make use of and adapt to care, legal services and education. This includes making Education, Health and Care Plans more accessible and easier to implement, such as by using a single assessment process.

This act also works to support the needs of families going through separation or the needs of children living in care or are about to leave care. This act helps to hold professionals and the government accountable for the outcomes of these children and recognises where changes need to occur.

The ten most important parts of the Children and Families Act 2014 are:

- Adoption and contract
- Family justice
- Children with special educational needs and disabilities
- Childcare Act
- The welfare of children
- The children's commissioner
- Statutory rights to leave and pay
- Time off work
- Rights to request flexible working
- General provisions

(Webster, 2022)

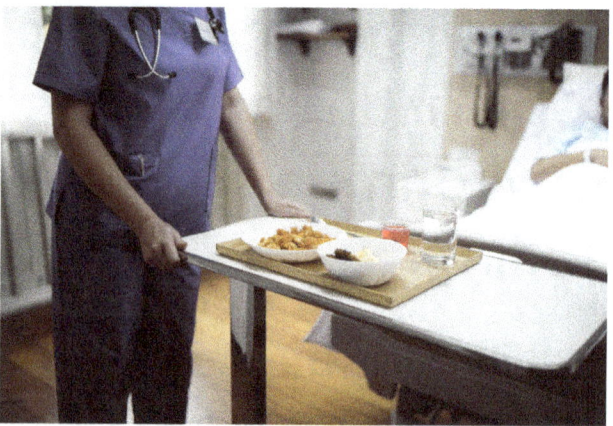

Activity

Look again at the Care Quality Commission 14 fundamental standards. Choose five of the standards and explain the kinds of things the CQC are looking for in these areas during their inspections. Think about:

- What would be a good way for professionals to show this?
- What might poor practice look like?
- The roles of professionals, managers and service users in upholding the standard.

Recap questions

1. Name two principles of safeguarding from the Care Act 2014.
2. How many fundamental standards do the CQC aim to uphold within health and social care services?
3. Why was the Children and Families Act 2014 introduced?

Control of Substance Hazardous to Health 2002 (COSHH)

The **COSHH regulations** were put in place to ensure that any substances that may be hazardous to health are stored and used in a way to limit the risk to those working with these substances, as well as people around them. In health and social care services, this could mean patients in a hospital, residents in a care home or visitors to a setting for example.

Examples of substances that could be hazardous to health include:

- Paint
- Cleaning products
- Blood or waste
- Medications

If these are not stored, disposed of or used in a safe manner, it could lead to the spread of infections, allergic reactions or injuries.

COSHH regulations ensure that employers and those working with these substances:

- Have risk assessed the use of the substance.
- Have assessed whether it is the best substance to use, is there a safer one?
- Are trained in how to use them safely and how to minimise the risk of harm.
- Know where the safest place to store the substances – usually a locked cupboard away from vulnerable individuals.
- Know to always keep these substances in their original container, to reduce the risk of contamination and have the information printed on the label to hand if needed.
- Understand what to do in the event of an emergency using this substance.

(Health and Safety Executive, 2019)

Manual Handling Operations Regulations 1992 (MHOR)

There may be many times within health and social care services where manual handling is needed. For example, this could be:

- To lift an individual out of a wheelchair.
- To sit an individual up in bed.
- To lift an individual who has fallen.
- To put a mobility aid into a vehicle.
- To move equipment needed to support an individual.

The **MHOR (1992)** issues a rank order to follow when considering the use of manual handling procedures. These are:

First – try to avoid manual handling as much as possible. If it isn't needed, don't use it.

> Safeguard – A measure taken to protect someone.
> Accountable – To be able to justify their actions.
> Induction – A formal introduction to a new role or job.

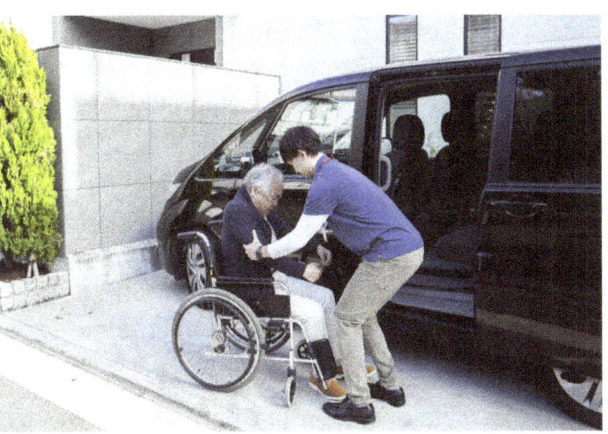

Second – make an assessment of any manual handling that may need to take place – what might the risks be?

Third – use the techniques as directed, following all procedures to minimise the risk of harm.

(Health and Safety Executive, 2018)

The regulations state that all employers need to complete a risk assessment for any manual handling operations that may need to take place in a particular service or setting. These should then be shared with employees during their induction or continued training to ensure they can undertake these tasks safely. This will help to protect vulnerable individuals, the employees themselves, and the employer.

Recap questions

1. What does COSHH stand for?
2. Name three of the CQC fundamental standards.
3. When might manual handling be needed?

Health and Safety at Work Act 1974

The **Health and Safety at Work Act 1974** is what most of the health and safety policies within workplaces are based on. It helps to give employers the guidance they need regarding what they need to do to protect everyone who enters their setting, and how to manage this on a day-to-day basis. It also helps to outline the different responsibilities of individuals, depending on their role. For example:

- It ensures employers know what their responsibilities are to prevent accident and injuries for their employees and everyone who visits. This could include creating policies, giving training and maintaining the building to prevent accidents.

- It also sets out the role of employees in protecting themselves and everyone who visits. This could include following their training and the policies, cleaning up spills, reporting trip hazards, and ensuring people sign in and out of the building.

(Health and Safety Executive, 2024)

The Act supports employees of health and social care services as they will be aware of their responsibilities and can use this to support the daily tasks they take part in. This can also be used by employees to report incidents to the employers when things aren't being done the way they should, which can then reduce the chance of accidents and increase safe ways of working.

This act can also support individuals using health and social care services as it helps to keep them safe, whether they are service users or visitors, to help them understand what they should expect from the professionals and how to report incidents if they occur.

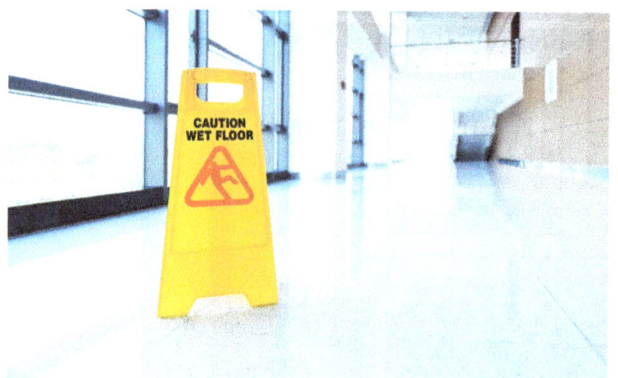

Management of Health and Safety Regulations 1999

The **Management of Health and Safety Regulations 1999** work alongside the Health and Safety at Work Act 1974 and require all employees, including those of health and social care organisations to create and manage a workplace that is safe for all.

One of the main ways to do this is for employers to assess and manage any risks that may arise and reduce or remove the chances of this happening. The process to achieve this is as follows:

Identify the hazards – Employers need to do this by looking around the area used for specific tasks, considering the size of the space and the state of the area. They should also consider whether hazardous substances are used in the space and observe working practices that occur there, recognising the hazards that may occur.

Assess the risks – Once potential hazards have been identified, assessing the risks might include who might be at risk, how the risk can be mitigated and who needs to take control of that role.

Control the risks – Once the risk has been identified, employers should explore whether the task or activity needs to exist or are there alternative ways to complete a task with less risk. This could include completing a task in a different space or using different equipment for example.

Record the findings – Any particularly notable risks identified will need to be recorded to reduce the risk of harm and ensure action is taken when needed. This could include a risk assessment and plan of action. This forms part of the Regulations for any services which employ five or more people, and also includes the reporting that occur due to any serious incidents.

Review the controls – Once risk assessments have been created and the actions implemented, it is important that these are reviewed. This is to ensure that positive changes are being made and that any control measures are actually reducing risk and hazards. If it is found that this is not happening, it will give the employer evidence to make changes to the risk assessment and perhaps adapt the roles of employees.

(Health and Safety Executive, 2019)

Identifying risks in health and social care environments

The best way to identify risks in a health and social care environment is through completing risk assessments. A **risk assessment** helps to make everyone aware of the potential risks that could occur and what action may need to be taken to minimise these.

There are some key details a risk assessment should include, such as:

- The name of the company/service,
- The date the assessment was carried out,
- Who the risk assessment was carried out by,
- The date the risk assessment should be reviewed,
- The potential hazards,
- What is being done to reduce the risk and what else could be done,
- Who could be at risk of harm,
- Whose responsibility it would be to take action regarding the hazard.

Risk assessments will be used to enable health and social care services to fulfil the requirements of the Health and Safety at Work Act (1974) and the Management of Health and Safety Regulations (1999). This is because it gives employers an opportunity to identify, assess, control, record findings and review controls put in place regarding different hazards and make everyone aware of these.

Reporting of injuries, diseases and dangerous occurrences regulations 2013 (RIDDOR)

RIDDOR is a law that makes certain that reports and made and records are kept when:

- An individual dies or is injured at a workplace
- People are diagnosed with a reportable illness
- A dangerous occurrence has happened (HSE, 2013)

The reports made would need to be shared with the relevant individuals to ensure action can take place. This could be the local authority where an incident happens or the Health and Safety Executive.

Mitigated – Making something bad less severe.
Implemented – To put a decision or plan into action.
Dangerous occurrence – An incident with the potential to cause serious harm.

Recap questions

1. How can professionals control the risks?
2. How can the Health and Safety at Work Act 1974 support employers?

Examples of injuries that need to be recorded and reported include:

- Death
- Injuries that affect their ability to work and get around for more than 7 days
- Diseases that have occurred due to the working environment
- Injuries to 'other' people in the service – such as visitors. (HSE, 2013)

Personal Protective Equipment at Work Regulations 1992

Personal Protective Equipment (**PPE**) is defined as 'all equipment intended to be worn...at work which protects the person against one or more risks....' (HSE.gov.uk).

Examples of PPE include:

- Shoe covers
- Face covers
- Eye protection/goggles
- Overalls
- Gloves
- Respirators

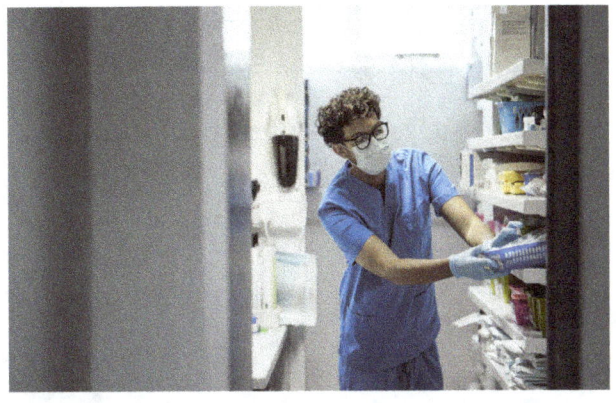

The regulations state that the use of PPE should be a last resort, and that all other possibilities to eliminate the risk should be taken into consideration first. The following controls need to be considered, in this order:

- Elimination – can the risk be completely eliminated?
- Substitution – can the hazardous product/idea be replaced with something else?
- Engineering controls – can the risk be isolated from individuals to reduce risk?
- Administrative controls – Can the regulations and processes be changed to adapt the way people work?
- PPE – if no other options are available, use PPE to protect individuals as much as possible. (HSE.gov.uk).

When the Health and Safety Executive inspect different services, the use of PPE and strategies used to prevent hazards form part of the investigation. They can then give actions and advice to services if they see poor practice being used to improve the care given to vulnerable individuals. It is then the responsibility of employers to take reasonable steps to implement these actions and create a safe environment for employees and vulnerable individuals.

> Ailments – An illness, usually a minor one.

Recap questions

1. What does RIDDOR stand for?
2. What does it mean to 'identify the hazards'?
3. In two sentences, summarise the Health and Safety at Work Act 1974.

Apply your understanding

Shaun is the manager of a residential home in Yorkshire. It cares for 24 service users at a time, some with dementia, some with other ailments, but all are elderly and vulnerable. The building is quite old and often has leaks from windows or the roof, and the kitchen is right next to the sitting area that the residents spend quite a lot of time in. There are stairs and a stair lift and some of the rooms have a bathroom, some have a shared bathroom. There is an outside space but the home is on a main road, limiting the time residents can spend outdoors. The home has always had a good number of staff, but recently there have been shortages.

Complete a risk assessment for Shaun for the residential home. What could the hazards be? What strategies could be used and who would do those?

What are the hazards?	Who might be harmed and how?	What are you already doing to control the risks?	What further actions do you need to take to control the risks?	Who needs to carry out the action?	When is the action needed by?	Done

Legislation relevant to promoting the rights of all individuals

Human Rights Act 1998

The **European Convention on Human Rights** was created to protect the human rights of all countries who are part of the European Council. From this, the Human Rights Act 1998 was created to bring the rules of the convention into British Law and ensure they were upheld for all people in the UK.

In this Act, each right is seen as an 'article', and these are listed below:

- Article 1: States must secure the rights of the convention
- Article 2: Right to life
- Article 3: Freedom from torture and inhuman or degrading treatment
- Article 4: Freedom from slavery or forced labour
- Article 5: Right to liberty and security
- Article 6: Right to a fair trial
- Article 7: No punishment without law
- Article 8: Respect for your private family life, home and correspondence
- Article 9: Freedom of thought, belief and religion
- Article 10: Freedom of expression
- Article 11: Freedom of assembly and association
- Article 12: Right to marry and start a family
- Article 13: Right to an effective remedy
- Article 14: Protection from discrimination in respect of these rights and freedoms

(Equality and Human Rights Commission, 2018)

The **Human Rights Act 1998** helps to ensure that all individuals in the UK are treated fairly and protected from harm. This ensures that all public services work to uphold the rights of individuals, such as hospitals or government agencies, therefore supporting the health and wellbeing of all. This could support the health and wellbeing of vulnerable individuals in particular as they will have the care and support needed, and professionals working with them will understand their role and how to put this into practice.

> **Degrading** – Causing someone to lose self-respect and feel humiliated or disrespected

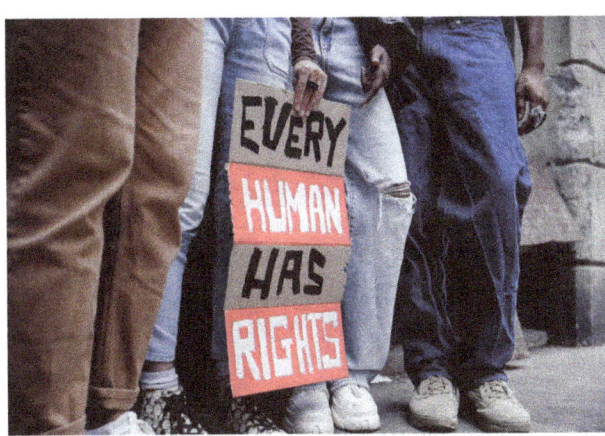

Equality Act 2010

The **Equality Act 2010** aims to protect all individuals who may be subject to discrimination based on protected characteristics. The nine **protected characteristics** are:

- Age
- Disability
- Gender reassignment
- Marriage and civil partnership
- Pregnancy and maternity
- Race
- Religion or belief
- Sex
- Sexual orientation.

The act protects these individuals by making the law easier to understand and informs people what they should be protected from. The act brought together many previous legislations and acts, including:

- The Equal Pay Act 1970
- The Sex Discrimination Act 1975
- The Race Relations Act 1976
- The Disability Discrimination Act 1995
- The Employment Equality (Religion or Belief) Regulations 2003

- The Employment Equality (Sexual Orientation) Regulations 2003
- The Employment Equality (Age) Regulations 2006
- The Equality Act 2006
- The Equality Act (Sexual Orientation) Regulation 2007

The Equality Act helps to promote the rights of all individuals by creating a safe environment for individuals to be themselves and have a fair chance at things such as employment, leisure activities and relationships. This would support positive health and wellbeing, such as promoting opportunities for progression and education and supporting positive self-worth and confidence.

Mental Health Act 2007

The **Mental Health Act 2007** defines a mental health disorder as 'any disorder or disability of the mind'. (NHS, 2018) This could include anxiety disorders, eating disorders or depression and can be used for any individuals, regardless of their age.

The Act helps individuals dealing with poor mental health to have a good understanding of their rights and be able to access the help and support they need. This act makes clear that individuals can be admitted, detained and treated in hospital without their consent if professionals feel there is a need to safeguard them from harm. Professionals may use their powers to do this if they feel the individual is at risk of harming themselves or to protect the public from risk of harm. Once detained, individuals will be able to receive treatment to enable them to return to making informed decisions for themselves.

Admitted – Allow someone to enter a place such as a hospital.

Detained – To keep someone in a place to support them.

Advocate – Someone, usually a professional, who speaks on behalf of a vulnerable individual.

Mental Capacity Act 2017

The intention of the Mental Capacity Act 2017 is to empower individuals over 16 years old who do not have the mental capacity to make their own decisions and to ensure they are protected. These decisions could include financial decisions, decisions about care or treatment and decisions about who they want supporting them. However, just because an individual may struggle with one type of decision, it doesn't mean they will struggle with them all. This means professionals will need to assess vulnerable individuals on a case-by-case basis to ensure the rights of all are upheld.

An advocate could be useful here to support an individual to make decisions and to help them to understand the choices available to them. They could also help other professionals to see things from the individual's point of view and give them confidence to be honest.

There are many reasons why individuals may lack the mental capacity to make decisions about their care. These include:

- People who have had a stroke
- People who have been diagnosed with dementia
- People who are unconscious
- People with poor mental health

(NHS, 2024)

Here are the guidelines of the Mental Capacity Act 2017:

- Professionals need to assume a person has the mental capacity to make decisions until proven otherwise.
- Professionals should help individuals to make decisions when possible.
- Professionals must not assume an individual lacks capacity just because they make a decision using poor judgement.
- If professionals need to make decisions for an individual, it must be in the individual's best interests.

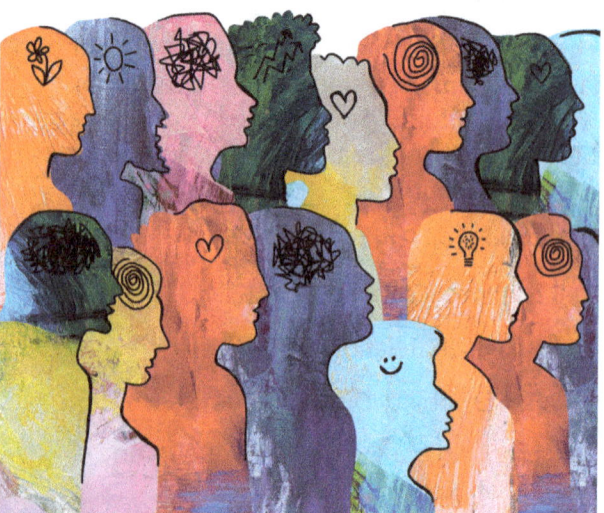

- Any decisions made need to be the least restrictive possible.

(NHS, 2024)

If the guidelines are followed, it would ensure that individuals lacking mental capacity are kept safe, but also that their needs and wishes are understood. Independent advocates would be able to confirm that their best interests had been a followed and that they haven't been discriminated against.

> **Recap questions**
>
> 1. What age of individuals does the Mental Capacity Act 2017 support?
> 2. Name four protected characteristics.
> 3. The Mental Capacity Act 2007 says that individuals can be admitted, _____ and _____ against their will.

> **Activity**
>
> Research the Mental Capacity Act 2017. Find out the following pieces of information:
>
> - How will professionals know whether a person can make their own decisions? What might be done to find out?
> - Who might act as an advocate?
> - Why might an individual's ability to make decisions for themselves change over time?

B2 How a duty of care contributes to safe practice

A duty of care is a 'legal obligation to provide a reasonable standard of care .... and act in ways that protect their safety', (Chartered Society of Physiotherapy, 2020). This contributes to safe practice in many ways as it ensures professionals are aware of their roles and responsibilities and will promote the welfare of vulnerable individuals at all times.

Legal obligation to protect wellbeing and prevent harm

All professionals working in health and social care should understand their **legal obligation to protect the wellbeing and welfare** of individuals using their services. Doing this helps to uphold their physical, mental and emotional health.

Upholding the rights and promoting the interests of vulnerable individuals

To uphold individuals' rights means to ensure they have control over their own lives and are not discriminated against or treated negatively based on factors such as their age or ability.

This serves as a reminder that the Human Rights Act 1998 applies to all, meaning that professionals need to ensure vulnerable individuals have a right to life and a right to marry and have a private life for example. Wherever possible, individuals need to be able to do these, albeit with support from professionals.

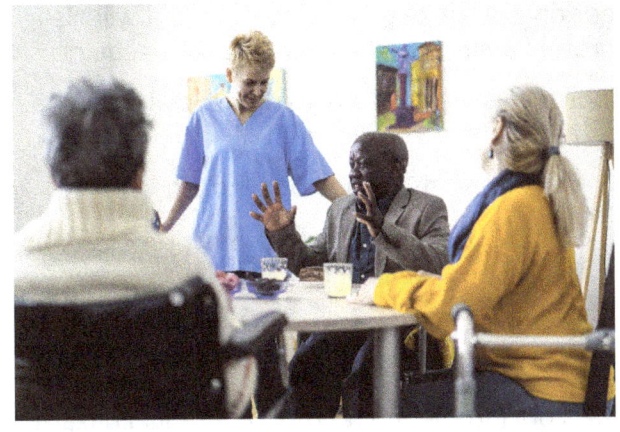

In order to promote the interests of vulnerable individuals, it is important that professionals build up a good relationship with the individual. This could be through informal conversations or working on activities together. If a good relationship is built up, professionals will be able to have a good understanding of:

- Their likes
- Their dislikes

- What they want to happen with their care
- Who they trust or like
- Their concerns and worries

By understanding these, professionals can promote their interests through creating activities they know they would enjoy and support them in creating friendships with others with similar interests. Also, by building good relationships, professionals can help them to explore and enjoy new things which can support their development.

Professionals can also promote their interests by discussing what they want to happen with their care. If a vulnerable individual feels comfortable, they will open up about their feelings. This can be shared in multi-agency meetings with other professionals, so that individuals' interests are made paramount. This will create a safe environment for individuals, helping to build up confidence and trust in others.

Protecting health, safety and wellbeing

If professionals show a duty of care, it can **protect the health, safety and wellbeing of vulnerable individuals**. Professionals in all health and social care services and beyond have a legal obligation to prevent harm coming to any individuals in their care such as from accidents, injuries, abuse or illness. By doing this not only will it keep individuals safe, it will also protect their mental and emotional wellbeing.

Individuals' health, safety and wellbeing can be protected by professionals:

- Following their code of conduct.
- Undergoing training to protect physical and emotional wellbeing.
- Building up trusting relationships with vulnerable individuals.
- Looking for and reporting potential hazards.
- Following safeguarding and health and safety policies and procedures.
- Having a good understanding of the needs of individuals requiring care.

Protecting health, safety and wellbeing contributes to safe practice as it will instil a culture of positive, effective working, where individuals will trust professionals and want to work with them. Showing a duty of care should be a collective effort of all professionals, who all have the same obligations.

Duty of candour

Professionals showing a **duty of candour** means a professional has a duty to be transparent and open with the individuals they are supporting (NHS, 2022).

A duty of candour is one of the CQC standards, which shows it is an important aspect of healthcare.

The CQC (2022) explain that it is the responsibility of the health and social care provider to ensure their service operates with the utmost concern for others, and that they ensure there is a culture of openness and transparency across all roles. This includes all professionals, including those working with service users directly, those working behind the scenes, such as kitchen staff, and managers. This will ensure staff know they can be open and honest with other staff and management, as well as with individuals and their families.

Being open and honest with individuals is a legal obligation professionals must uphold this, however, this can also support the relationships between service providers and individuals who feel they have not been treated appropriately. If an individual and their family receive a meaningful apology when poor treatment has been given, this can go a long way to repairing relationships and securing changes for the future.

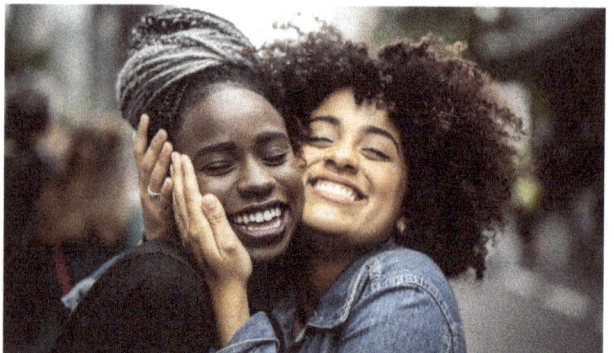

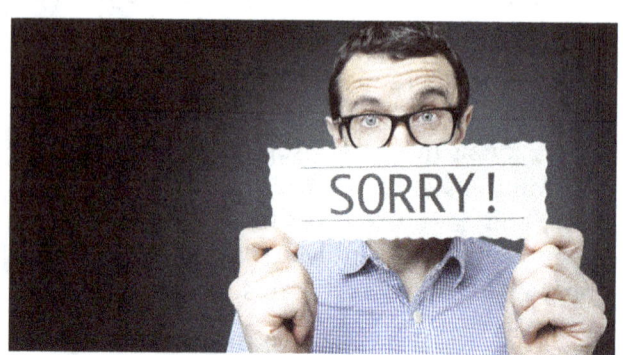

The CQC requires that all notifiable incidents are dealt with through showing a duty of candour. A notifiable incident is when it meets all of the following 3 criteria:

- The result was unexpected or unintended
- It occurs during an activity the CQC regulate, such as surgery, diagnostic assessments, treatment for an illness or personal care
- This has or might result in death, or moderate or severe harm.

(Care Quality Commission, 2022)

If a notifiable incident occurs, it is the duty of the health and social care services to show a duty of candour. This might include:

- Apologising for the treatment of an individual.
- Being clear and honest about the potential outcome and the reasons for this.
- Liaising with other services who might have been included in the incident.
- Being clear about all the options an individual now has.
- Making clear the changes that will now be made following this negative outcome.

Multi-agency – Professionals from different services or agencies working together to support an individual.

Paramount – More important than anything else.

Liaising – To cooperate on a specific matter.

Transparent – Making sure everything can be seen.

Legal obligation – A duty to do something as required by law.

Recap questions

1. What is multi-agency team working?
2. How do we know whether an incident is a 'notifiable incident'?
3. How can professionals show a duty of candour?

If a duty of candour is shown, it will support professionals in upholding their duty of care and ensure safe practice. This is because they will be aware of how their actions impact the health of vulnerable individuals and will know their responsibilities within this. They will also work to protect the safety of individuals and hold others to account through openness and transparency.

Apply your understanding

Look at the following scenarios. Assess whether you think these fall into the category of 'notifiable incidents' as described above.

An individual is taking medication that is known to cause low mood and increase the chance of developing depression. This is shared with the individual at the time of prescribing, but the individual decided that the benefits of taking the medication outweighed the risks. Now the individual has been suffering from extreme depression and recently tried to take their own life.

Is this a notifiable incident? Explain your reasons.

An individual was having dental surgery and the dental surgeon was unaware that the individual was allergic to latex gloves. The individual then had a severe anaphylactic reaction and spent some time in hospital afterwards.

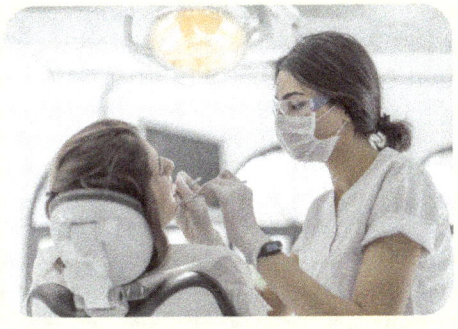

Is this a notifiable incident? Explain your reasons.

Maintaining expected standards of care

It is important that all professionals in health and social care understand their roles and responsibilities when it comes to the care they provide. All professionals need to be aware of the minimum standards of care expected in their profession and strive to do even better than this; the better the standard of care given, the better the outcomes for the individuals using the service.

It is important to be aware that all professionals need to maintain the expected standard of care regardless of their role within a service, such as care workers or practice managers. Seniority and experience, or lack of thereof, does not exclude a professional from maintaining positive care standards, as this is expected by all.

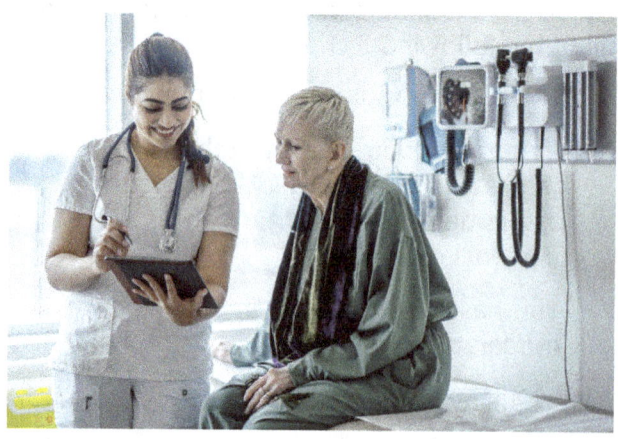

If standards of care are maintained, it can lead to:

- **Good relationships** being built up between the professionals and the individuals using the service.
- Individuals and their families **understanding the care** they can expect to receive.
- Professionals **knowing what their role is** and how to succeed in that role.
- Services being able to **hold professionals accountable** for their actions.
- **Minimal complaints**.
- A **positive culture** around the service.

The Care Quality Commission (CQC) Fundamental Standards

In Learning Aim B1: The Influence of Legislation, you were introduced to the Health and Social Care Act 2008, which was built on the CQC's 14 fundamental standards, but here they are in a little more detail:

1. **Person-centred care**

   This is when services put the individuals using the service at the heart of decision making and they are empowered to make their own choices.

2. **Visiting and accompanying**

   This is when individuals are enabled to have visitors and are able to go and visit other family members, if health allows. This also means that individuals can have someone accompany them to appointments.

3. **Dignity and respect**

   This includes having privacy, being treated equally and individuals having support to remain independent.

4. **Consent**

   This ensures that before treatment is given, the individual or a family member gives their consent.

5. **Safety**

   This is when risks are assessed and any potential hazards in a care environment are dealt with.

6. **Safeguarding from abuse**

   This means that individuals must not suffer any abuse under the care of professionals.

7. **Food and drink**

   This means that individuals must have enough food and drink to stay healthy while in the care of professionals.

8. **Premises and equipment**

   This means that the buildings and areas where care is given must be clean and free from hazards.

9. **Complaints**

   This means that there must be a complaints procedure in place and if a complaint is made, it should be thoroughly investigated.

10. **Good governance**

    This means that services must have senior staff in charge who are aware of their responsibilities and have plans to meet the standards of care needed.

11. **Staffing**

    This means there must be the appropriate number of staff within services who are trained and competent to do the job.

12. **Fit and proper staff**

    This means that all checks must be made before hiring staff, to ensure they are capable of the job they are being employed to do and that they will not cause harm, such as Disclosure and Barring Service (DBS) checks.

13. **Duty of candour**

    This means to ensure services work in a transparent and open way regarding an individual's care.

14. **Display ratings**

    This means that all services must provide their CQC rating in the building and on the website so individuals can make informed decisions about their care.

Being part of the Health and Social Care Act 2008 means these standards are now a legal obligation for professionals in health and care services to abide by. When the CQC complete inspections of services, they are judged against these 14 standards and given a rating, which is to be displayed. This will give individuals looking for services the information they need to make informed decisions about whether they accept care from that particular service, or whether they look elsewhere. These inspections will help to ensure the standards expected of the service are upheld and maintained over time and that the professionals leading these services are aware of what to do to support their staff in doing this.

Care Certificate Standard 3

The **Care Certificate Standards** help to ensure that people in professional roles have the skills and knowledge to offer high-quality care to all who need it. There are 15 of these standards, developed by Skills for Care and Health Education England, which should be adhered to and included as part of an induction package for new professionals. This means they will be informed of these standards at a very early stage in their career to enable them to incorporate them into their positive working culture.

The 15 standards in the Care Certificate are as follows:

Induction – Prepare someone for a role/position.

Recap questions

1. What could happen if standards of care are not maintained?
2. Why is it important that services uphold the CQC standard of 'Display Ratings'?

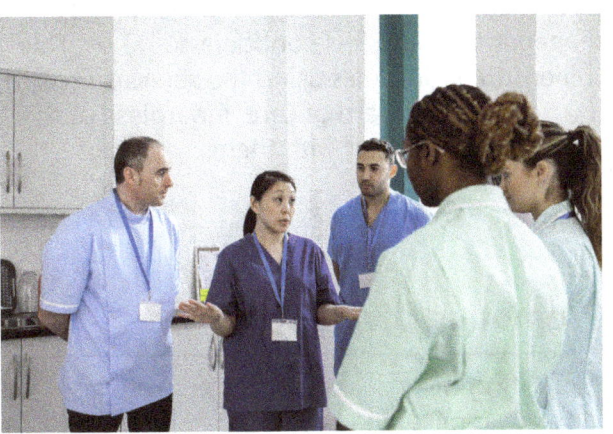

- Understanding your role
- Your personal development
- Duty of care
- Equality and Diversity
- Working in a person-centred way
- Communication
- Privacy and dignity
- Fluids and nutrition
- Awareness of mental health, dementia and learning disability
- Safeguarding adults
- Safeguarding children
- Basic life support
- Health and safety
- Handling information
- Infection prevention and control

(Skills for Care, 2015)

Standard 3: Duty of care, helps to maintain expected standards of care. This is because it encompasses important information that a professional can use throughout their work, right from the beginning. This can help them to maintain their own professional standards as they will have understood the expectations clearly and how to deal with complaints, incidents and difficult situations, as well as the importance of equality and how to work in an inclusive way.

When all professionals follow this standard, it can ensure there is a culture of maintaining positive standards of care, that helps to keep individuals safe from harm, abuse or injury. This is because professionals will be held accountable for their actions in regard to this standard, and professionals will feel supported to uphold these positive ways of working by management, and feel confident to do so. This will ensure individuals using the services receive a consistent standard of care, regardless of the professional working with them.

Safer recruitment processes

Promoting diversity

Promoting diversity means to remove bias, raise awareness, and have clear policies and procedures to prevent discrimination.

- It can support safer recruitment processes as it means all professionals will feel able and empowered to apply for jobs within their skill set, recognising they will be treated equally regardless of their race, gender, sexual orientation or religious beliefs for example.

- It can also protect the wellbeing of the professionals and also show individuals using the services that diversity is celebrated. For example, if an individual from a specific culture felt uncomfortable accessing services, seeing that they are promoting diversity will help the individual to feel more positive about asking for support, which will lead to more positive health outcomes in the long term.

The **Equality Act 2010** requires that in any job role, all potential candidates are considered, regardless of whether the protected characteristics are evident. This can ensure fair and equivalent access to all job roles as well as a more diverse workforce, enabling them to offer specialised support as and when needed.

> **Activity**
>
> Choose three of the CQC fundamental standards. For each, explain in detail:
> - How this could be shown/implemented in two different services?
> - The negatives that could occur for service users if the fundamental standard is not upheld.
> - The role of managers and the role of employees in upholding the standard.

Recap questions

1. What can good standards of care lead to?
2. What Act supports the CQC fundamental standards?
3. How many standards are there in the Care Certificate?
4. Why is Standard 3 so important to individuals using services?

Disclosure and Barring Service Regulations (DBS)

The Disclosure and Barring Service came about due to the amalgamation of two other services doing similar things, the Criminal Records Bureau and the Independent Safeguarding Authority. It was thought that this would save money and time in finding out the safety of prospective professionals when working with vulnerable individuals.

Before an individual is offered a job, a DBS check may be applied for. There are four different types of DBS check:

- **Basic DBS certificates** – this shows any unspent convictions and cautions.
- **Standard DBS certificates** – this shows any unspent and spent convictions and cautions.
- **Enhanced DBS certificates** – this shows any unspent and spent convictions and cautions as well as other information relevant from the police.
- **Enhanced DBS checks with barred lists** – this includes everything on the enhanced

DBS certificates, as well as checks on the Barred list. (A guide to DBS checks 2 3, n.d.)

These are applied for by prospective employers to ensure the individuals they are aiming to employ will be safe to work in their service. This will reduce the chances of poor care being given and will ensure vulnerable individuals are not at risk of harm or abuse, helping to maintain expected standards of care.

> Consistent – Something happening in the same way.
>
> Protected characteristics – Specific attributes protected from discrimination.
>
> Equivalent – The same or similar.
>
> Amalgamation – Combining two things together.
>
> Prospective – Something that might happen.
>
> Justified – Given good or legitimate reasons.
>
> Isolation – Being alone.

Balancing the rights of others and a duty of care

It is important to balance an individual's rights and a duty of care when professionals work with vulnerable individuals. This is to ensure the safety of others and prevent conflict in professional relationships. If the rights and a duty of care are balanced, it will lead to good relationships being built as well as the needs of individuals being met.

Balancing the rights of individuals and a duty of care can be achieved through:

Liaising with the individual, the carer and their family when completing risk assessments

It is important when professionals carry out risk assessments that they liaise with the individual involved, their carer and their family. This is important to ensure that the needs of the individual are understood and that any plans put in place to protect them are valid and justified. This will lead to the individual working well with professionals as they will feel understood and the family will be able to offer their own advice due to having a clear idea of their needs and wishes. By liaising with family members, the individual, and their carers, it will help to balance an individual's rights and a duty of care as professionals will know what risks the individuals they are caring for may face and by showing a duty of care, it will help professionals to uphold their rights.

Promoting choice, control and empowerment and enabling service users' ownership of their own care journey

This can be achieved through positive communication and through building a positive relationship with the individuals needing care and support. If individuals are able to make their own choices and feel in control of their own life, they will feel more empowered to discuss what they want and have their rights upheld. This can support professionals to balance their rights and a duty of care by giving them the confidence to take risks with their life to make positive changes, such as taking up new opportunities or developing new relationships.

Protecting the individual without unnecessary restricting their freedom

It is important when making decisions about the care of individuals that the least restrictions possible are put in place. This will help to ensure that individuals are accepting of their care and don't feel that they are being forced into isolation or are unable to take part in activities they are interested in. By listening to the individual, professionals can put in place only the restrictions needed to ensure their safety. This will demonstrate a duty of care, as there will have been lots of things considered to ensure an individual's safety.

Effective communication

It is important that the communication needs of individuals are understood and implemented so that information can be shared effectively, ensuring their rights can be upheld. A duty of care will be shown here by using effective communication skills, such as:

- Makaton
- British sign language
- Enhanced facial signals and gestures
- Using shorter sentences
- Speaking to individuals in a quiet space
- Using the help of an advocate

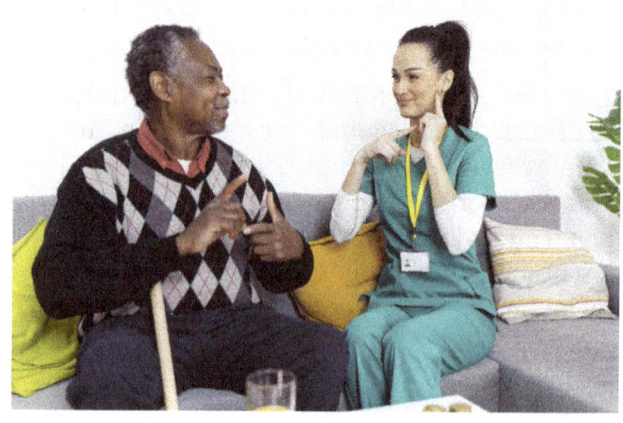

Recap questions

1. What does DBS stand for?
2. Why is it important for professionals to ensure that individuals are empowered to make decisions?
3. Name some examples of effective communication.

Apply your understanding

Fortina Day Centre has found themselves short staffed at short notice. One member of staff has recently left for a new job and two members of staff have gone off sick. This has left the manager panicking and without more staff, the day centre would have to close. The manager has some friends who have shown an interest in the day centre, and she has asked them to help out until she manages to hire more staff. These have not been DBS checked and have not been given copies of any processes and procedures, such as fire evacuation procedures or safeguarding procedures. The children are often left with the workers at the day centre while the parents took part in discussions with health and social care professionals, such as midwives or health visitors.

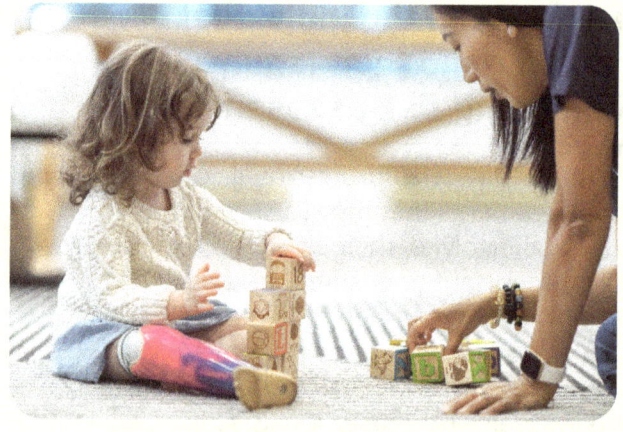

Answer the following questions:

1. What could be the dangers of having volunteers without a DBS check?
2. How could these volunteers make the trained staff feel?
3. What might parents say about this?
4. What might this do to the reputation of the day centre?
5. What should the manager have done to rectify the situation?

B3 Duty of care and working with vulnerable individuals

Applying All Our Health (2022)

All Our Health was created in 2022 to help professionals to understand the needs of individuals more clearly and to ensure wellbeing is being promoted across all services. The aim of this was to provide guidance and recommendations to improve the services professionals offer and provide information for professionals in charge.

In the All Our Health (2022) document, a definition of being vulnerable is given:

'Being vulnerable is defined as in need of special care, support, or protection because of age, disability, risk of abuse or neglect.'

(Office for Health Improvements and Disparities, 2022)

Understanding this definition should help professionals to distinguish between individuals who are vulnerable and those who might not be, in order to prioritise the help and support they are offering. More information is also offered when defining vulnerable adults and vulnerable children.

Risk factors

There are many **risk factors** that can affect whether an individual has more chance of being classed as being vulnerable. This means they have more chance of needing care, support and protection. These risk factors could directly impact the vulnerability of an individual or could be a contributing factor alongside others. Risk factors can be at individual, family and environmental levels.

Individual risk factors include:

- Going through trauma or traumatic injuries
- Genetic conditions
- Learning disabilities
- Alcohol or substance abuse

Family risk factors include:

- Low income
- Poor parenting
- Family size
- Abuse
- Neglect
- Family violence or breakdown

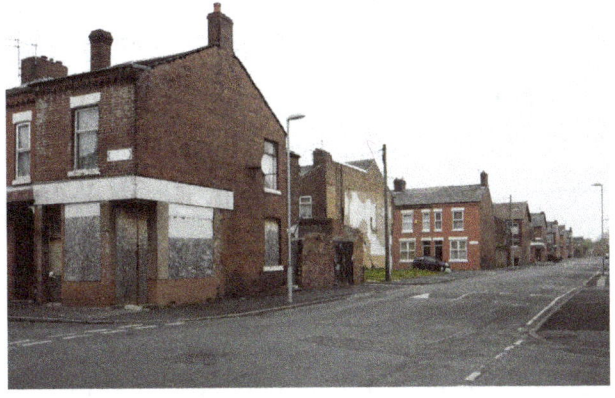

Deprivation is a risk factor for vulnerability

Environmental risk factors include:

- Living in unsafe communities
- Poor social mobility
- Living in a deprived area
- Discrimination
- Difficulties accessing services

(Office for Health Improvements and Disparities, 2022)

Protective factors

Protective factors help to decrease the potential impact of risk factors. Protective factors can therefore reduce the risk of a person becoming vulnerable, improving their independence and life chances. Protective factors can also exist at individual, family and environmental level.

Individual protective factors include:

- Healthy problem-solving skills
- Emotional intelligence
- Having a caring family
- Good communication skills

Family protective factors include:

- Having a stable family
- Having positive relationships
- Having financial security
- Having consistent parenting

Environmental protective factors include:

- Living in a safe environment
- Having good housing
- Having access to resources for hobbies
- Having a sense of belonging

(Office for Health Improvements and Disparities, 2022)

The impact of vulnerability

There are many things that having increased vulnerability can lead to. The longer an issue goes unnoticed or if treatment and support is delayed, the worse the issue can become. This can lead to higher costs to implement intervention. If vulnerability is ignored, it can lead to:

- Social exclusion
- A lack of continuing support
- A potential for repeated impacts of trauma.

(Office for Health Improvement and Disparities, 2022)

The impact of pandemics

When COVID-19 hit the UK in March 2020, no one knew how this would impact their lives. In reality, it led to repeated lockdowns, separation from family, an inability to work and the fear of ill health, which was hard on everyone across the country.

This pandemic, as an example, was even harder on vulnerable individuals. This is because they may have been on the 'shielding list'. This was a list of individuals who were at even more risk of serious illness from COVID-19, and these individuals were given even more restrictions to

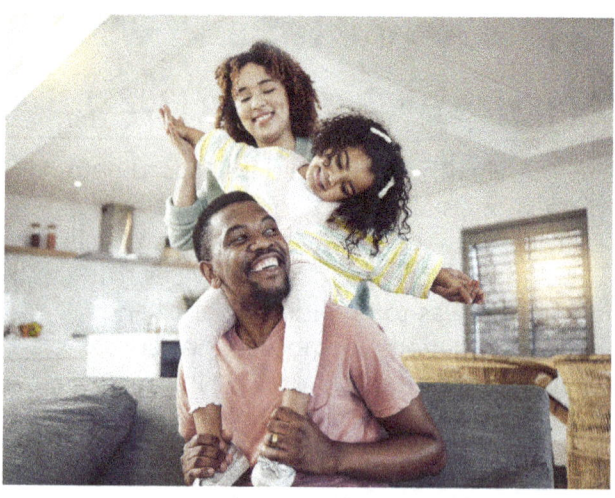

A stable family and consistent parenting is a protective factor for vulnerability

Trauma – A deeply distressing experience.

Social mobility – How a person's socio-economic status changes.

Resilience – The ability to recover quickly from difficult situations.

Recap questions

1. Name two protective factors.
2. Name two risk factors.
3. When was All Our Health guidance created?

follow in their every day life.

For the vulnerable individuals in particular, the impact of the pandemic included:

- Increased levels of loneliness
- Social isolation
- Reduced emotional resilience

Apply your understanding

Jeremy has been diagnosed with heart disease and COPD. He has been overweight for years and this is showing no signs of improving. He is very intelligent, but has recently lost his job due to his health, so is now struggling for money. He lives in a very nice house in a nice neighbourhood with his family, who have been very supportive, however, due to the location of the house, he is struggling to be able to go to all his appointments to improve his health.

1. Explain which risk factors Jeremy is facing and which protective factors would help him the most.

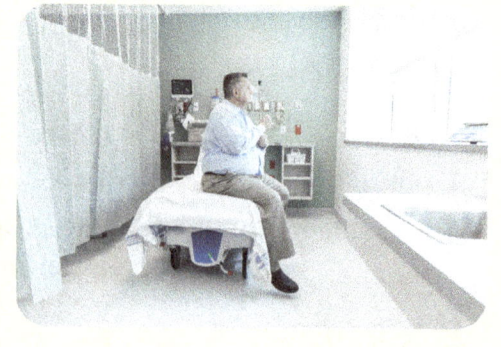

Cultural considerations when working with vulnerable individuals

All professionals need to understand and follow any specific cultural considerations when working with vulnerable individuals. This is to ensure their physical safety as well as maintaining their emotional and mental wellbeing.

Treating individuals with dignity

When professionals work with vulnerable individuals, they need to ensure they **respect their dignity**. This includes making them feel worthy and that their opinions matter, such as what they want to be called and how they want to be treated. Also, it is important that professionals respect the beliefs and culture of individuals so that they feel comfortable to ask for things to support these, such as to celebrate a particular event. Making sure their opinions matter includes following their opinions when it comes to their care, such as who they want to receive their care from and what medication they wish to take.

Professionals having an open, non-judgemental attitude and accepting cultural differences

Professionals need to make sure they have an open, **non-judgemental** attitude, this means that they do not judge others or criticise them for their decisions. If this is evident when professionals are working with vulnerable individuals, it will lead to positive relationships being built as well as professionals feeling able to work with each other in respectful ways. Professionals accepting cultural differences leads to non-discriminatory practice and celebrations and events being used to create a positive environment.

> Non-discriminatory practice – Treating people fairly and in the same way as others.
>
> Dominant – Having power over the others.

Professionals expanding on their own cultural awareness

It is important that professionals working with vulnerable individuals make time to **understand the cultural differences** of the individuals they are caring for. This will help to make sure that professionals have a deeper understanding of the requirements of individuals' cultures and are aware of how to meet the needs of these individuals. This can lead to vulnerable individuals being catered for when it comes to dietary requirements or cultural festivals, outside of the dominant group within the service. If professionals make time to do this, it can show vulnerable individuals that their needs are understood and can create a positive culture within different settings.

Responding to concerns about vulnerable individuals

It is important that when there are concerns about the safety or wellbeing of vulnerable individuals, professionals are aware of their roles and responsibilities to ensure they are protected.

Following organisational policies and procedures

Each different health and social care service will have appropriate policies and procedures to protect the wellbeing of vulnerable individuals. Some of the policies and procedures include:

- Safeguarding
- Health and safety
- Equal opportunities
- Record keeping
- Confidentiality
- First aid

Following these policies and procedures will ensure that professionals are aware of the signs of abuse and neglect or harm that vulnerable individuals may be going through. They will also make sure that when these are noticed, professionals know what to do to protect their wellbeing according to the service type. This will ensure that all professionals in the service are following the same policies and procedures, which will give the individuals confidence in the care they are being given and help the employers to put their faith in the employees to work according to the agreed guidelines.

Report concerns to a senior person in charge

The safeguarding policy will state that concerns need to be reported to a senior person. This is important to reduce the risk of breaking vulnerable individual's confidentiality, which would lead to them no longer sharing important information. Therefore, by sharing vital information with the senior person in charge, it helps to make sure it is only given to others on a 'need to know' basis, and professionals and vulnerable individuals will be sure that the most appropriate intervention is given.

Documenting concerns

Policies such as the safeguarding policy will outline how professionals should document their concerns when they occur. This could include everyday concerns, such as how much an individual has had to eat, or serious safeguarding issues, such as signs and symptoms of abuse.

Concerns should be documented as soon as possible after concerns have been raised. This should be done in the way required by the safeguarding policy of the service and be given to the senior person in charge. Documenting concerns should include:

- The date, location and time of any concerns.
- Basic relevant information about the individual.
- The facts seen – such as any physical marks.
- The facts told – anything the individual has said that leads to concern.
- Any actions taken by professionals to help.
- Any immediate danger the individual might be in.

Make use of whistleblowing policies

Whistleblowing is when professionals report wrongdoing that they see or know about. This can be done regarding things that happen in the past, present, or things they may feel will happen in the future if changes don't happen. Whistleblowing happens when professionals report:

- A criminal offence.
- When someone's health and safety is in danger.
- Damage to the environment.
- A company or service breaking the law.
- When someone is covering up wrongdoing.

All health and social care services need to have whistleblowing policies that professionals are made aware of and have access to. This helps to ensure services and professionals are aware of their accountability to employees and vulnerable individuals, which can lead to positive ways of working.

Recap questions

1. Name two policies and procedures that can help to support vulnerable individuals.
2. What does 'whistleblowing' mean?
3. Why should professionals expand their own cultural awareness?

Activity

Use the internet to look up a health and social care service of your choosing that is local to you, and consider the policies and procedures that will be used in that service

Then complete the following table in as much detail as possible from the information you have found out:

Policy/Procedure	Key points of this in this service	How this can support vulnerable individuals
Safeguarding		
Health and safety		
Equal opportunities		
Record keeping		
Confidentiality		
First aid		

End of Topic Practice Activity

You will be using the same health and social care service that you discussed in the practice activity for Learning Aim A.

Write down your ideas about the following:

- Choose a relevant piece of legislation. How can it support safe practice in your chosen health and social care service?
- How can a duty of care can be shown to protect vulnerable individuals in your chosen health and social care service?
- Can you analyse how legislation and duty of care can ensure safe practice in your chosen service?
- Can you evaluate, using balanced arguments, how effective duty of care and health and safety legislation are at ensuring safe practice in your chosen service?

This practice task will help you prepare for the following assessment criteria:

B.P3 Describe how health and safety legislation supports safe practice in a selected health and social care setting.

B.P4 Describe how duty of care supports safe practice and protects vulnerable individuals in a selected health and social care setting.

B.M2 Analyse how health and safety legislation and duty of care influence safe practice in a health and social care setting.

B.D2 Evaluate the effectiveness of health and safety legislation and duty of care to ensure safe practice in a selected health and social care setting.

Learning Aim C: Examine aspects of monitoring and maintaining safe practice in health and social care environments

C1 Standards setting and regulation of health and social care environments in England

Regulation and standards to measure, monitor and improve quality of care and outcomes

There are many regulations and standards that should be followed by professionals to improve the quality of care given by different services. If these are followed, it will ensure that professionals and employers understand their role and that services are able to offer a sustained quality of care.

Care Quality Commission (CQC)

The **CQC** is an independent regulatory body for the quality and safety of the care delivered in health and social care environments in England.

The CQC:

- Registers
- Monitors
- Inspects
- Rates services

After these have taken place, the CQC take action to ensure improvements are made if necessary and publish their views to enable informed choices to be made by vulnerable individuals and their families. The CQC also outline 15 fundamental standards they expect to be followed to uphold good standards of care, these are outlined in Learning Aim B2. When inspecting services, these are the standards which the CQC make recommendations on and determine their ratings against. Due to this, it helps to improve the quality of care services give to vulnerable individuals as they understand their accountability against these standards, ensuring these are followed and maintained.

(Care Quality Commission, 2023)

Professional regulation

Professional regulators have a responsibility to ensure that professionals within health and social care services are registered with the appropriate regulated body and that they are able to practise in their area of expertise. Each of the nine regulatory bodies should give reassurance to individuals that they will be treated with respect and fairness and that ethical standards will be upheld. If individuals feel they have not been treated in this way, complaints can be made about them to the regulatory body. Whistleblowing by professionals can also be made with these bodies. (NHS employers, 2021)

The regulatory bodies include:

- **General Medical Council (GMC)** - These are the regulatory body for registering doctors in the UK. These ensure doctors maintain professional standards and where doctors fall short, they can place restrictions on their ability to work until improvements have been made. (NHS Employers, 2021)

- **Health and Care Professions Council (HCPC)** - These regulate 15 different health and social care professionals, including chiropodists, occupational therapists, paramedics, physiotherapists and radiographers. The HCPC keeps a register of these professionals and takes action if standards are not met. (NHS Employers, 2021)

- **Nursing and Midwifery Council (NMC)** - These regulate nurses and midwives across the UK as well as nursing associates in England. These promote education amongst these professionals and hold them to account through investigations when issues or complaints arise. (Nursing and Midwifery Council, 2023)

- **Social Work England (SWE)** - These regulate social workers through values and principles that promote collaboration to protect vulnerable individuals. They hold professionals to account against the social work professional standards and promote the use of education and training among its members. (Social Work England, 2024)

Codes of practice

Codes of practice are statements that describe the standards of professional conduct and practice required by professionals across all health and social care services. This helps to give employers confidence that their employees are aware of their role and their duty of care to themselves, other professionals and vulnerable individuals. It also gives professionals a good understanding of what to do in specific situations and who to seek help and guidance from when needed.

There are different codes of practice depending on the role of regulated professionals, but they have common goals. When professionals become part of their regulatory body, they are also agreeing to their codes of conduct. This helps to show their competence in their role by giving professionals opportunities to showcase their abilities.

Codes of practice can help service providers to ensure that the professionals have all the equipment and knowledge to maintain safety and enable revalidation of their registration annually. This is a statutory requirement for these professionals to continue working in their field. (NMC, 2018)

> **Ethical standards** – Principles that promote fairness and trust.

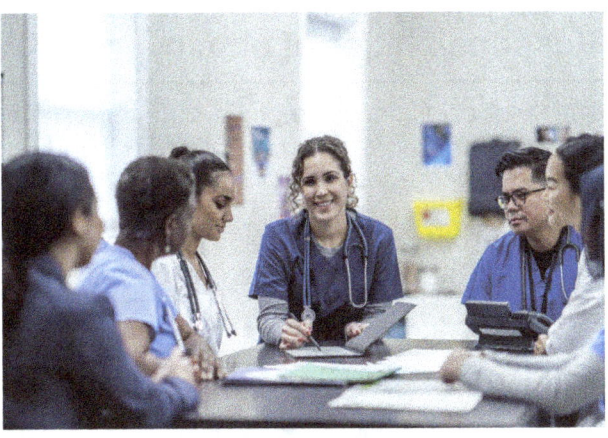

Recap questions

1. Name two of the regulatory bodies.
2. How many fundamental standards does the CQC promote?
3. Why is a code of practice good for employers?

Activity

Choose one of the regulatory bodies discussed above. Complete some research, finding out the following:

- Which professionals does the regulatory body support?
- When was the regulatory body set up?
- How often do professionals need to revalidate their registration?
- What standards are expected of the regulated professionals?

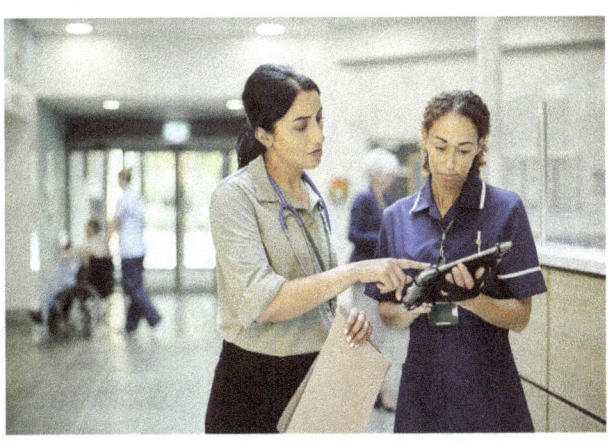

C2 Responsibilities for maintaining safe environments

Both employers and employees have responsibilities to maintain a safe environment for themselves and for the vulnerable individuals they care for and their families.

Responsibilities of employers

The responsibilities of employers are important to ensure the employees who work for them can do their job well and that they are protected from harm. These include:

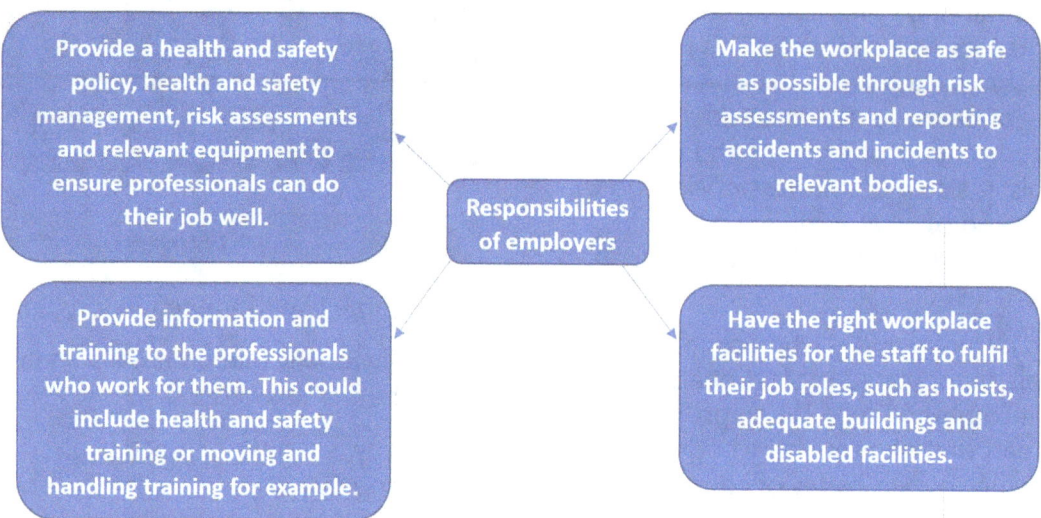

- Provide a health and safety policy, health and safety management, risk assessments and relevant equipment to ensure professionals can do their job well.
- Make the workplace as safe as possible through risk assessments and reporting accidents and incidents to relevant bodies.
- Provide information and training to the professionals who work for them. This could include health and safety training or moving and handling training for example.
- Have the right workplace facilities for the staff to fulfil their job roles, such as hoists, adequate buildings and disabled facilities.

Responsibilities of employees

Employees have many responsibilities to ensure they follow the requirements of their job role and follow the policies and procedures set out for them. Their responsibilities include:

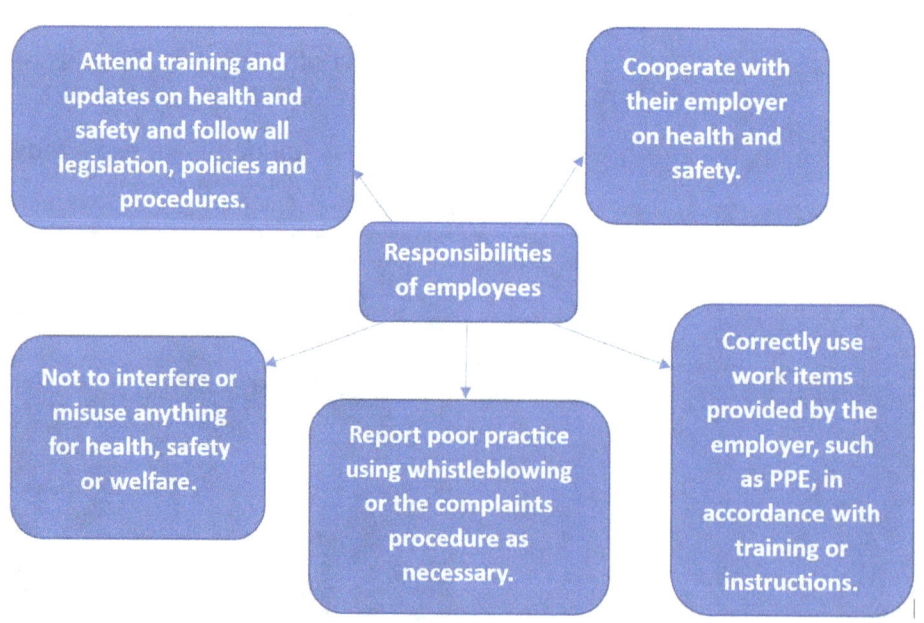

- Attend training and updates on health and safety and follow all legislation, policies and procedures.
- Cooperate with their employer on health and safety.
- Not to interfere or misuse anything for health, safety or welfare.
- Report poor practice using whistleblowing or the complaints procedure as necessary.
- Correctly use work items provided by the employer, such as PPE, in accordance with training or instructions.

> **Activity**
>
> Think about the responsibilities of employees outlined above. Then consider the following:
>
> - Explain what might be the best way for employers to share these responsibilities with employees?
> - Explain how employers would check these responsibilities are being followed.
> - Assess how these responsibilities could be used for holding professionals accountable for their actions.
> - Analyse what you think employees should do if they feel their employers are not upholding their responsibilities.

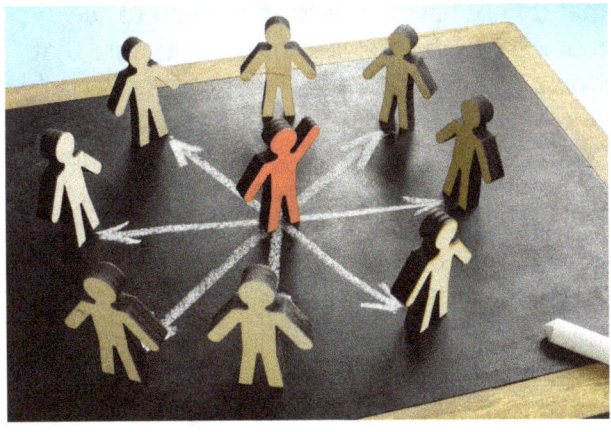

Recap questions

1. How would employers and employees following their responsibilities ensure a safe environment is created?
2. How could employees report poor practice?
3. Give an example of a policy that should be created by employers.

C3 Effective record keeping in health and social care environments

Purpose of records in health and social care

Effective record keeping is vital in health and social care services to maintain safe practice and support vulnerable individuals. The main purpose of record keeping is to communicate information clearly and effectively, and ensure this gets to the right people in a timely manner.

Records kept can include a great deal of information about an individual, which can be of great use to other professionals or family members supporting them. This could include:

- test results
- care plans
- treatment plans
- recovery information
- basic information such as date of birth, weight and allergies.

If records are kept and shared when necessary, it can reduce workload of other professionals and lead to better outcomes for individuals seeking support from services. It can also ensure information is shared in the most appropriate way, which can reduce the risk of confidentiality leaks and also reduces the risk of misunderstandings.

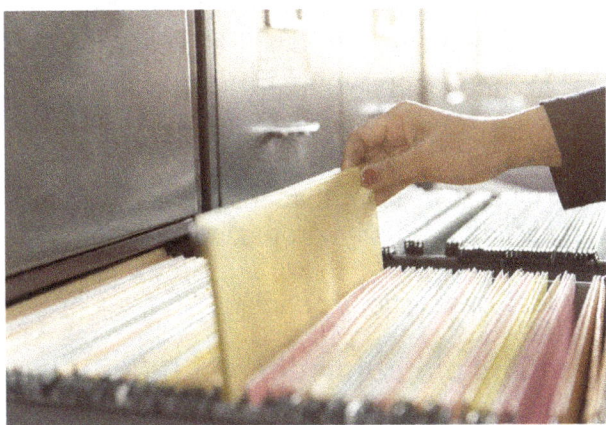

Legal and ethical obligations for record keeping

There are many legal and ethical obligations that professionals and services need to follow to maintain accurate records. This is to protect confidentiality and ensure they are fit for purpose. Many of the legislations and procedures that need to be followed outline the importance of maintaining full, clear, accurate records which are completed in a timely manner after care or treatment has been given.

It is important that when keeping records, they are stored in a way that maintains confidentiality and prevents unauthorised access by professionals or visitors to the service that do not have permission or need to see them. To do this, services must make sure that where records are kept is large enough to hold the records needed, such as filing cabinets that can be locked, to reduce the chances of files being left out of the cabinet. Any electronic storage also needs to be large enough to hold all of the files necessary and only be accessed by those who 'need to know'.

The legislation supporting this include:

General Data Protection Regulations (2018)

The **Data Protection Act 2018** outlines the way professionals in the UK follow GDPR rules. This states that Data Protection is the responsibility of all professionals, not just those who work in safeguarding or data.

There are 6 data protection principles which explain that professionals must ensure that information is (UK Government, 2018):

- Used fairly, lawfully and transparently,
- Used for specific purposes,
- Used in a way that is adequate, relevant and limited to only what is necessary,
- Accurate and up to date,
- Kept for no longer than is necessary,
- Handled in a way that ensures appropriate security, including protection against unlawful or unauthorised processing, access, loss, destruction or damage.

Freedom of Information Act (2000)

The **Freedom of Information Act 2000** gives individuals the right to information held by public authorities, such as the NHS or Local Authorities. This means that services and professionals must keep records safe until such time as it might be asked for and needs to be kept in a way where it can be found or accessed when needed.

The Freedom of Information Act states that the public can access the information through:

- Individuals formally requesting it straight from the service,
- The authorities publishing information, such as inspection reports or activities being undertaken.

(Information Commissioner's Office, 2023)

Legislation – A law passed by parliament.
Unauthorised – Not having permission.

Health and Social Care Act (2008)

The **Health and Social Care Act 2008** led to the creation of the **Care Quality Commission**, which inspects and regulates health and social care services, as well as reviews and investigates them if issues arise. One of the areas the CQC is responsible for regulating is the maintenance of records across each service.

Regulation 17 of the Health and Social Care Act 2008 states that 'health and social care providers must securely maintain accurate, complete and detailed records for patients or service users, employment of staff and overall management', (NHS, 2021).

Therefore, if effective record keeping measures are implemented, it will lead to positive inspections by the CQC and approving reports, as this will enable the service to offer safe and effective care.

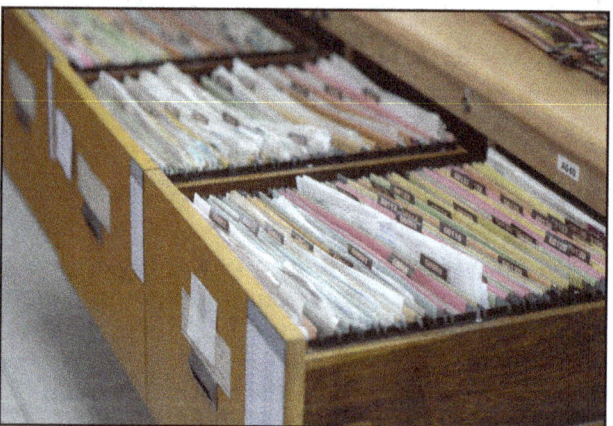

Recap questions

1. How many data protection principles are there?
2. Name one of them.
3. Why is it important that the storage used for records is appropriately sized?

Apply your understanding

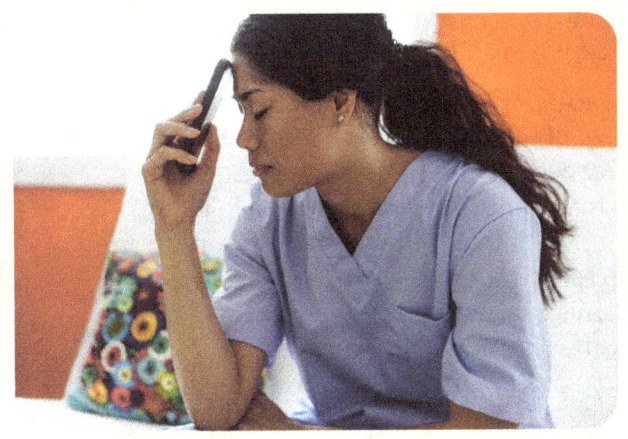

Katrina works at a residential care home. She has worked in the office for around 10 years and really enjoys her job. However, a new care manager, Zara, has recently joined the home. She has previously worked in homes with negative CQC reports and has brought along a negative working culture, leading to conflict amongst professionals. When Zara started the role, she said she wanted to learn about positive practices and make positive changes. However, it didn't take long before many negative and lazy actions began. These included:

- Zara leaving vulnerable individuals paper records out in the open, such as in the staff room or in their rooms.
- Zara leaving the file room unlocked, saying 'it takes too much effort to open it every time'.
- In meetings with individuals and their families, Zara has been saying she has made notes of changes to their health or care to update their records, but hasn't done this.
- Zara using patient records of those who have passed away to gather statistics without the family's knowledge. When confronted with this by Katrina, Zara stated that 'they won't mind as they are not here to complain'.

This has left Katrina feeling like she is in an impossible situation.

Which of the legislation and ethical obligations is Zara not following?

What do you think Katrina should do to maintain the safety of the individuals in the home and also ensure she is meeting her duty of care?

Types of records kept for individuals using health and social care services

There are many different types of information needed to be able to offer the most effective support to individuals needing care. This means there may be a variety of records held on them that needs to be kept safe.

Patient identifying information

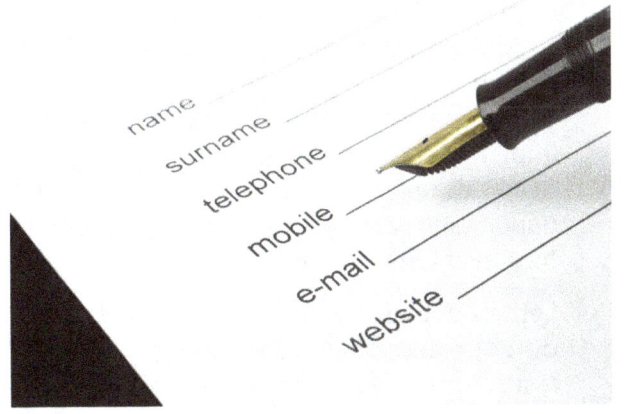

This includes any type of information that could identify an individual using services. This could include:

- Name
- Address
- Telephone number
- Date of birth
- NHS number
- Email address
- Images

It is therefore important that any identifiable information is kept and stored safely and appropriately, where access is only available to a select number of professionals.

Health and care records

Every time an individual visits a service, there will be a record made. This could include:

- **Notes from the professional** - such as what was discussed or what the individuals concerns were. This is important so that any professionals giving follow-up appointments are aware of previous discussions and any treatment given. This can reduce time wasting and ensure effective suggestions are made.

- **Test results** – such as results from blood tests or scans for example. This is important as these could inform further discussions between individuals and professionals and could increase or reduce any treatment being given.

- **Medication** – such as any medication prescribed by the professional or any medication regularly taken. This is important so professionals can prescribe any further treatment safely, as they will have knowledge of any contraindications or limitations due to current or past medication.

- **Medical history** – such as prior illnesses, family history of an illness or condition, or previous medication taken and their effects. This is important as a diagnosis may be reached quicker and with less invasive procedures.

- **Care plans** – which will include what treatment and support is to be given, when, and by whom. This is important so professionals are aware of their own responsibilities to an individual receiving care, and can be held accountable for their implementation of the care they are giving. Also, this helps individuals and their families understand how they will be receiving care, to prevent any confusion.

- **Letters between GPs, specialists and other professionals** – such as referrals, test results or professionals requesting advice or guidance. Letters and other correspondence need to be held and kept safe alongside other records for long-term reference. This can help professionals give the most effective care and make further referrals if needed.

> Prescribed – A medical professional authorising the use of.
>
> Contraindications – A reason for an individual not to receive a particular medication.
>
> Prior – Something that has happened before.
>
> Invasive – Procedures involving medical instruments which are inserted into the body, such as a needle.
>
> Deterioration – Something becoming progressively worse.

Observation records

There are many records that need to be kept regarding individuals who are using long-term care, such as in residential homes or long-term hospital wards. This is because there are many individuals who may not be able to speak for themselves or understand questions they may be asked, and so professionals recording observations is vital to the care of many. For example, this could be important for individuals with dementia or using medication which affects their memory or ability to complete tasks.

Any observations made will need recording in the appropriate way for the service and reporting to professionals in charge, such as shift leaders or care managers. This will ensure that intervention is given where necessary to protect the health of individuals.

Observations that need recording include:

- Any deterioration in health – such as a specific symptom worsening.
- Slips, trips or falls – as this could need further investigation.
- Nutrition intake – such as how much has been eaten by an individual.
- Medication compliance – to make sure medication is being taken and having the desired effect.

Recap questions

1. Name three things that would be classed as 'identifying information'.
2. Why is it important that letters between GPs and other professionals are recorded?
3. Why is it important to record any observations regarding an individual's nutrition intake?

Digital records

Digital records have become commonplace in the health and social care sector.

- They are much easier to store, protect and share when required.
- They enable health and social care services to store much more information without the need for physical storage, freeing up more space to use as treatment areas or offices.
- Being able to share digital records saves time and money – services can access the records more easily, without having to look through paper records, and sending them electronically saves time and postage costs.
- This also means that professionals receive important information quicker, to enable more timely support or treatment.

The use of digital technology to monitor health

Due to the technology we now have available, it is much easier for professionals to monitor health from afar and take action where needed.

Electronic patient records (EPR)

One key way digital technology is used is through **electronic patient records (EPR)**. This is an electronic version of an individual's medical record and contains any information regarding their health. This information is kept electronically by services, such as the NHS, and is usually accessible to individuals through the NHS app. This means it is accessible almost anywhere and can help to improve multi-agency working, supporting health, care, safety and efficiency. (NHS England, 2023)

Electronic patient records may hold information such as (NHS England, 2023)

- Name
- Date of birth
- NHS number
- Investigations completed by professionals
- Test/investigation results
- Information/advice given to individuals
- Treatment
- Prescribed medication
- Decisions made

Telehealth and telemedicine

- **Telemedicine** is a branch of telehealth, but telemedicine is only used by clinical healthcare professionals, such as GPs. This gives professionals an opportunity to communicate with individuals in electronic ways to support the introduction of new medication or monitor long-term health conditions.
- **Telehealth** on the other hand, is used on a larger scale. This enables individuals to communicate and have consultations with many different professionals in clinical and non-clinical roles. Telehealth also includes the use of remote patient monitoring, where electronic devices are used to monitor, collect and transmit data regarding health, such as the use of smart wearables. These then create electronic data that can be added to electronic patient records and seen in almost immediately by professionals such as GP's or health specialists, enabling action to be taken quickly if needed.

The use of telehealth and telemedicine for virtual appointments can be of great help to many. In times where health services are stretched, such as during the COVID-19 pandemic, virtual telehealth calls ensured individuals could be seen quickly without any further risk to the health of the individuals or professionals. Also, these can be used to enable appointments to fit into individuals' schedules, due to work or family responsibilities, as well as enabling faster appointments to be given and more choice regarding the professional being seen. This can help to build an individual's confidence in professionals and help health care to fit into today's fast-paced world.

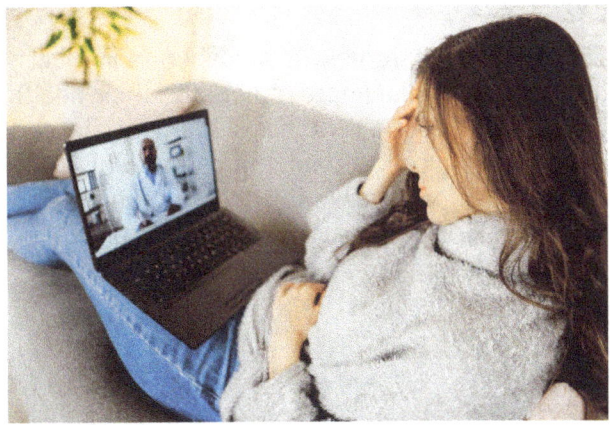

15.

Smart wearables and apps

These can be used as part of telehealth discussed above to send vital information to healthcare professionals regarding an individual's health and allows action to be taken if a condition deteriorates.

Smart wearables can monitor things such as:

- Heart rate
- Oxygen levels
- Breaths per minute
- Temperature
- Movement
- Blood glucose levels
- Sleep patterns

As the data from these will go directly to the professionals, it can enable swift action to be taken in the event of an issue, and follow-up consultations will be more focused due to the amount of data available for discussion. These wearables can also be monitored through a smartphone app for the individuals themselves to monitor.

Apps on smartphones or smartwatches have become a key component for many individuals monitoring their health, enabling them to have key data when seeking medical advice. This can include:

- Step counters
- Weight monitoring (gains or losses)
- Calorie intake
- Heart rates
- Oxygen levels
- Sleep patterns

(Cover, 2024)

These can be extremely useful when individuals are trying to make improvements to their health or monitor existing conditions. Many of these apps not only collect data, but can also give advice and tips to make further improvements, such as recipe suggestions or exercise tips for example, creating a digital record of any progress made.

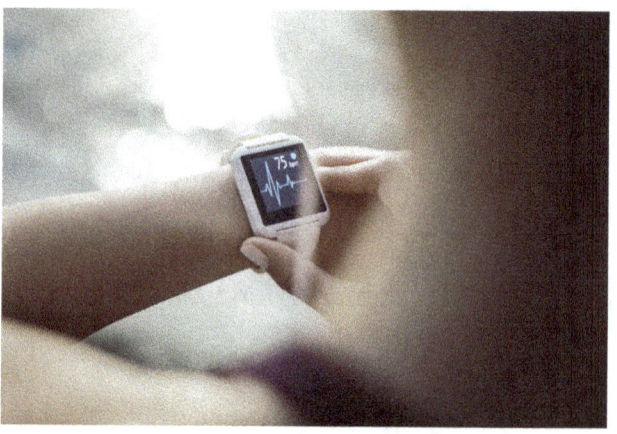

Recap questions

1. Explain the difference between telehealth and telemedicine.
2. What information might be kept in electronic patient records?

Inefficiencies – Failure to make the best use of resources.

Accessible – To be able to be used easily.

The reduction of inequalities

Due to the use of digital records, it can help to reduce many of the inequalities often faced by individuals accessing health and social care services. This is because it can reduce the need for physical appointments, enabling more appointments and therefore, can lead to earlier diagnosis and treatment.

By reducing inequalities, it can lead to:

- Improved access to the care available
- Improved quality of care
- A reduction in the costs associated with providing care
- A reduction in inefficiencies
- More personalised care

This can lead to individuals having more confidence when accessing services and understand that steps are being taken to make support more accessible, reducing inequalities further. These individuals are also usually the most hard to reach, so by changing ways of working, it can improve the health and wellbeing of many.

Benefits of digital records

There are many benefits for the professionals and individuals using services to have access the digital records. These include:

- Having instant access to up-to-date information.
- The ability to share information quickly and accurately.
- Changes in health status and needs can be noticed and responded to quickly.
- The chances of missed visits, sudden changes, number of falls and medication errors being minimised.
- Support staff to perform their role more effectively due to effective time planning and prioritisation.

Cybersecurity

Cybersecurity is how organisations, such as the NHS or local authorities, protect the data they hold against threats from unauthorised individuals or cyber-attacks. Maintaining cybersecurity can mean that organisations need to ensure they have policies and procedure regarding the following:

- Making sure professionals **use strong passwords** when accessing sensitive data and digital records.

- Making sure professionals **log out of all computers and systems** when they have finished using them to prevent unauthorised access of data.

- Making sure all professionals are **aware of what a data breach might look like**, how to prevent it and what to do if signs show there has been a cyber-attack.

If professionals are aware of these and follow them, it can help to reduce the risk of a data breach or cyber-attack, and will help individuals to feel confident in professionals and services. This will help them to seek help and support when needed and allow them to be open and transparent about their needs. This in turn will lead to effective care and support being offered, leading to improved health of individuals.

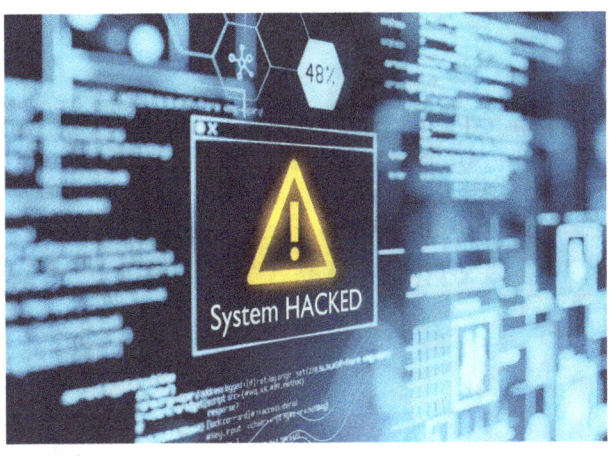

Cyber-attacks – Any attempt to steal or expose electronic data.

Recap questions

1. What is an electronic patient record?
2. What is the difference between telehealth and telemedicine?
3. Name two benefits of services having digital records.

> **Activity**
>
> Imagine there has been a cybersecurity breach at a local NHS trust and that the following has happened:
>
> 1. The records of over 300,000 people had been stolen and released onto the internet.
> 2. This data included clinical information, contact details, medical history and financial information.
> 3. This also included information from the mental health services, putting many individuals at risk of their mental status being made public.
> 4. The spokesperson from the NHS trust told patients to not worry and that this kind of leak rarely results in actual harm.
>
> Once you have read through these facts, consider:
>
> 5. How the individuals using the services in this area may have felt.
> 6. What they might be worried about.
> 7. How they might feel about using the service again in the future – especially those previously using mental health services.

C4 Poor practice and its impact in health and social care

Poor practice is a failure to provide a good standard of care and support, which usually leads to negative outcomes for the individuals accessing this care. This could be because their concerns have not been listened to or their needs have not clearly been understood. It could also be due to the pressures on the service itself, such as poor staffing levels or inadequate training. Whatever the reason, poor practice can lead to a loss of interest in the service and a negative working culture for staff.

The impact on individuals using the service

If poor practice is given to vulnerable individuals and their family, there can be many negative consequences. These include:

- **A lack of person-centred care** being given, which could lead to individuals not feeling able to access the care or services needed.

- A **denial of basic rights**, restriction of choices and fear of retribution. This could lead to fear of voicing their opinion and being the victim of abuse or neglect.

- **Poor experiences** leading to mistrust and non-compliance due to negative relationships with professionals.

- Reluctance to accept services as they may not feel able to trust the professionals offering them or fear a repeat of poor practice given in the past.

- A **breakdown in partnership relationships**, leading to conflict and information not being shared or given effectively.

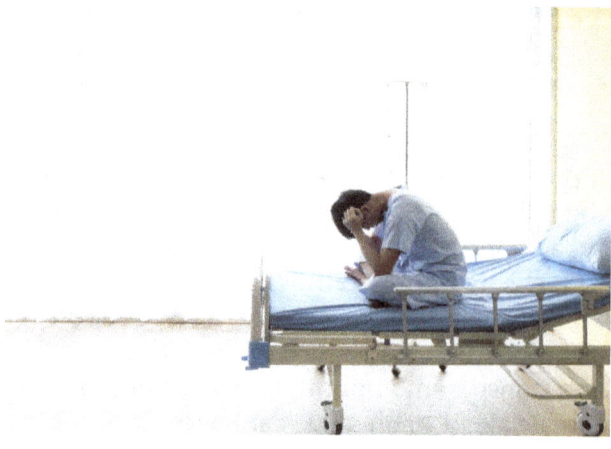

The impact on staff

If staff work in a culture of poor practice, they are likely to feel negative towards their employer and feel as though they cannot do their job effectively. This is likely to lead to:

- Retention and recruitment challenges as professionals will not want to stay in their role long term. If specific services also have a bad reputation, it will prevent professionals from wanting any roles within it, leading to professionals who already work there being put under even more pressure.
- **Low morale and a negative impact on mental health and wellbeing.** This could lead to professionals taking sick leave and suffering from mental health issues such as anxiety or depression, which will have an impact on the care they can give to individuals.
- **Poor staff wellbeing and high sickness levels** as professionals feel overwhelmed and overworked, which will make it even harder for employers and other professionals to maintain a good standard of care.
- **Increased serious case reviews** which may lead to dismissal or removal of fit to practise registration. This is more likely to happen if poor practice is given as individuals are more likely to feel unsatisfied with the care they are given and mistakes are more likely to be made.
- **Training gaps** which may lead to an increase in accidents, injuries or fatalities. It can also increase the risk of infection, medication errors and poorly maintained equipment, leading to professionals feeling unable to complete their roles, negatively impacting professional relationships.

The impact on employers/organisations in health and social care

The consequences to employers or organisations can be severe if they are found to be in charge of delivering and encouraging poor practice. These can include:

- Inadequate selection and recruitment processes of staff. This could include staff not being DBS checked or undertaking the appropriate training for the role. This could lead to an increase in mistakes being made and professionals feeling an ethical burden.
- **Breach of legislation and regulations,** which could lead to legal challenges. This will impact the employer or organisation as it could lead to constant conflict with families and professionals, leading to a negative atmosphere for all involved.
- Reputational damage, such as poor CQC ratings, which could lead to potential closure or prosecution.

> Retribution – A punishment given to individuals for the choices they've made.
>
> Non-compliance – Refusal to follow.
>
> Reluctance – Unwillingness to do something.
>
> Retention – Keeping the use of something or someone.
>
> Recruitment – Finding people to work in a particular role.
>
> Inadequate – Not good enough.
>
> Reputational damage – A loss that impacts an organisation negatively along with the relationships with others.

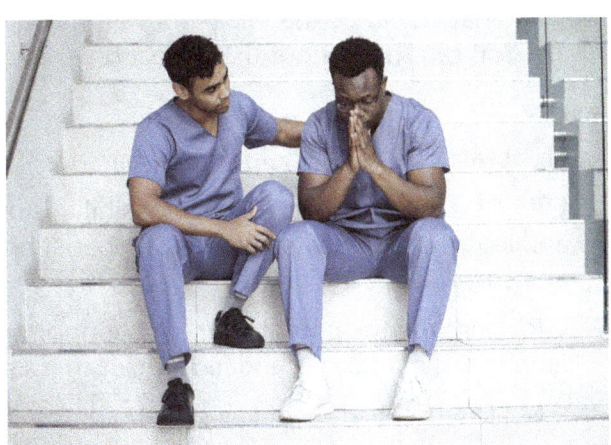

Recap questions

1. One of the impacts of poor service is them being reluctant to accept help. What could this lead to?
2. How could the impact on staff of poor staff wellbeing affect others working in the organisation?
3. What could poor ratings by the CQC lead to?

End of Topic Practice Activity

You need to think about safe practice and record keeping, and the impact this has on service users. You need to use the same service as used in the Learning Aim B practice activity.

Write down your ideas about the following:

- What roles and responsibilities do a) employers and b) employees have to maintain safe practice in your chosen service? You can think about their legal and ethical requirements.

- Discuss how employees, employers, service users and their families are involved in developing safe practice in your chosen service. How can the effectiveness of safe practice be improved?

- Can you justify your recommendations above to improve safe practice in your setting? How would they make a difference? You will need to back up your arguments with evidence.

- What would be the impact of not maintaining safe environments in your chosen service? You can think about the impact on employers, employees and vulnerable individuals.

This practice task will help you prepare for the following assessment criteria:

C.P5 Describe the roles and responsibilities of employers and employees to meet regulatory and legal requirements and ethical obligations to maintain safe practice in a selected health and social care setting.

C.P6 Describe the potential impact of poor practice in maintaining safe environments on employers, employees and individuals in a selected health and social care setting.

C.M3 Discuss the role of key stakeholders in maintaining safe practice and make recommendations to improve the effectiveness of safe practice in a selected health and social care setting.

C.D3 Justify recommendations for effective safe practice in a selected health and social care setting.

Unit 7 Health science

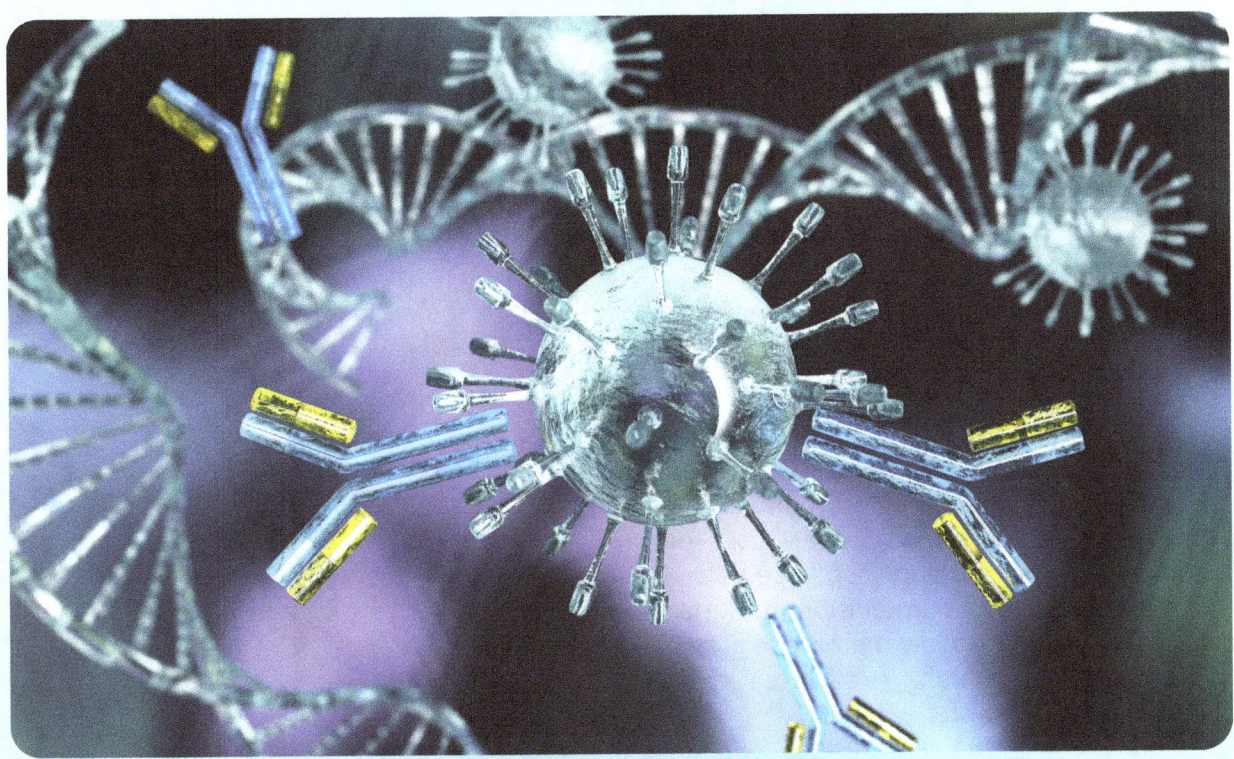

In this unit you will understand important ideas about microbiology and how they relate to heath science. You will also understand the impacts of infectious disease on wider society.

In this unit you will learn about:

- Different microorganisms that cause disease.
- How the human body protects itself against pathogens.
- Factors that contribute to certain diseases.
- Epidemiology and the role of organisations in controlling disease.

How will I be assessed?

In this unit you will be assessed through an internal assessment consisting of a series of tasks, covering Learning Aims A, B, C and D. The assignment is set by the awarding body and marked by your tutor.

Learning Aim A: Understand the concepts of microbiology relevant to health science

Learning Aim B: Examine the role of microorganisms in human health and disease

Learning Aim C: Understand the factors that can influence the development of diseases and infections

Learning Aim D: Investigate the impact of diseases and their treatment in a global context

Learning Aim A: Understand the concepts of microbiology relevant to health science

Microbiology is the study of microorganisms. These microscopic organisms, including viruses, bacteria, fungi, and protozoa, impact on various aspects of human health. Having a good knowledge of the concepts of microbiology allows healthcare professionals to understand the causes, diagnosis, prevention, and treatment of infectious diseases.

A1 Structure and reproduction of microorganisms

Microorganisms include viruses, bacteria, fungi and protozoa. They have an incredibly diverse range of structures. The individual structures play vital roles in their survival, reproduction, and ability to cause disease. In Section A1 you will learn about the different structures of these microorganisms. Understanding their structures allows scientists to develop methods for their detection, identification, and control.

Viruses

Viruses are the smallest known infectious agents. In their simplest form they are made of a genetic material, either DNA or RNA, surrounded by a protein coat called a capsid. Some viruses may also have an outer envelope composed of lipids and proteins. The glycoproteins on the surface act as antigens and they allow the virus to attach to host cells. Viruses can only reproduce within the cells of a host organism.

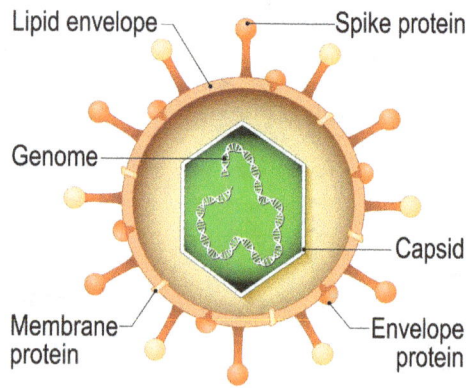

The structure of a virus

There are several different types of viruses, including:

- **Retroviruses** are a type of RNA virus. Their genetic material is single-stranded RNA. They use an enzyme called reverse transcriptase to convert their RNA into DNA. The DNA is then integrated into the host cell's genome. This allows the virus to replicate its genetic material along with the host cell's DNA. HIV is an example of a retrovirus.

- **Bacteriophages** are viruses that infect bacteria. Bacteriophages have a complex structure, consisting of head and tail fibres. The head contains the genetic material of the virus, while the tail fibres are involved in attaching to and infecting the bacterial cell.

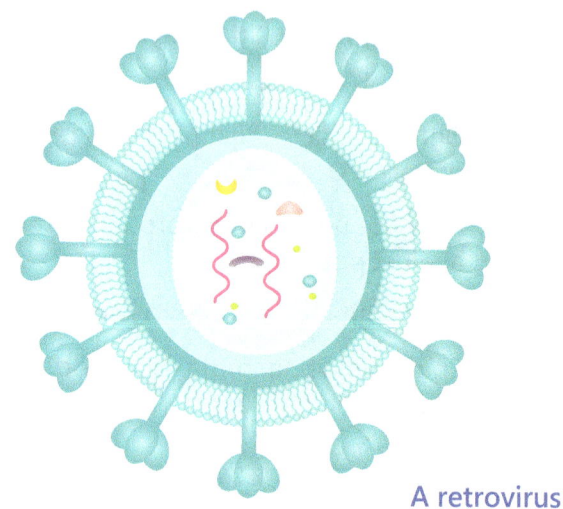

A retrovirus

The structure of a virus is closely related to its ability to infect and replicate within a host cell. The capsid protects the viral genetic material and allows attachment to the host cell. The envelope is a similar structure to animal cell membranes and helps the virus to enter the host cell. The viral genetic material contains the instructions for the virus to reproduce and assemble new viruses.

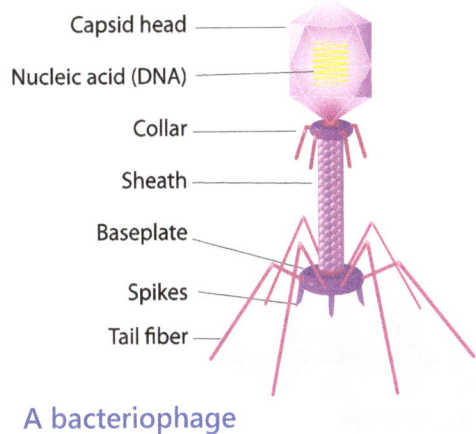

A bacteriophage

> Antigens – Any substance that triggers an immune response in the body, such as the production of antibodies.
>
> Complementary – The specific pairing of molecules based on their shapes and chemical properties. This allows them to fit together precisely, like a lock and key.
>
> Host cells – A living cell that is invaded by a virus or another type of microorganism. The invading microorganism uses the host cell's resources and machinery to replicate itself.

Viral reproduction

Viruses are only able to reproduce inside a host cell. The process of viral reproduction involves several key steps:

1. **Attachment**: The virus attaches to specific receptors on the surface of the host cell. The antigens on the virus's surface attach to complementary proteins on the host cell membrane.

2. **Penetration**: Once attached, the virus enters the host cell. The mechanism of entry varies depending on the type of virus. Some viruses inject their genetic material into the host cell, while others enter the cell as a whole.

3. **Replication**: The viral genetic material takes over the host cell's machinery and directs the synthesis of new viral proteins and genetic material.

4. **Assembly**: The newly synthesised viral components are assembled into new virus particles.

5. **Release**: The new virus particles are released from the host cell. This occurs through **lysis**, where the host cell bursts open, destroying the host cell.

Recap questions

1. What are the two main components of a virus in its simplest form?
2. What is the role of the capsid in a virus?
3. What enzyme do retroviruses use to convert their RNA into DNA?
4. What is a bacteriophage?
5. List the five stages of viral reproduction.
6. How are new virus particles released from the host cell?

While the specific details of viral reproduction can vary depending on the type of virus and the host cell involved, these general steps are common to all viruses. Understanding the process of viral reproduction is essential for developing new antiviral drugs and vaccines.

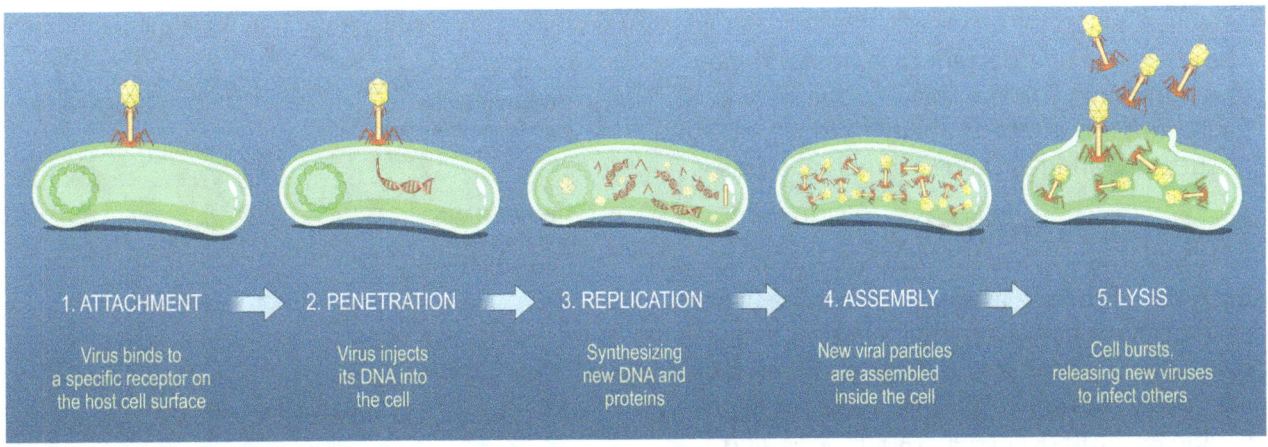

Diagram of a bacteriophage infecting and replicating inside a host cell

Bacteria

Bacteria are **prokaryotic** organisms, meaning they are single-celled organisms that lack a nucleus and other membrane-bound organelles. Despite their simple structure, bacteria show a huge diversity of shapes and functions.

The basic structure of a bacterial cell consists of a cell wall, cell membrane, cytoplasm, ribosomes, and genetic material (DNA and RNA).

The **cell wall** is a rigid structure that surrounds and protects the bacterial cell. It is composed of a polymer called peptidoglycan.

The **cell membrane** is a thin, flexible barrier that separates the inside of the cell from the outside environment. It is composed of a phospholipid bilayer.

Some bacterial cells have additional features:

- **slime capsule** to prevent them from drying out
- **flagellum** (or multiple flagella) which are tail-like structures that allow for movement
- **pili** which help in attaching to host tissues

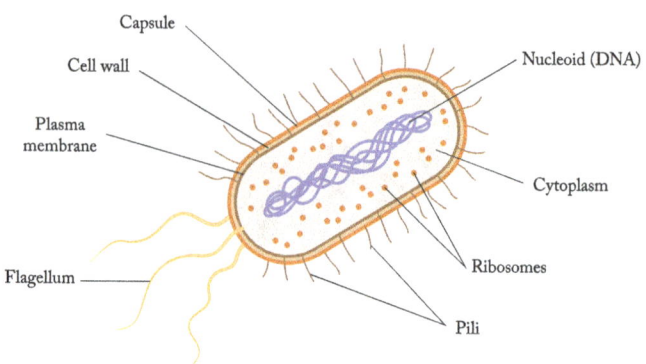

The structure of a bacterial cell

Bacteria can be classified based on their shape. There are four main shapes of bacteria:

- **Cocci:** Cocci are spherical bacteria. They can be arranged in pairs (diplococci), chains (streptococci), or clusters (staphylococci).
- **Bacilli:** Bacilli are rod-shaped bacteria. They can be arranged in pairs (diplobacilli) or chains (streptobacilli).
- **Spirilla:** Spirilla are spiral-shaped bacteria.
- **Vibrio:** Vibrio are comma-shaped bacteria. They are similar to spirilla but have a single curve.

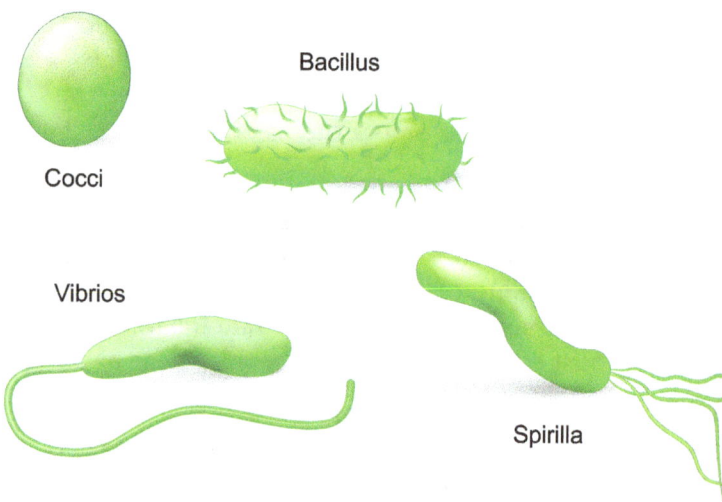

The four main types of bacteria

The **structure** of a bacterium is closely related to its **function**. For example, the shape of a bacterium can affect its ability to move, attach to surfaces, and resist environmental stresses.

Bacterial reproduction

Bacteria reproduce asexually through a process called **binary fission**. In binary fission, a single bacterial cell replicates its DNA and then divides into two daughter cells. This process is relatively simple and can occur very rapidly, allowing

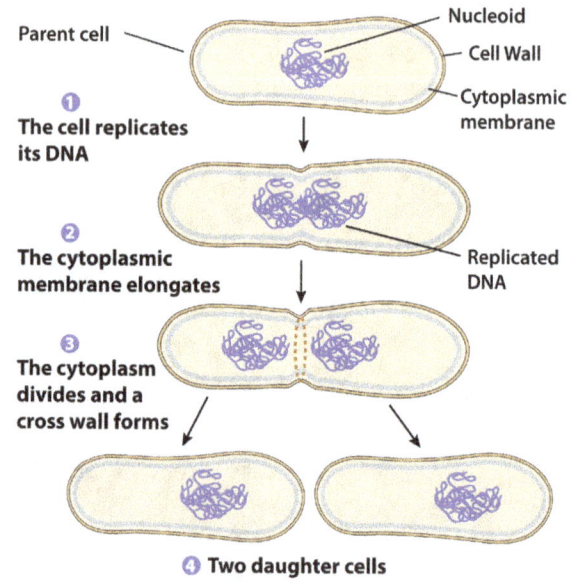

Binary fission

bacteria to reproduce large numbers of offspring in a short period of time.

Under favourable conditions, bacteria can divide every 20-30 minutes. This rapid growth rate is one of the reasons why bacterial infections can spread so quickly. However, bacterial growth can be influenced by various factors, including:

- temperature
- pH
- nutrient availability
- antibiotics.

While binary fission is the primary method of bacterial reproduction, some bacteria can also exchange genetic material through **horizontal gene transfer**, in a process called **conjugation**. This process involves the transfer of DNA between bacterial cells, which can lead to the bacteria acquiring new genes and traits. Horizontal gene transfer can contribute to the spread of antibiotic resistance.

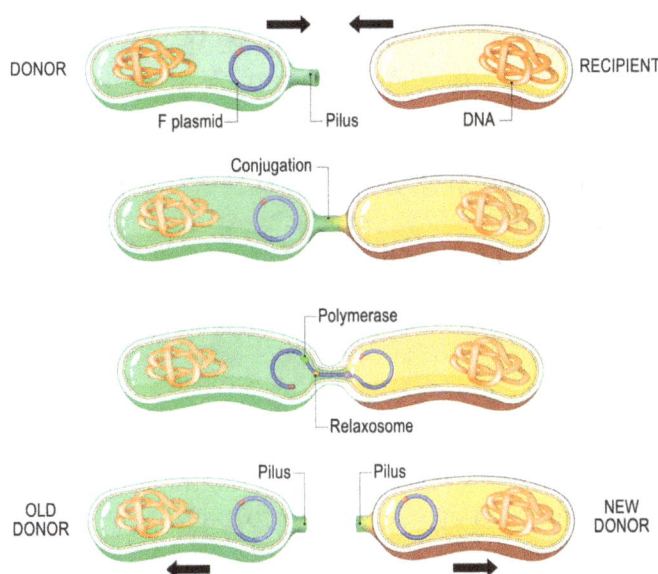

Conjugation

> **Phospholipid bilayer** – A double layer of phospholipid molecules that forms the primary component of cell membranes.

Fungi

Fungi are **eukaryotic** organisms, meaning they have a nucleus and other membrane-bound organelles. They are distinct from plants and animals, and they have their own kingdom, Fungi.

Fungi are **heterotrophs**, meaning they obtain nutrients from other organisms. They can be found in a variety of environments, including soil, air, water, and decaying matter.

There are two main types of fungi: yeasts and moulds.

- **Yeasts** are single-celled fungi that are typically spherical or oval (see diagram of basic fungal cell). They can reproduce by budding, where a small outgrowth forms on the parent cell and eventually separates to become a new daughter cell.

Recap questions

1. What are prokaryotic organisms?
2. Name two structures found in all bacterial cells.
3. What is the function of the bacterial cell wall?
4. List three additional structures that some bacterial cells may possess.
5. What is the shape of cocci bacteria?
6. What is the main method of bacterial reproduction?

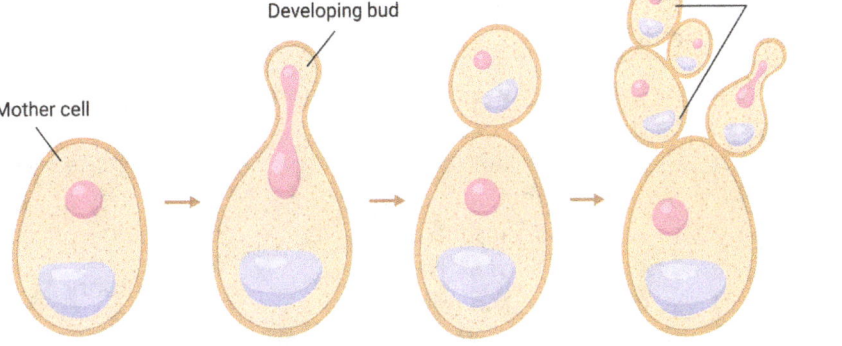

Yeast budding

Moulds are **multicellular** (made up of many cells) fungi that are composed of filaments called hyphae. Hyphae can grow into networks called mycelium, which can be seen as a fuzzy or cottony mass. Moulds reproduce by producing **spores**, which are tiny reproductive structures that can be dispersed by wind, water, or other means.

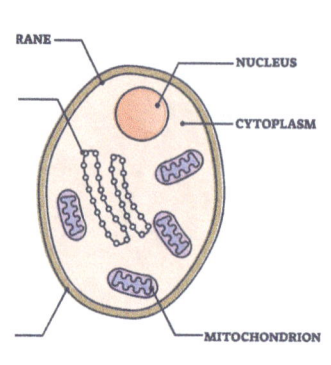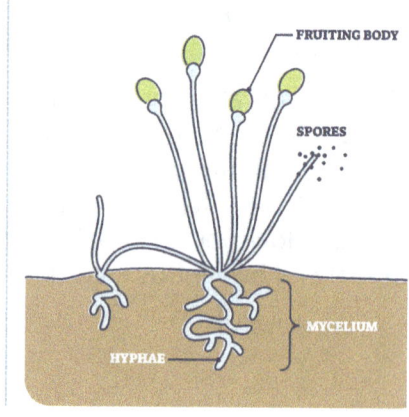

The structure of a fungal cell (left) and a multicellular fungus (right)

Protozoa

Protozoa are single-celled eukaryotic organisms. They are typically larger and more complex than bacteria. Protozoa have a variety of structures, depending on the species. Some protozoa have cilia or flagella, which are hair-like structures that enable them to move.

Several examples of protozoa include:

- **Plasmodium:** Plasmodium is a type of protozoa that causes malaria. It is a parasitic organism that is transmitted to humans through the bite of an infected mosquito. The reproductive cycle of plasmodium is complex and involves two hosts — humans and the female Anopheles mosquitoes.

- **Trypanosome:** Trypanosomes are protozoa that are transmitted to humans by insects, such as the tsetse fly. They can cause serious diseases, such as African trypanosomiasis (sleeping sickness) and Chagas disease. The life cycle of trypanosomes can be complex and may involve different hosts, depending on the species. For example, the African trypanosome, which causes sleeping sickness, has a complex life cycle that involves both humans and the **tsetse fly**. The parasite reproduces asexually in the human bloodstream, and then sexually in the tsetse fly.

- **Unicellular green algae:** Unicellular green algae are a group of photosynthetic protozoa. They are similar to plants in that they contain chlorophyll and can produce their own food through photosynthesis. They are important primary producers and play a vital role in the food chain. **Unicellular green algae** reproduce primarily through **asexual reproduction**. This involves the division of a single cell into two or more daughter cells.

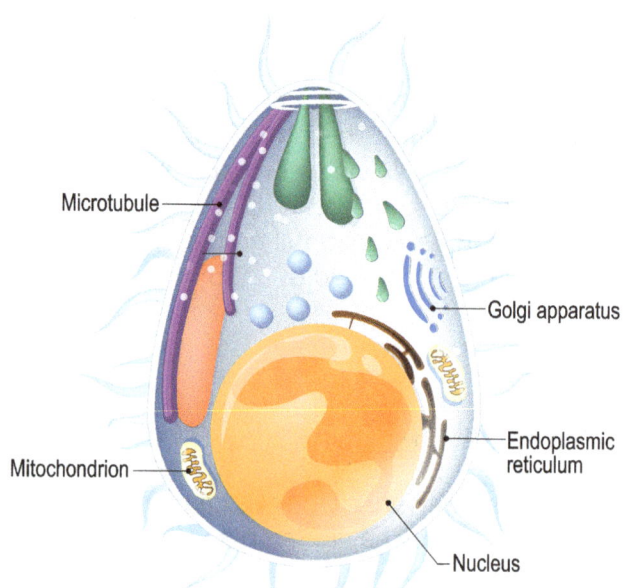

The structure of plasmodium

Plasmodium, the parasite that causes malaria, has a complex life cycle that involves both sexual and asexual reproduction. The life cycle takes place in two hosts: humans and female Anopheles mosquitoes.

In the female Anopheles mosquito:

1. **Sexual reproduction:** In the mosquito's gut, **gametocytes** (see stage 4 below) fuse to form sporozoites. These sporozoites move to the mosquito's salivary glands, where they are ready to infect another human when the mosquito bites again.

In humans:

2. **Asexual reproduction:** When a female Anopheles mosquito infected with Plasmodium bites a human, it injects **sporozoites** (the infective stage of the parasite) into the bloodstream.

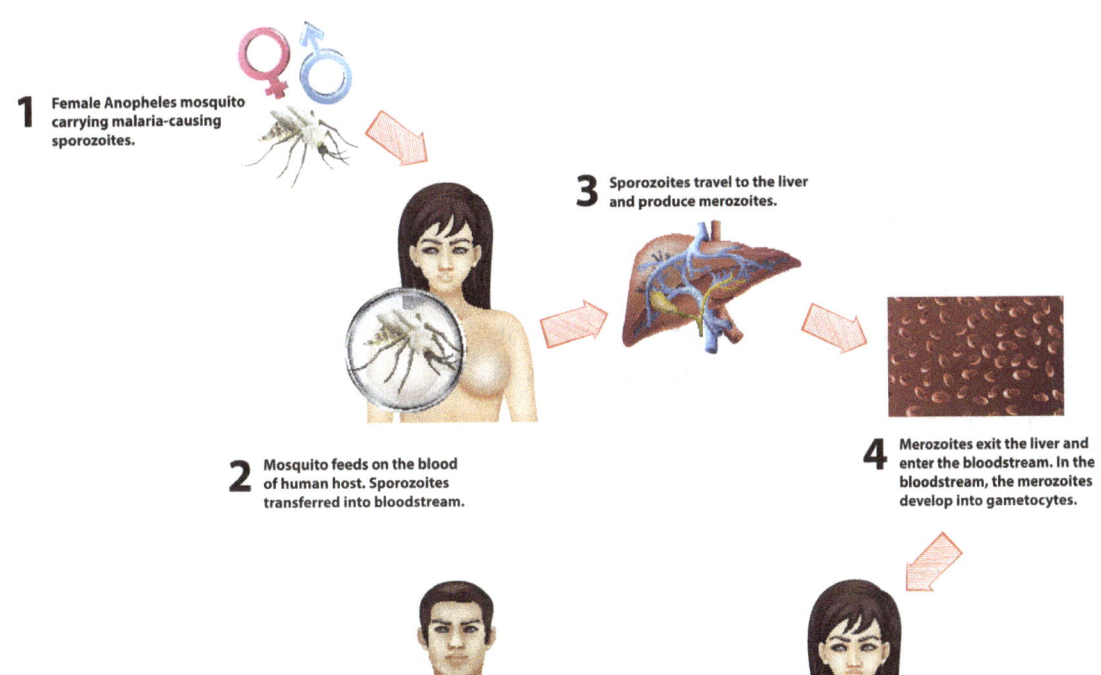

Malaria transmission

> Asexual – Reproduction that does not involve the fusion of gametes (sex cells) from two different parents.

3. **Merozoites**: These sporozoites travel to the liver, where they multiply asexually and form merozoites.

4. **Gametocytes**: The merozoites eventually burst out of the liver cells and enter the bloodstream, where they invade red blood cells. In the bloodstream some of the merozoites develop into gametocytes, which are male and female sex cells.

5. **Gametocytes in mosquito**: If a female Anopheles mosquito bites an infected human, it ingests gametocytes along with the blood.

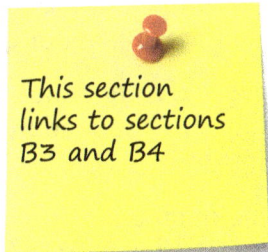

This section links to sections B3 and B4

Recap questions

1. Are fungi prokaryotic or eukaryotic organisms?
2. How do fungi obtain their nutrients?
3. How do yeasts reproduce?
4. What are the filamentous structures that make up moulds called?
5. Are protozoa prokaryotic or eukaryotic organisms?
6. Name two structures that may enable some protozoa to move.
7. What disease is caused by the protozoan Plasmodium?
8. What is the role of the tsetse fly in the transmission of some trypanosome infections?
9. How do unicellular green algae obtain their food?
10. In the human host, what is the name of the stage of the Plasmodium life cycle that invades red blood cells?

> **Apply your understanding**
>
> A small village in rural India has been experiencing an unusual outbreak of illness. Symptoms include fever, chills, fatigue, and in some cases, severe headaches and vomiting. Local health officials suspect a possible infectious disease outbreak. Interviews with villagers indicate that many of the affected individuals have been bitten by mosquitoes recently.
>
> 1. Based on the information provided, what type of microorganism is most likely causing the outbreak?
> 2. What disease is most likely responsible for the outbreak?
> 3. How is this disease typically transmitted?
> 4. What preventative measures could be taken to control the spread of this disease in the village?

> **Activity**
>
> 1. Describe two key differences between prokaryotic and eukaryotic cells.
> 2. Describe the life cycle of a typical virus. Include the key stages involved and explain the significance of each stage.

A2 Environmental conditions for the growth of microorganisms

Requirements for microorganisms that infect humans

Microorganisms that infect humans have specific requirements to survive and thrive within their host environment. These requirements include:

- **Host organisms**
  - **Humans**: While some microorganisms can infect other animals, the primary host for human pathogens (disease-causing microorganisms) is humans. Pathogens must be able to evade or overcome the human immune system to establish an infection.
- **Nutrients**
  - **Organic compounds**: Microorganisms require organic compounds, such as carbohydrates, proteins, and lipids, as sources of energy and building blocks for growth.
  - **Vitamins and minerals**: Some pathogens may also require specific vitamins and minerals for their metabolic processes.
- **Optimum temperature**
  - **Body temperature**: Most human pathogens have an optimum temperature that closely matches human body temperature (around 37°C). This allows them to grow and multiply efficiently within the host.
  - **Temperature tolerance**: Some pathogens may have a wider temperature tolerance, allowing them to survive in environments outside the body, such as on surfaces or in water.
- **Water**
  - Microorganisms require water for their metabolic processes and growth. Pathogens often thrive in moist environments, such as mucous membranes, skin folds, and bodily fluids.

> **Recap questions**
>
> 1. Name three organic compounds that microorganisms require for growth.
> 2. Besides organic compounds, what other nutrients may be required by some pathogens?
> 3. What is the optimum temperature for most human pathogens?
> 4. Why is water essential for microorganisms?
> 5. Where do pathogens often thrive due to the presence of moisture?

A3 Methods of controlling microorganisms

Microorganisms can pose significant threats to human health and wellbeing. To minimise these risks, various methods have been developed to control their growth and spread. These methods can be physical or chemical, and target microorganisms in different ways, aiming to prevent their spread and reduce their harmful effects.

Control techniques

Microorganisms can be controlled using various techniques to prevent their growth and spread. These techniques can be classified into physical and chemical methods:

Physical methods	Chemical methods
Refrigeration: This slows down microbial growth by reducing the metabolic rate. It's commonly used to preserve food and biological samples.	**Disinfectants**: These are chemical agents used to kill or inactivate microorganisms on inanimate (non-living) objects and surfaces. Common disinfectants include bleach and alcohol.
Freezing: This can stop microbial growth by forming ice crystals that disrupt cellular structures. It's used for long-term storage of food, biological samples, and vaccines.	**Antibiotics**: These are drugs that kill or inhibit the growth of bacteria. They are used to treat bacterial infections.
Autoclaving: This involves using high temperature and pressure to sterilise materials. It's commonly used in healthcare settings to sterilise surgical instruments and laboratory equipment.	**Antiseptics**: These are chemical agents used to kill or inhibit microorganisms on living tissue. They are commonly used to clean wounds and prevent infections.
Radiation: This can be used to kill microorganisms by damaging their DNA. It's used in food preservation and medical sterilisation.	
Drying: This removes moisture, which is essential for microbial growth. It's used to preserve food and other products.	

The choice of control technique depends on the specific application and the type of microorganisms being targeted. For example, sterilisation is required for medical equipment, while disinfection is sufficient for non-living surfaces.

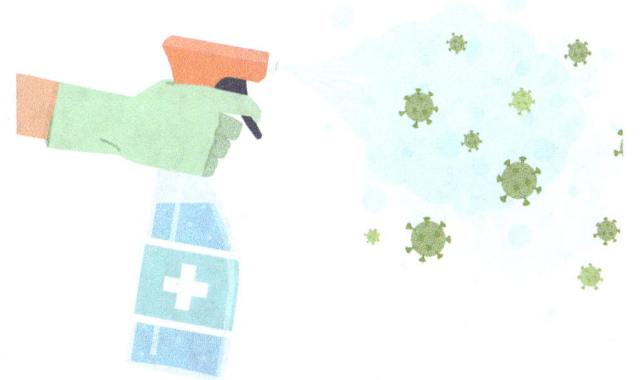

> **Recap questions**
>
> 1. What is the primary goal of microbial control techniques?
> 2. Name two physical methods of microbial control.
> 3. How does refrigeration control microbial growth?
> 4. What is the difference between disinfectants and antiseptics?
> 5. Explain how autoclaving achieves sterilisation.
> 6. Why is drying an effective method for controlling microbial growth?

Vector control

Vector control is a public health strategy to prevent the transmission of diseases by insects and other animals. These disease-carrying organisms, known as vectors, can spread a variety of illnesses, including malaria, dengue fever, sleeping sickness, and Lyme disease.

Two of the most significant vectors are mosquitoes and tsetse flies.

Mosquito control

- **Habitat reduction**: This involves eliminating or modifying breeding grounds for mosquitoes, such as stagnant water in ponds, ditches, or containers.
- **Larvicides**: Chemical or biological agents are used to kill mosquito larvae before they mature into adults.
- **Adulticides**: Insecticides are applied to kill adult mosquitoes, often through spraying or fogging.
- **Personal protection**: Using mosquito nets, repellents, and long-sleeved clothing can help individuals avoid mosquito bites.

Tsetse fly control

- **Livestock management**: Livestock (animals like sheep and cows) are hosts for tsetse flies. Reducing the number of livestock in an area can help limit the populations of tsetse flies.
- **Trapping and targeting**: Using traps and targeted insecticide applications can reduce tsetse fly populations.
- **Habitat modification**: Clearing vegetation and improving access to areas where tsetse flies breed can also be effective.

By controlling the population of these and other disease-carrying insects, public health officials can significantly reduce the incidence of vector-borne diseases.

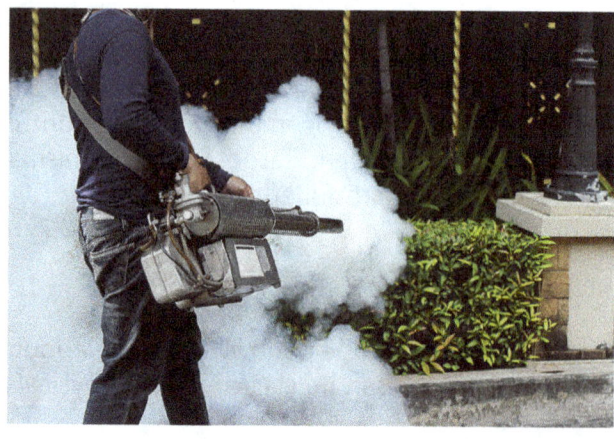

The picture shows fogging being used to kill adult mosquitoes

Policies and procedures for infection control in the UK

The UK has implemented comprehensive policies and procedures to prevent and control the spread of infections within healthcare settings. These guidelines are in line with evidence-based practices and are regularly updated to address emerging threats.

Protective clothing

- **Standard precautions**: Healthcare workers are required to wear gloves, aprons, and masks for all patient interactions, regardless of the patient's diagnosis.
- **Transmission-based precautions**: For patients with known or suspected infections, additional protective equipment may be required, such as gowns, respirators, and eye protection.

Isolation

Patients with infectious diseases may be placed in **isolation** to prevent the spread of pathogens. This can involve isolating patients in a single room, using ventilation systems with a HEPA filter, or restricting visitors.

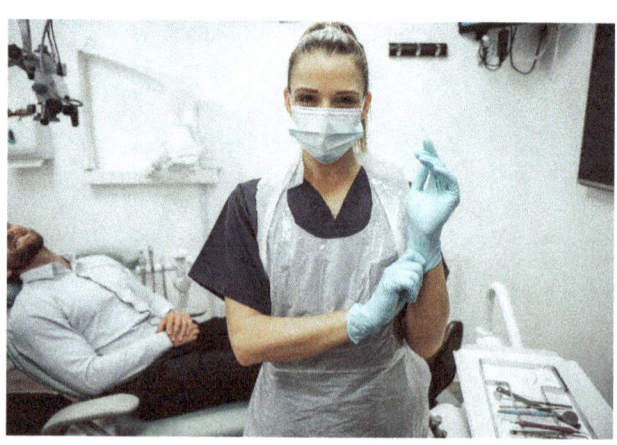

Barrier nursing

Barrier nursing is a set of infection control procedures used in healthcare settings to minimise the spread of infectious diseases. It involves the use of physical barriers, such as gloves, gowns, masks, and other protective equipment, to prevent the transmission of pathogens between patients, healthcare workers, and visitors.

Barrier nursing also includes environmental cleaning and waste management. Patient rooms and shared spaces are regularly cleaned and disinfected to reduce the presence of infectious agents. The proper disposal of contaminated materials, such as sharps and soiled linens, is essential to prevent the spread of infection.

Barrier nursing is also used to prevent the introduction of microorganisms into a sterile field, such as during surgery or invasive procedures.

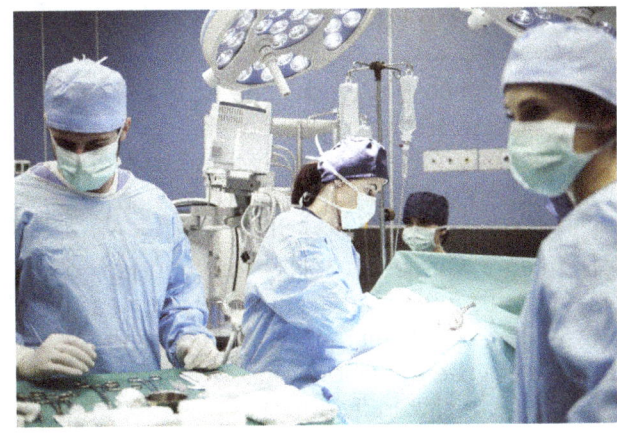

HEPA filter – A HEPA filter (High-Efficiency Particulate Air filter) is a type of air filter designed to capture a high percentage (up to 99.9%) of airborne particles, including dust, pollen, mould, bacteria, and even some viruses.

Antimicrobial action

Soaps play an important role in antimicrobial action by controlling the spread of microorganisms through disrupting their cell membranes.

How soaps work

Microbial disruption: When soap comes into contact with microorganisms, it disrupts their lipid bilayer, the outer membrane that protects them from the environment. This disruption can lead to **cell lysis** (bursting of the cell) resulting in the death of the microorganism.

Emulsification: Soaps are surfactants, meaning they have both hydrophilic (water-loving) and hydrophobic (water-hating) properties. When soap is mixed with water, it forms structures called micelles, which are spherical structures that can trap small pieces of pathogen.

Mechanical removal: In addition to their antimicrobial properties, soaps can also mechanically remove microorganisms from the skin surface through scrubbing.

Solid versus liquid soaps

While both solid and liquid soaps are effective in controlling microorganisms, there are some differences between them:

- **Lather**: Liquid soaps generally produce a richer lather than solid soaps, which can be more effective at removing dirt.
- **Convenience**: Liquid soaps are often more convenient to use, especially for people with mobility limitations. In a healthcare setting, using a liquid soap prevents contact with other surfaces.
- **Ingredients**: The specific ingredients in solid and liquid soaps can vary, but both types typically contain surfactants, fragrances, and preservatives.

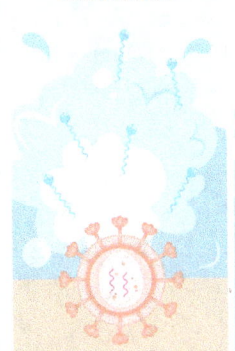
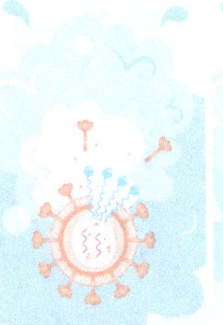
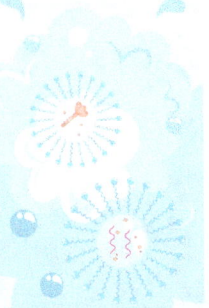

How soap works

Importance of handwashing

Proper handwashing with soap is one of the most effective ways to prevent the spread of infectious diseases. By removing harmful microorganisms from the hands, we can reduce the risk of transmitting them to others or infecting ourselves. It is recommended to wash hands with soap and water for at least 20 seconds, particularly before preparing food, after using the bathroom, and after coming into contact with sick individuals.

Apply your understanding

Ward 4 at a local hospital is experiencing an outbreak of a highly contagious gastrointestinal illness. Symptoms include vomiting, diarrhoea, and fever. Initial investigations suggest the outbreak may be linked to a norovirus.

1. Based on the information provided, what infection control measures should be implemented immediately on Ward 4?
2. What specific types of personal protective equipment (PPE) should healthcare workers wear while caring for patients with suspected norovirus infection?
3. Explain the importance of environmental cleaning and waste management in controlling the outbreak.
4. How can the implementation of barrier nursing principles help prevent the spread of the norovirus to other wards within the hospital?

Recap questions

1. What are vectors?
2. Name two diseases that can be transmitted by vectors.
3. How can habitat reduction be used to control mosquito populations?
4. What are larvicides used for in vector control?
5. How can livestock management help control tsetse fly populations?
6. What is the primary goal of infection control procedures in healthcare settings?
7. What are standard precautions in the context of healthcare?
8. When might transmission-based precautions be implemented?
9. What is the purpose of isolation in healthcare settings?
10. What are two examples of physical barriers used in barrier nursing?
11. How does soap disrupt microbial cells?
12. Explain the role of mechanical removal in the action of soap.
13. Why is proper handwashing with soap important for public health?

Find out more

www.eboru.com/BTEC-HSC-links

YouTube video on Malaria – Plasmodium

YouTube video about WHO Handwashing techniques

Activity

Microbial control techniques - fill in the gaps

Microorganisms can be controlled using various techniques to prevent their growth and spread. These techniques fall into two main categories: (1) _____ and (2) _____ methods.

(3) _____ methods include techniques such as refrigeration, which slows down microbial growth by reducing their (4) _____. Freezing can stop microbial growth by forming ice crystals that disrupt cellular structures. (5) _____ utilises high temperature and pressure to sterilise materials. Radiation can kill microorganisms by damaging their (6) _____. Finally, drying removes moisture, which is essential for microbial growth.

(7) _____ methods include the use of disinfectants, which are chemical agents used to kill or inactivate microorganisms on (8) _____ objects and surfaces. Examples of disinfectants include bleach and alcohol. (9) _____ are chemical agents used to kill or inhibit microorganisms on living tissue. Antibiotics are drugs specifically designed to kill or inhibit the growth of (10) _____.

End of Topic Practice Activity

In this practice activity you will focus on microorganisms and how they spread.

- Complete a table like the one below to explain some of the features of a microorganism of your choice. There is some guidance below to help you work through this task.

Type	Specific type	Diagram	Reproductive method	Survival needs
E.g. Virus	E.g. Bacteriophage			

- Create a mind map about the transmission and effective control measures for a microorganism.
- Once you have created the mind map can you discuss with a partner why you have included your chosen control measures.
- Produce a scientific report analysing the effectiveness of control methods for your selected microorganism. You will need to think about the effectiveness of control methods, how these methods target the specific microorganism and potential limitations or side effects. Use credible sources to back up your ideas.

This practice task will help you prepare for the following assessment criteria:

A.P1 Describe the structure and reproductive methods of four different microorganisms and their requirements for growth.

A.M1 Discuss how four different microorganisms are transmitted and how their requirements for growth can be controlled.

A.D1 Justify the methods used to control two different microorganisms.

Learning Aim B: Examine the cause and spread of disease in humans

Diseases can be caused by a variety of factors, including infectious agents, genetic abnormalities, environmental toxins, and lifestyle choices. This section looks at infectious disease and how it is transmitted from one individual to another. This transmission can occur through various means, such as direct contact, airborne transmission, or through contaminated food or water.

B1 Methods of non-specific defence used by the human body

The human body has evolved a variety of **non-specific defence mechanisms** to protect itself from a wide range of pathogens. These mechanisms are effective against a variety of pathogens regardless of their specific type.

> Mucous membranes – Cells that line organs and cavities in the body and which secrete mucus.

Skin

The **skin** is the body's first line of defence, forming a physical barrier that prevents microorganisms from entering. It is also slightly acidic, creating an environment that is unfavourable for many pathogens. The sebaceous glands secrete sebum, an oily substance that helps to moisturise the skin and create a protective barrier.

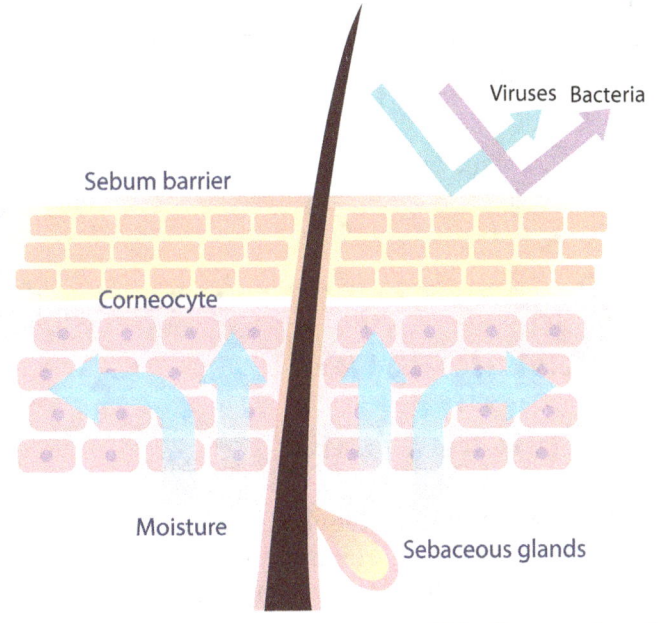

Skin forms a barrier

Mucous membranes

Mucous membranes line the respiratory, digestive, urinary, and reproductive tracts, providing a physical barrier against pathogens. They produce mucus, a sticky substance which traps microorganisms. In the respiratory tract, **cilia** (tiny hairlike structure on the surface of cells) move mucus and trapped microorganisms upward, where they can be expelled through coughing or sneezing.

Tears

Tears contain **lysozyme**, an enzyme that can break down the cell walls of bacteria. This helps to protect the eyes from infection. Tears also help to flush away microorganisms from the eyes.

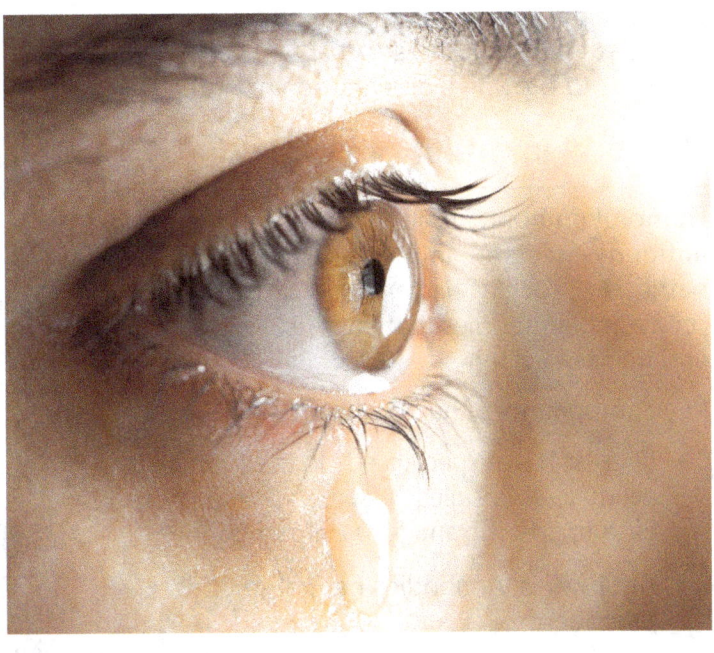

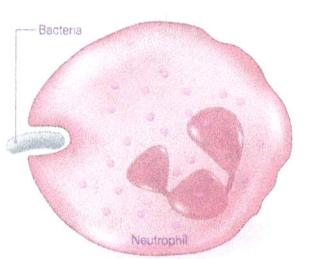
Endocytosis

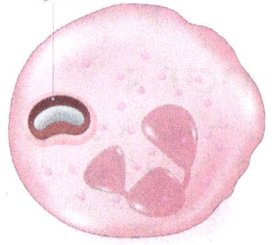
Phagosome formation

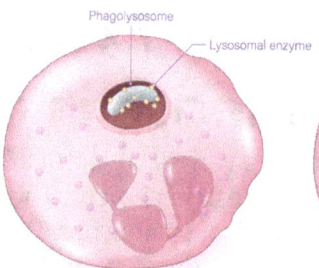
Digestion

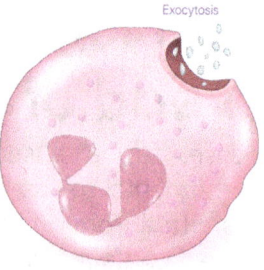
Release of microbial product

Phagocytosis

Phagocytes

Phagocytes are white blood cells that engulf and destroy foreign particles, including microorganisms. There are two main types of phagocytes: neutrophils and macrophages. Phagocytes use a process called phagocytosis to engulf and destroy pathogens.

> **Recap questions**
>
> 1. What is the body's first line of defence against pathogens?
> 2. Name two ways the skin acts as a barrier to pathogens.
> 3. Where are mucous membranes found in the body?
> 4. What are phagocytes and what is their function?

B2 Role of the immune system as a defence against infection

Adaptive immunity

The **adaptive immune system** consists of different types of cells working together to protect the body from pathogens. It can respond to and remember specific pathogens. The adaptive immune system is broadly divided into two branches – humoral immunity and cell-mediated immunity. These two branches work together to provide a defence against infection.

Humoral immunity

Humoral immunity is also known as the **antibody-mediated immune system**. It targets pathogens, such as bacteria and viruses, by producing antibodies that specifically bind to and neutralise them.

Key components of humoral immunity:

- **B-cells**: These specialised white blood cells produce antibodies, Y-shaped proteins that bind to specific antigens on pathogens.
- **Antibodies**: Antibodies neutralise pathogens by:

  * **Binding to antigens**: This prevents the pathogen from infecting cells.
  * **Opsonisation**: Coating pathogens with antibodies to make them clump together. This flags them up to phagocytes so they will be destroyed through phagocytosis.

Role of humoral immunity:

- **Primary response**: When a pathogen first enters the body, B-cells differentiate into plasma cells, which produce antibodies specific to the invading antigen.
- **Secondary response**: Upon subsequent exposure to the same pathogen, memory B-cells rapidly produce large amounts of antibodies, providing a more rapid and effective immune response.
- **Neutralising toxins**: Antibodies can also neutralise toxins produced by bacteria.

Cell-mediated immunity

While humoral immunity is effective against extracellular pathogens, it is less effective

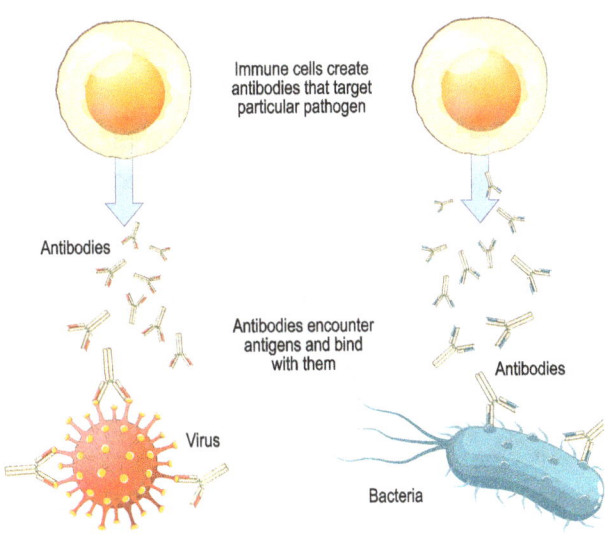

Y-shaped antibodies can attack viruses and bacteria

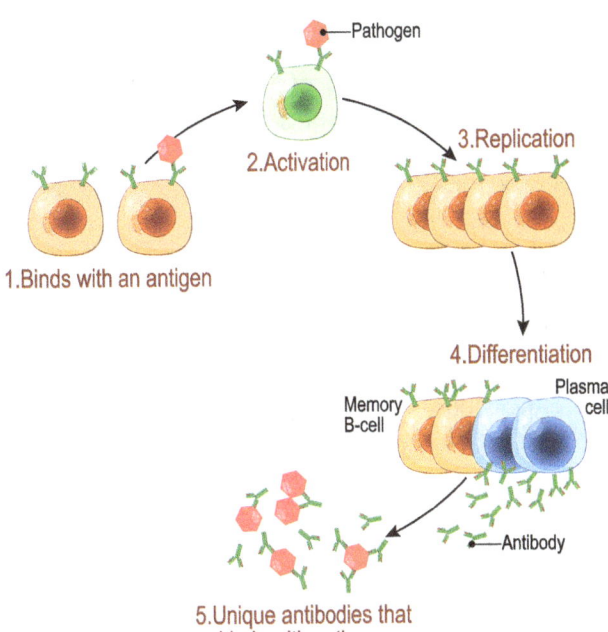

Humoral immunity. 1. Y-shaped antibodies on B-cells bind to an antigen on a pathogen. This activates the B-cell, causing it to replicate and produce memory B-cells and plasma cells. The plasma cells create antibodies for the specific pathogen, which are released to destroy it. The memory B-cells can react more quickly to the pathogen in the future.

against **intracellular pathogens**, such as viruses that have already infected cells. This is where **cell-mediated immunity** comes into action. This type of immunity involves T-cells, another type of white blood cell. T-cells recognise and attack cells infected with pathogens. There are two main types of T-cells:

- **Helper T-cells**: These cells coordinate the immune response by activating other immune cells, including B-cells and macrophages. They also release signalling molecules that help to stimulate the production of antibodies.

- **Cytotoxic (killer) T-cells**: These cells directly kill cells infected with viruses or other intracellular pathogens. They do this by releasing toxic substances that destroy the infected cell.

Leukocytes

Leukocytes, also known as white blood cells, are the main cells of the immune system. They are responsible for recognising and eliminating pathogens. There are different types of leukocytes including macrophages and T-lymphocytes.

- **Macrophages** are large, specialised white blood cells. They are a type of phagocyte and are responsible for engulfing and destroying foreign particles, such as bacteria, viruses, and cellular debris. This process is known as phagocytosis. Macrophages also play a vital role in initiating the immune response by releasing signalling molecules that attract other immune cells to the site of infection.

- **T-cells** (also called T-lymphocytes) play a central role in cell-mediated immunity, as described previously.

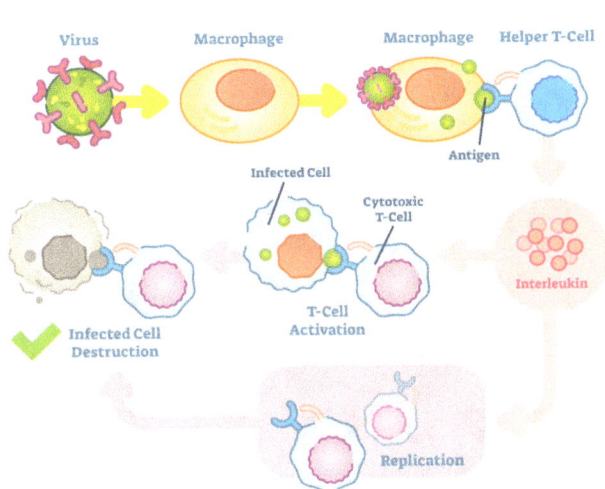

Cell-mediated immunity. If a pathogen infects cells, then Antigen Presenting Cells (APCs) show the virus's antigen to a T-cell. The APC in this diagram is called a macrophage. When the T-cell receptor recognises the pathogen, and creates cytotoxic T-cells, to kill the infected cells, and helper T-cells, to help coordinate the immune system response.

Inflammation

Inflammation is a process that occurs in response to tissue damage or infection. It is a protective mechanism that helps to isolate and eliminate harmful substances. It promotes healing and restores tissue function.

Key mechanisms of inflammation:

1. **Increased blood supply**

- **Vasodilation**: Blood vessels dilate, increasing blood flow to the injured or infected area. This brings oxygen, nutrients, and immune cells to the site of injury.
- **Hyperaemia**: The increased blood flow causes redness and warmth in the affected area.

2. **Increased capillary permeability**

- **Gaps between endothelial cells**: The walls of capillaries become more permeable, allowing fluid, white blood cells, and other immune cells to leak into the surrounding tissues.
- **Swelling**: This increased permeability leads to swelling (**oedema**) as fluid accumulates in the tissues.

3. **Immune cell migration**

- **Chemotaxis**: Chemical signals called cytokines attract immune cells, such as neutrophils and macrophages, to the site of inflammation.
- **Phagocytosis**: Immune cells engulf and destroy foreign particles, such as bacteria and damaged tissue.

4. **Tissue repair**: Once the infection or injury is cleared, immune cells help to promote tissue repair and regeneration.

Signs of inflammation

Signs	Reason
Redness	Increased blood flow causes redness.
Swelling	Fluid accumulation in the tissues leads to swelling.
Pain	Inflammation stimulates nerve endings, causing pain.
Heat	Increased blood flow and metabolic activity raise the temperature of the affected area.

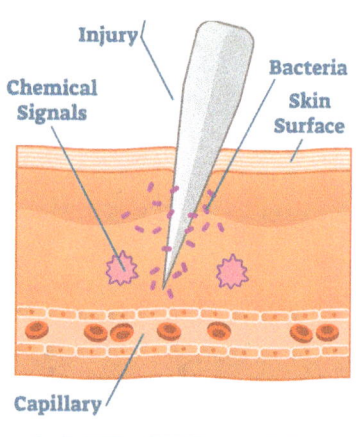

Tissue Injury
Release of chemical signals (Histamine)

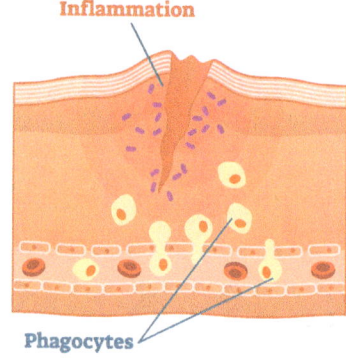

Dilation and Increased Leakiness of Capillary
Phagocytes Migrate to the Area

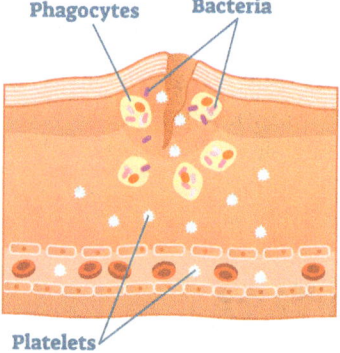

Phagocytes Consume Bacteria and Cell Debris
Platelets Move Out of the Capillary to Seal the Wounded Area

Community immunity

Community immunity, also known as **herd immunity**, is a concept in epidemiology where a significant portion of a population is immune to a contagious disease. This immunity can be achieved through either vaccination or natural infection. When a high percentage of the population is immune (ideally over 95%), the spread of the disease is significantly reduced, protecting even those who are not immune.

Community immunity protects individuals who cannot be vaccinated due to medical reasons or who have not developed immunity through natural infection.

By reducing the spread of a disease, community immunity helps to prevent outbreaks and epidemics. Community immunity is therefore a powerful tool for controlling the spread of infectious diseases.

> **Epidemiology** – The study of the distribution and cause of health and disease conditions in defined populations.

Recap questions

1. What are the two main branches of the immune system?
2. What is another name for humoral immunity?
3. What type of cells produce antibodies?
4. What is the role of memory B-cells in the immune response?
5. What are the two main types of T-cells?
6. Which branch of the immune system is more effective against intracellular pathogens?
7. What is inflammation?
8. What is vasodilation and why is it important during inflammation?
9. What causes swelling during inflammation?
10. What is chemotaxis?
11. What are the four signs of inflammation?
12. Why does the affected area become warm during inflammation?
13. What are leukocytes?
14. What are macrophages?
15. What is phagocytosis?
16. What is the main role of T-cells in the immune system?
17. What are the two main types of T-cells?
18. What is the function of cytotoxic T-cells?
19. What is community immunity?
20. How can community immunity be achieved?

Vaccination

Vaccination is a preventive measure that involves the administration of a vaccine to stimulate the body's immune system to develop immunity against a specific disease. Vaccines contain either weakened or inactive forms of pathogens, or part of the pathogen, which triggers the immune system to produce antibodies.

Vaccine development

The development of vaccines has advanced public health and prevented countless deaths and illnesses. The process of vaccine development involves several stages:

1. **Research and development**:
   - **Pathogen identification:** Scientists identify the specific pathogen causing a disease.
   - **Pathogen understanding:** Researchers study the pathogen's structure, reproduction and how it interacts with the human body.
   - **Antigen identification:** Scientists identify the antigens on the pathogen that trigger an immune response.

2. **Vaccine design**:
   - **Vaccine platform selection:** Scientists choose a suitable vaccine platform. This

can be live attenuated (a weakened version of the pathogen), inactivated pathogen, protein subunit (like an antigen), or genetic material like mRNA.

- **Preclinical testing:**
  * **Animal testing:** The vaccine is tested on animals for safety and efficacy.
  * **Immunogenicity:** Scientists evaluate the vaccine's ability to induce an immune response.

3. **Clinical trials:**

- **Phase I:** Small groups of healthy volunteers are given the vaccine to assess safety.
- **Phase II:** Larger groups of volunteers are given the vaccine to assess efficacy and safety in different populations.
- **Phase III:** Thousands of volunteers are given the vaccine in randomised controlled trials to confirm efficacy and safety.

4. **Regulatory approval:**

- **Submission to regulatory agencies:** The vaccine developer submits clinical trial data to regulatory bodies. In the UK it is the Medicines and Healthcare Products Regulatory Agency (MHRA) that approves vaccines for use.
- **Review and approval:** Regulatory agencies review the data to ensure the vaccine is safe and effective.

5. **Manufacturing and distribution:**

- **Large-scale production:** The vaccine is manufactured on a large scale.
- **Distribution:** The vaccine is distributed to healthcare providers for administration to the public.

6. **Ongoing monitoring:**

- **Continued monitoring** of the vaccine's safety and effectiveness after it is administered to the general population.
- **Addressing adverse events:** Any potential side effects or adverse events are investigated and addressed.

The development of the COVID-19 vaccine

The development of COVID-19 vaccines was a remarkable achievement, setting new records

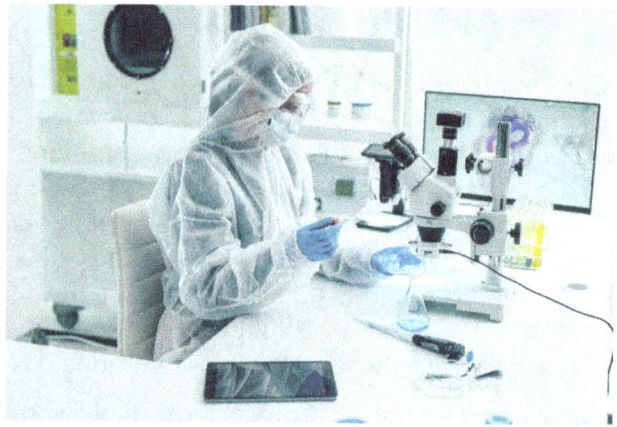

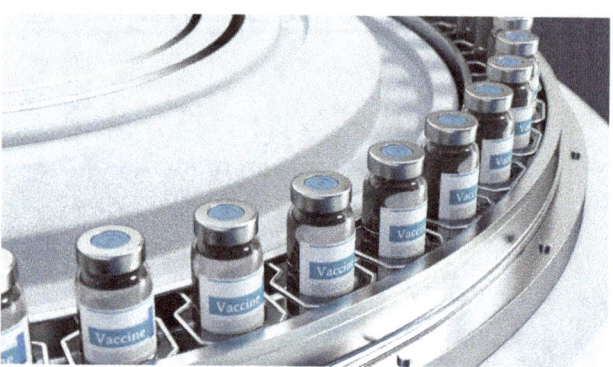

Vaccines begin with research and development and end in large-scale manufacturing and distribution

for speed and efficiency. Several factors contributed to the rapid development of these vaccines:

- **Pre-existing research:** decades of research on related coronaviruses provided valuable insights and gave scientists a head start in understanding the structure of the virus.
- **Global collaboration:** Scientists and researchers from around the world collaborated to accelerate vaccine development. Resources were shared between pharmaceutical companies and clinical trials were conducted simultaneously on a global scale.
- **Innovative technologies:** Newer vaccine technologies, such as mRNA vaccines, were used as they were highly effective and could be rapidly adapted to target the SARS-CoV-2 virus.
- **Emergency use authorisation:** Regulatory agencies granted emergency use authorisations, allowing vaccines to be administered before full regulatory approval.

Live attenuated and inactivated vaccines

> **Efficacy** – The ability of a drug to produce the desired beneficial effect in ideal conditions.
>
> **Randomised controlled trials** – A type of drug trial that compares the effects of two or more treatments by randomly assigning participants to different groups.

Vaccines work by exposing the body to a weakened or inactive form of a pathogen, stimulating the immune system to produce antibodies that can fight off the disease. There are two main types of vaccines: live attenuated and inactivated. The choice between a live attenuated and an inactivated vaccine depends on several factors, including the specific disease, the age and health of the individual, and the risk of adverse reactions.

	Live attenuated vaccine	Inactivated Vaccine
How do they work?	Contain live, but weakened, forms of the pathogen. The weakening process, known as attenuation, reduces the pathogen's ability to cause disease.	These vaccines contain a killed or inactivated form of the pathogen.
Advantages	Produce a stronger immune response compared to inactivated vaccines, as they mimic natural infection.	Inactivated vaccines are generally considered safer for immunocompromised individuals as there is no risk of the pathogen reverting to its virulent form.
Disadvantages	Small risk that the weakened pathogen could revert to its virulent form, causing disease. Therefore, these vaccines are generally not recommended for immunocompromised individuals.	Inactivated vaccines typically produce a weaker immune response compared to live attenuated vaccines, often requiring multiple doses or boosters.
Examples	Vaccines for measles, mumps, rubella, chickenpox, and polio are examples of live attenuated vaccines.	Vaccines for hepatitis A, hepatitis B, influenza, rabies, and tetanus are examples of inactivated vaccines.

Role of vaccines in herd immunity

Herd immunity, also known as community immunity, is a concept in epidemiology where a significant portion of a population is immune to an infectious disease. This immunity can be acquired through either vaccination or natural infection. When a high percentage of the population is immune, the spread of the disease is significantly reduced, protecting even those who are not immune.

Vaccines play an important role in achieving herd immunity. Vaccination can significantly reduce the number of susceptible individuals in a population. Because vaccines trigger an immune response, it stimulates the production of antibodies, giving protection against that disease. This makes it more difficult for the disease to spread, protecting those who cannot be vaccinated due to medical reasons or who have not developed immunity through natural infection.

Recap questions

1. What is the primary purpose of vaccination?
2. What are the two main types of components that vaccines can contain?
3. What is the role of regulatory agencies in vaccine development?
4. What is the primary function of vaccines in the human body?
5. How do live attenuated vaccines work?
6. What is the main advantage of inactivated vaccines?

Role of vaccines in eliminating disease

Vaccines have played a key role in eradicating several infectious diseases. One of the most notable examples of a vaccine eliminating a disease is the eradication of smallpox.

Smallpox was a highly contagious and often fatal viral disease. In 1796, a scientist named Dr Edward Jenner developed the smallpox vaccine. This was the first use of a vaccine against disease. Edward Jenner noticed that people who had been infected with cowpox were immune to smallpox. Cowpox is a milder virus which is similar in structure to smallpox. Jenner then inoculated an 8-year-old boy with a small amount of the virus which he had collected from an infected sore on a milkmaid's hand. The boy developed immunity against smallpox.

Through widespread vaccination campaigns, smallpox cases were gradually reduced, resulting in the World Health Organisation (WHO) declaring smallpox as being eradicated worldwide in 1980.

The eradication of smallpox is as a powerful reminder of the potential of vaccines to eliminate infectious diseases.

Recap questions

1. What is herd immunity?
2. How can herd immunity be achieved?
3. How do vaccines contribute to herd immunity?
4. What disease was eradicated through widespread vaccination?
5. Who is credited with developing the smallpox vaccine?
6. What is the significance of the eradication of smallpox?

Activity

1. Explain the role of B-cells in the humoral immune response.
2. Describe the key features of inflammation and its role in the body's defence.
3. Discuss the importance of herd immunity in controlling the spread of infectious diseases. Include in your answer how vaccination contributes to achieving herd immunity.
4. Describe the stages involved in the development of a new vaccine.

Apply your understanding

In a small, rural community, there has been a recent outbreak of measles. Health officials are investigating the cause of the outbreak and are working to contain its spread.

Background information:

Measles is a highly contagious viral infection that can cause serious complications, including pneumonia and encephalitis.

Vaccination is the most effective way to prevent measles.

The community has a history of low vaccination rates, particularly among children.

1. What is measles, and what are its potential complications?
2. What is the most effective way to prevent measles?
3. Why might low vaccination rates contribute to an outbreak of measles?
4. What steps can health officials take to contain the outbreak and prevent further spread?
5. How can the community increase vaccination rates to prevent future outbreaks?

B3 Transmission routes

Disease transmission routes are the pathways through which infectious agents, such as bacteria and viruses, spread from an infected individual to a susceptible host. These routes can be direct, involving physical contact, or indirect, using vectors (like mosquitoes) or via contaminated surfaces. By understanding the routes, we can help to prevent the spread of diseases and maintain public health.

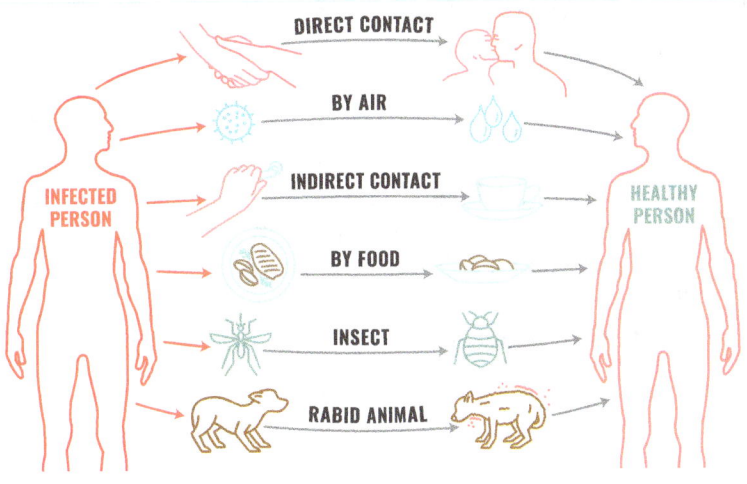

Disease transmission routes

Direct contact

Disease transmission by direct contact occurs when there is physical contact between an infected person and a susceptible person. This can happen through a variety of ways, including:

Person-to-person contact

This is the most common type of direct contact transmission. It can occur through direct transfer of bacteria, viruses, or other pathogens from one person to another. This can happen through touching, kissing, sexual contact, or contact with infected bodily fluids. Examples include:

- **Skin-to-skin contact**: Diseases like scabies, impetigo, and ringworm are spread through direct contact with infected skin lesions.

- **Droplet transmission**: Respiratory illnesses like influenza, measles, and COVID-19 are transmitted through droplets expelled when an infected person coughs, sneezes, or talks. These droplets can land directly on the mucous membranes of a susceptible person's eyes, nose, or mouth.

- **Sexual contact**: Sexually transmitted infections (STIs) like HIV, chlamydia, and gonorrhoea are spread through sexual contact with an infected person.

Animal-to-person contact

This type of transmission occurs when a person comes into contact with an infected animal or its waste. This can happen through direct contact with the animal, such as petting or kissing, or through indirect contact, such

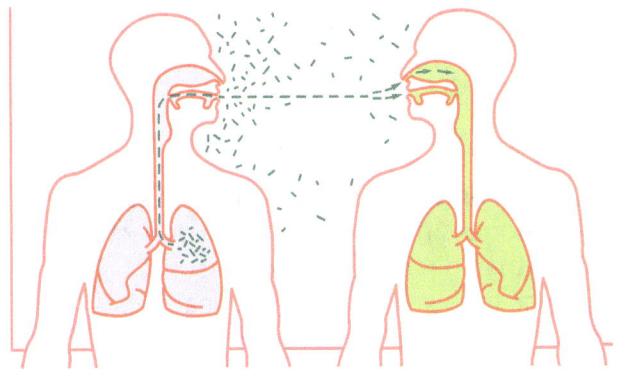

Droplets released during coughing and sneezing can spread certain diseases

> **Lesion** – An area of abnormal tissue caused by injury or disease.

as touching a contaminated surface. Some examples of diseases that are transmitted through animal-to-person contact include:

- Rabies
- Ringworm
- Leptospirosis
- Toxoplasmosis

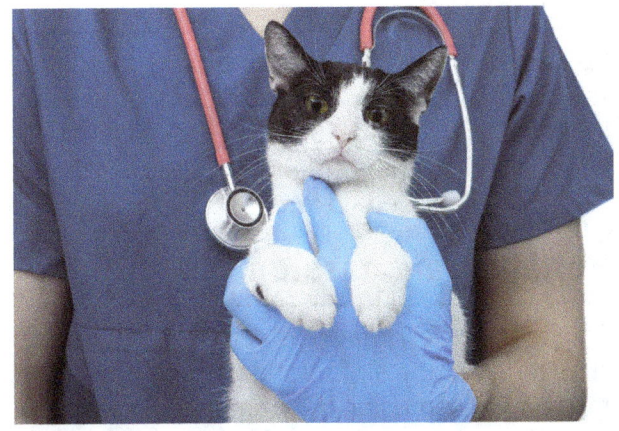

Animals can spread disease through biting

Infected animal bites or handling animal waste:

- **Infected animal bites**: This type of transmission occurs when a person is bitten by an infected animal. Examples include rabies, which is transmitted through the saliva of infected animals, and cat scratch disease, which is caused by bacteria present in the mouths of cats.

- **Handling animal waste**: This type of transmission occurs when a person comes into contact with the faeces or urine of an infected animal. Contact with infected animal faeces can lead to the transmission of diseases like toxoplasmosis, which is caused by a parasite found in cat faeces.

Mother-to-unborn child

A mother can pass an infectious disease on to her unborn child via the placenta or during delivery.

- **Through the placenta**: Certain pathogens can cross the placental barrier and infect the developing foetus. Examples include HIV and toxoplasmosis.

- **During delivery**: During delivery the baby passes down through the vagina. Group B streptococcus is a bacterium that can colonise the vagina and rectum of pregnant women. During childbirth, the baby can be exposed to Group B streptococcus and become infected.

Indirect contact

Indirect contact involves the transmission of pathogens through a medium or vector rather than direct person-to-person contact. In this section you will learn about some common modes of indirect contact transmission:

Surface contamination

Pathogens can survive on surfaces for varying periods, depending on factors like temperature, humidity, and the specific type of pathogen. When a susceptible person touches a contaminated surface and then touches their mouth, nose, or eyes, they can become infected.

Examples of bacteria commonly spread through surface contamination include Staphylococcus aureus and Salmonella. COVID-19 can survive on surfaces for up to 72 hours.

Droplet transmission

Respiratory droplets expelled during coughing, sneezing, or talking can transmit pathogens like influenza and COVID-19. These droplets can be inhaled by others or land on surfaces where they may be picked up later.

Particle transmission

Smaller particles, known as **aerosols**, can remain suspended in the air for long periods. This mode of transmission is common for diseases like tuberculosis and some fungal infections.

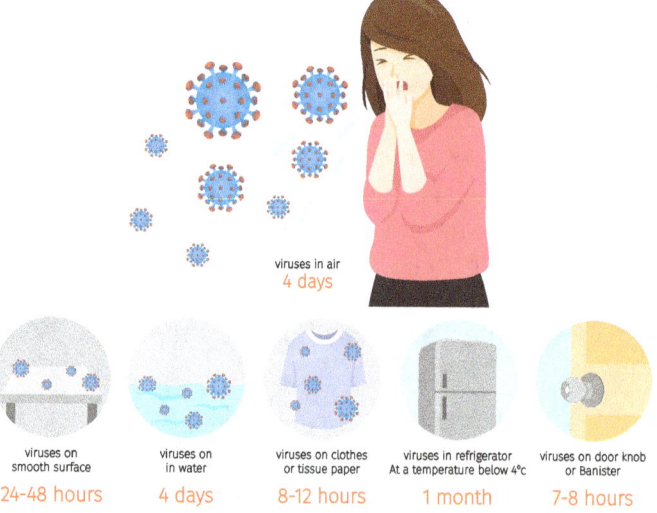

viruses in air
4 days

viruses on smooth surface
24-48 hours

viruses on in water
4 days

viruses on clothes or tissue paper
8-12 hours

viruses in refrigerator At a temperature below 4°c
1 month

viruses on door knob or Banister
7-8 hours

Pollution particulates can also contribute to the spread of respiratory illnesses by carrying pathogens or irritating the respiratory tract.

Vector-borne transmission

Vectors, such as insects and animals, can transmit pathogens from one host to another. Examples include:

- **Mosquitoes**: Mosquitoes can transmit diseases like malaria, dengue fever, and Zika virus.

- **Fleas**: Fleas can transmit diseases like plague.

- **Lice**: Lice can transmit diseases like typhus.

- **Ticks**: Ticks can transmit diseases like Lyme disease.

Food and water contamination

Consuming contaminated food or water can lead to various illnesses. Pathogens like E. coli, Salmonella, and norovirus can be present in contaminated food and water, causing gastrointestinal infections.

Activity

1. Explain how surface contamination can lead to the spread of disease. Provide two specific examples of pathogens that can be spread this way.
2. Describe the role of vectors in the transmission of infectious diseases. Give one example of a vector-borne disease.
3. Explain the importance of hygiene practices and education in preventing the spread of infectious diseases. Give three specific examples of how these can be implemented in a school setting.

Recap questions

1. What is the most common type of direct contact transmission?
2. List two diseases that are spread through skin-to-skin contact.
3. How are respiratory illnesses like influenza typically transmitted?
4. What are two examples of diseases that can be transmitted through animal bites?
5. How can a mother transmit an infection to her unborn child?
6. What is the key characteristic of indirect contact transmission?
7. How can pathogens spread through surface contamination?
8. What are aerosols, and how are they related to disease transmission?
9. Name two diseases that can be transmitted by mosquitoes.

Apply your understanding

Riverside High School is experiencing an outbreak of a suspected contagious illness. Symptoms reported include fever, cough, fatigue, and muscle aches. School leaders are concerned about the rapid spread of the illness and are seeking guidance from public health experts.

1. What are the possible modes of transmission for this illness based on the reported symptoms?
2. What steps should school leaders take to contain the outbreak and prevent further spread?
3. How can school leaders identify and isolate infected students?
4. What role can education and hygiene practices play in preventing the spread of this illness?
5. What are some potential long-term consequences for students who contract this illness?

B4 Types of infectious disease

Infectious diseases are caused by microorganisms (bacteria, viruses, fungi, and protozoa) that invade the human body and disrupt its normal functioning. In this section you will learn about the different types of infectious disease.

Viral infections

Viral infections are caused by microorganisms called viruses. Viruses invade host cells and then hijack their cellular machinery to enable them to replicate and spread. The severity of a viral infection depends on various factors, including the type of virus, the strength of the host's immune system, and the specific cells targeted by the virus. There are many different types of viruses which can cause disease in humans.

	Colds (rhinovirus)	Influenza	HIV-related disease	Avian Flu in Humans
Structure	Small, non-enveloped viruses with single-stranded RNA	Enveloped viruses with RNA	HIV is a complex retrovirus with two copies of single-stranded RNA	Enveloped virus with RNA
Requirements for growth	Replicate best at temperatures around 33-37°C, which is the typical temperature of the human respiratory tract. It cannot replicate on its own and requires a host cell to reproduce.	Replicate best at temperatures around 33-37°C, which is the typical temperature of the human respiratory tract. It cannot replicate on its own and requires a host cell to reproduce.	Targets and infects immune cells, specifically Helper T cells. It cannot replicate on its own and requires a host cell to reproduce.	It cannot replicate on its own and requires a host cell to reproduce.
Transmission routes	Spread through direct contact with infected droplets or contaminated surfaces.	Spreads through respiratory droplets and can also be transmitted through contact with contaminated surfaces.	Spread through bodily fluids like blood, semen, vaginal fluids, and breast milk.	Human infections are often linked to close contact with infected birds (live or dead). It is rare for it to spread from human to human.
Effects on human health	Mild respiratory symptoms like a runny nose, sneezing, and congestion.	Can cause fever, chills, cough, sore throat, muscle aches, headache, and fatigue. Severe cases can lead to pneumonia and other complications.	Over time, HIV weakens the immune system, making individuals susceptible to opportunistic infections and cancers.	Can cause fever, chills, cough, sore throat, muscle aches, headache, and fatigue. Severe cases can lead to pneumonia and other complications.

Bacterial infections

Bacterial infections are caused by single-celled organisms called bacteria. These microorganisms can thrive in various environments, including the human body. They can cause a wide range of illnesses, from mild infections to life-threatening diseases.

- **Tuberculosis** (TB) bacteria are rod-shaped and have a waxy outer coating that makes them resistant to drying out. TB bacteria are slow-growing and require oxygen to survive. TB is primarily spread through the air when an infected person coughs, sneezes, or talks. TB initially affects the lungs, but it can also spread to other organs. Symptoms include cough, fever, night sweats, and weight loss. If left untreated TB can be fatal.

- **Salmonella food poisoning** is caused by Salmonella bacteria. These bacteria are rod-shaped and have flagella, allowing them to move. Salmonella bacteria grow best in warm, moist environments. Salmonella is often transmitted through contaminated food, such as poultry, eggs, and raw vegetables. Salmonella food poisoning causes diarrhoea, abdominal cramps, and fever. In severe cases, it can lead to dehydration and even death.

- **Streptococcal sore throat** is caused by streptococcus bacteria. Streptococcus bacteria are spherical and can form chains. Streptococcus bacteria are **aerobic**, meaning they require oxygen to grow. Streptococcus bacteria are spread through respiratory droplets. Streptococcal sore throat causes a sore throat, fever, and swollen lymph nodes. Complications can include ear infections, sinusitis, and rheumatic fever.

- **Meningococcal meningitis** is caused by the Neisseria meningitidis bacteria. These bacteria are spherical and often occur in pairs. Meningococcal bacteria are aerobic and grow best at body temperature. They are spread through respiratory droplets. Meningococcal meningitis is a serious infection that can cause inflammation of the meninges, the membranes surrounding the brain and spinal cord. Symptoms include fever, headache, stiff neck, and confusion. In severe cases, it can lead to brain damage, hearing loss, and death.

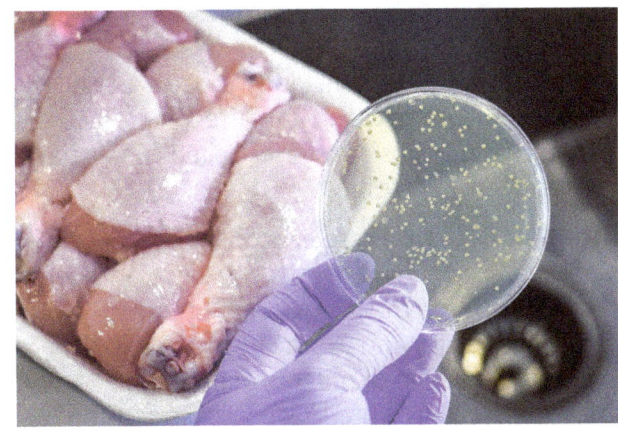

Salmonella is found on raw food such as chicken

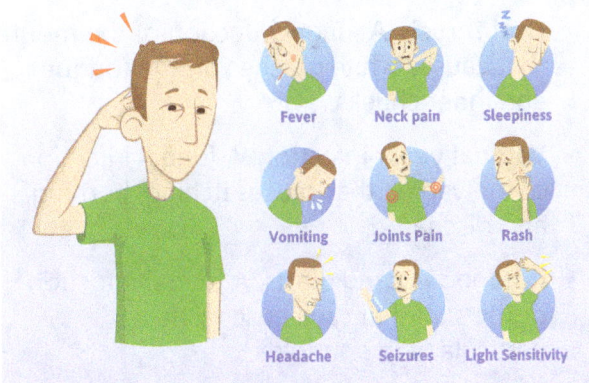

Recap questions

1. Name three different types of viruses that can cause disease in humans.
2. What are the requirements for a virus to grow and replicate?
3. Describe the typical transmission routes of viral infections.
4. Explain the relationship between HIV and the human immune system.
5. Describe the characteristics of the bacteria that cause Tuberculosis (TB).
6. How is Salmonella food poisoning typically transmitted?
7. What are the common symptoms of streptococcal sore throat?
8. What is meningococcal meningitis and how is it spread?

Fungal infections

Fungal infections, particularly those caused by yeasts, are common and can affect various parts of the body. Yeasts are single-celled fungi that reproduce by budding.

Candidiasis is a disease caused by yeasts. Candida are oval-shaped yeast cells. Candida thrives in warm, moist environments, such as the skin, mouth, and vagina. It can overgrow when the balance of microorganisms in these areas is disrupted. Candidiasis is often **opportunistic**, meaning it occurs when the body's defences are weakened. It can be transmitted through direct contact with infected individuals or surfaces. Candidiasis can cause a variety of infections, including:

- **Oral thrush**: A fungal infection of the mouth that causes white patches on the tongue and inner cheeks.
- **Vaginal yeast infection**: A fungal infection of the vagina that causes itching, burning, and discharge.
- **Cutaneous candidiasis**: A fungal infection of the skin that can cause rashes, particularly in skin folds.

Tinea infections (ringworm) are caused by dermatophytes, a type of fungus that feeds on keratin, a protein found in skin, hair, and nails. Like other fungi, dermatophytes thrive in warm, moist environments. Tinea infections can spread through direct contact with infected individuals or contaminated objects, such as towels and clothing. Tinea infections can cause ringworm infections all over the body. If it occurs on the feet, then it is commonly known as athlete's foot.

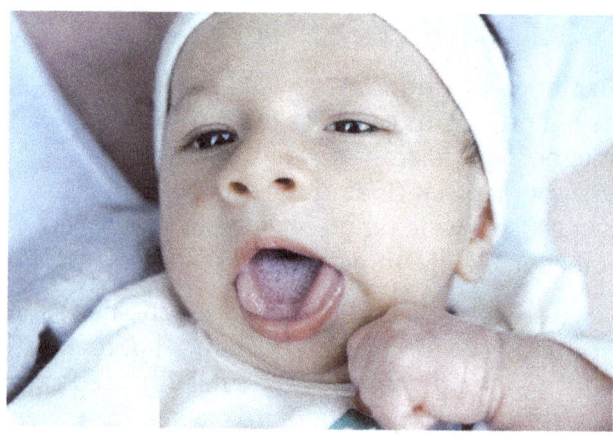

A baby with oral thrush

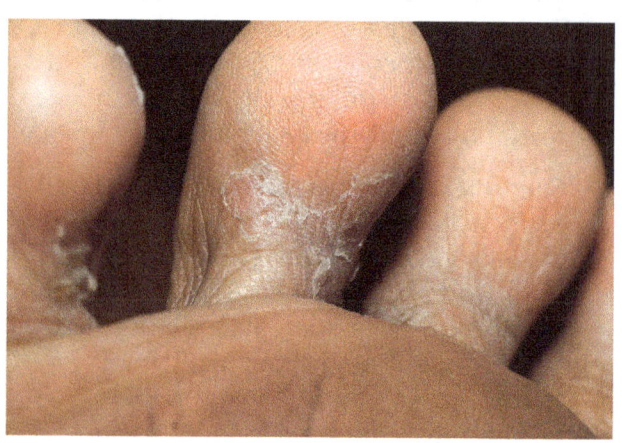

Athlete's foot

Protozoan infections

Protozoa are single-celled eukaryotic organisms that can cause a variety of infectious diseases in humans. These parasites have complex life cycles and often require specific conditions for their growth and development.

Malaria is an example of a protozoal infection. The malaria protozoa has a complex life cycle involving both human and mosquito hosts. They require specific conditions, such as temperature and humidity, to complete their life cycle. Malaria is transmitted to humans through the bite of an infected female Anopheles mosquito. Malaria can cause a range of symptoms, including fever, chills, headache, muscle aches, and fatigue. In severe cases, it can lead to organ failure and death.

Recap questions

1. What are yeasts and how do they reproduce?
2. What are the common sites of infection for Candida, the yeast that causes candidiasis?
3. What are dermatophytes and what do they feed on?
4. How are tinea infections typically transmitted?
5. What are protozoa and how do they cause disease in humans?
6. What are some key factors that influence the life cycle of malaria parasites?

Activity

1. Explain why the spread of some viral infections, such as influenza, can be difficult to control.
2. Describe the characteristics of the bacteria that cause Streptococcal Sore Throat.
3. Explain how HIV weakens the immune system and increases the risk of opportunistic infections.
4. Discuss the risk factors and potential complications associated with Candidiasis.

Apply your understanding

Joh is a 20-year-old university student. They present to the student health centre with a sudden onset of fever, headache, and stiff neck. They also report nausea and vomiting. Their flatmate mentions that Joh has been unusually sleepy and irritable over the past few days.

1. What are the most likely causes of Joh's symptoms, and why is meningitis a serious concern?
2. What diagnostic tests would you recommend for Joh?
3. How is bacterial meningitis typically treated?
4. What are the potential complications of meningitis, and how can they be prevented?

B5 The cause and spread of blood infections

Blood infections, also known sepsis, occur when harmful pathogens enter the bloodstream. These microorganisms can originate from various sources, including wounds, surgical sites, urinary tract infections, or lung infections. Once in the bloodstream, they can rapidly multiply, leading to a **systemic** (whole body) inflammatory response that can damage multiple organs.

Blood components

Blood is a fluid tissue composed of several components, each with a specific function. These components include plasma, red blood cells, white blood cells, and platelets.

- **Red blood cells**, also known as erythrocytes, are the most numerous cells in the blood. They have a biconcave disc shape and contain haemoglobin, a protein that binds to oxygen. Haemoglobin allows red blood cells to transport oxygen from the lungs to the body's tissues.

- **White blood cells**, also known as leukocytes, are part of the immune system and help fight infection. They are less numerous than red blood cells and come in distinct types, each with a specific function. Some white blood cells engulf and destroy bacteria and other pathogens, while others produce antibodies to help neutralise them.

- **Platelets**, also known as thrombocytes, are small cell fragments that play a vital role in blood clotting. When a blood vessel is damaged, platelets clump together and release clotting factors, which help to form a clot and stop bleeding.

- **Plasma** is the liquid component of blood, making up about 55% of its total volume. It is a complex mixture of water, proteins, electrolytes, and other substances. Plasma plays a vital role in maintaining blood pressure, regulating body temperature, and transporting various substances.

- **Serum** is the fluid portion of blood that remains after clotting. It lacks clotting factors as they are removed during the clotting process. In the body it helps to transport fatty acids and hormones.

Diseases/problems associated with blood components

While blood is essential for life, it can also be a source of various health problems and diseases. A change in the balance or function of its components, such as red and white blood cells, platelets, and plasma, can lead to a range of conditions, from mild to life-threatening. These disorders can affect oxygen transport, immune function, blood clotting, and overall bodily health.

Erythrocytic diseases

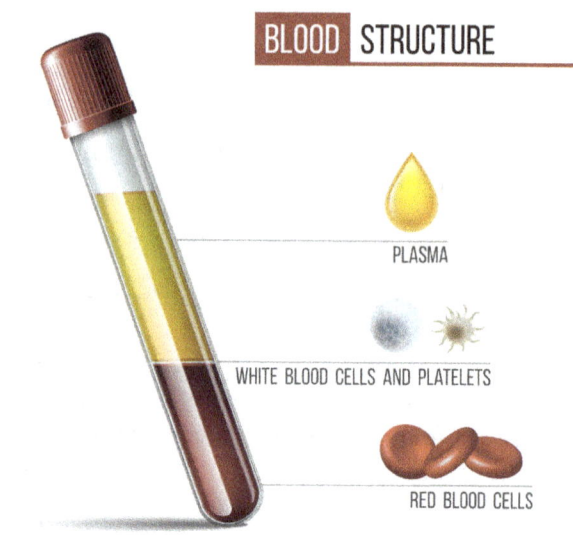

Erythrocytic diseases are a group of disorders that affect red blood cells (erythrocytes), which are responsible for carrying oxygen throughout the body. These diseases can disrupt the production, function, or lifespan of red blood cells, leading to a variety of symptoms and health complications.

- **Sickle cell anaemia** is an inherited disorder which causes red blood cells to become misshapen and rigid, resembling sickles (crescent-shaped). These abnormal red cells can block blood vessels, leading to pain crises and organ damage.

  There is no cure for sickle cell anaemia, but treatments are available to help manage the symptoms and complications of the disease. These treatments include medications to relieve pain, prevent infections, and reduce the number of sickle cell crises. In some cases, blood transfusions or bone marrow transplants may be necessary.

- **Thalassaemia** is an inherited blood disorder that affects the production of haemoglobin, the protein in red blood cells that carries oxygen around the body. People with thalassaemia don't produce enough haemoglobin, which can make them very **anaemic** (tired, short of breath and pale).

- **Haemolytic diseases of the newborn (HDN)** are a group of conditions that affect babies in the first few weeks to months after birth. HDN occurs when there is a blood group incompatibility between the mother and her baby. This incompatibility causes the mother's immune system to attack the baby's red blood cells, destroying them.

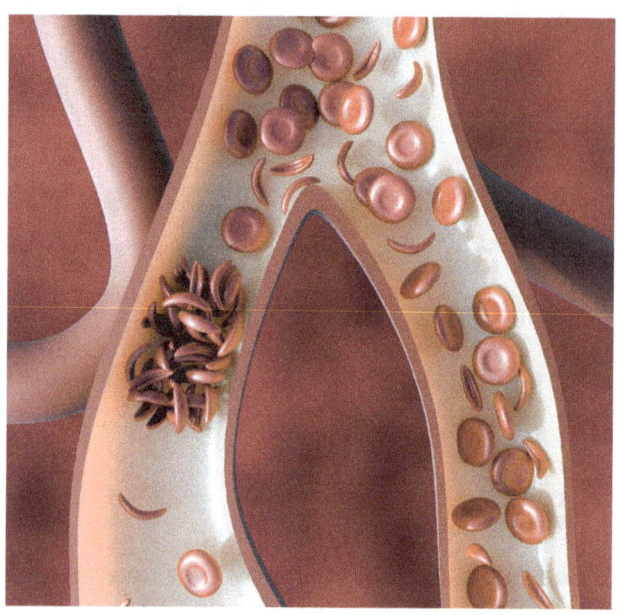

Sickle cell anaemia affects the shape of red blood cells, which can then block blood vessels

The most common type of HDN is **rhesus disease**. Rhesus disease occurs when the mother has rhesus negative blood (RhD negative), and the baby has rhesus positive blood (RhD positive). If the mother is exposed to the baby's RhD positive blood during pregnancy or delivery, her body will start to produce antibodies against the RhD factor. These antibodies cross the placenta and will start to destroy the baby's red blood cells. HDN can cause several problems for the baby, including jaundice, anaemia, and in severe cases, brain damage or death. In the case of Rhesus disease, HDN can be prevented by injecting the mother with RhD immunoglobulin during pregnancy.

Recap questions

1. What are the four main components of blood?
2. Which is the most numerous type of cell in the blood?
3. What is the function of red blood cells?
4. What is the function of white blood cells?
5. What is the function of platelets?
6. What is the liquid component of blood?
7. What are erythrocytic diseases?
8. What is the main characteristic of sickle cell anaemia?
9. What is thalassaemia?
10. What causes Haemolytic Diseases of the Newborn (HDN)?

Leukocytes and white blood cell diseases

Leukocytes (white blood cells) are part of the immune system and they defend the body against infections and diseases. However, abnormalities in their production, their function, or the number of white blood cells can lead to various health conditions:

- **Lymphocytosis** is a condition in which there are too many lymphocytes in the blood. It can be caused by a variety of things, including viral infections, bacterial infections, and autoimmune diseases. The symptoms of lymphocytosis are fever, fatigue, or swollen lymph nodes. In most cases, lymphocytosis is not a serious condition and goes away on its own. In some cases, it can be an early sign of leukaemia.

- **HIV/AIDS** is a more severe and complex condition affecting white blood cells. Human immunodeficiency virus (HIV) attacks the immune system, specifically targeting CD4 Helper T cells. CD4 cells play an important role in immunity as they recognise pathogens and produce cytokines (chemical messengers) which activate other immune cells. As the virus progresses, it weakens the immune system, making individuals susceptible to opportunistic infections and cancers. Untreated HIV infection can lead to acquired immunodeficiency syndrome (**AIDS**). AIDS is the final stage of HIV infection.

In the 1980s people could not survive HIV. However, advancements in medical care have dramatically improved things for people with HIV. Drugs known as antiretroviral therapy (ART) can be taken to suppress the virus, preventing it from progressing to AIDS and allowing people with HIV to live long, healthy lives.

> **Opportunistic infections** – Infections caused by pathogens that take advantage of a weakened immune system or other compromised bodily defences.
>
> **Bone marrow** – The soft, spongy tissue found inside the centre of bones that produces blood cells.

Leukaemia

Leukaemia is a type of cancer that affects the blood and bone marrow, leading to the uncontrolled production of abnormal white blood cells. These abnormal cells don't function properly and can crowd out healthy blood cells, impairing the body's ability to fight infection, transport oxygen, and clot blood.

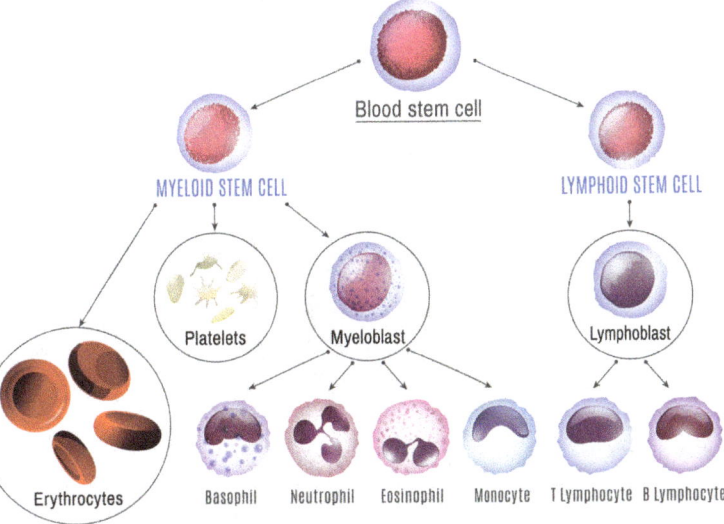

The different blood cells which develop from blood stem cells

Two common types of leukaemia are:

- **Acute Myelogenous Leukaemia (AML)** is a type of cancer that affects the bone marrow, the spongy tissue inside bones where blood cells are produced. In AML, the bone marrow starts producing abnormal white blood cells called **myeloid cells**. These myeloid cells don't function properly and can block the production and function of healthy blood cells.

  It is a fast-growing cancer (acute) and is more commonly found in adults. Symptoms include fatigue and weakness (due to low red cell numbers), frequent infections (impaired white cell function), bleeding and bruising (low platelet count).

- **Chronic Myelomonocytic Leukaemia (CMML)** is a slowly progressing type of leukaemia that affects two types of white blood cells - **myeloid** and **monocyte** cells. It is characterised by an overproduction of white blood cells, particularly **monocytes**. Symptoms of CMML include fatigue, frequent infections, easy bleeding or bruising and fever.

Treatment for leukaemia depends on the specific type, stage, and overall health of the patient. Common treatment options include chemotherapy, radiation therapy, and bone marrow transplantation.

Lymphomas

Lymphomas are a type of cancer that affects the **lymphatic system** – a network of vessels and glands that help fight infection. They develop when lymphocytes, a type of white blood cell, grow and multiply uncontrollably.

There are two main types of lymphoma:

- **Hodgkin lymphoma** develops when abnormal lymphocytes, called Reed-Sternberg cells, start to grow uncontrollably. It often starts in the lymph nodes of the neck, chest, or underarms and can spread to other parts of the body.

- **Non-Hodgkin lymphoma** is a more common type of lymphoma. It is a general term for a group of cancers that affect lymphocytes. It can develop in various parts of the lymphatic system, including the lymph nodes, spleen, bone marrow, and other organs.

Symptoms of lymphoma can include:

- Swollen lymph nodes
- Fever
- Night sweats
- Unexplained weight loss
- Fatigue

Common treatment options for lymphoma include chemotherapy, radiation therapy and immunotherapy. The type of treatment used depends on the type, stage (how far the disease has progressed), and overall health of the patient.

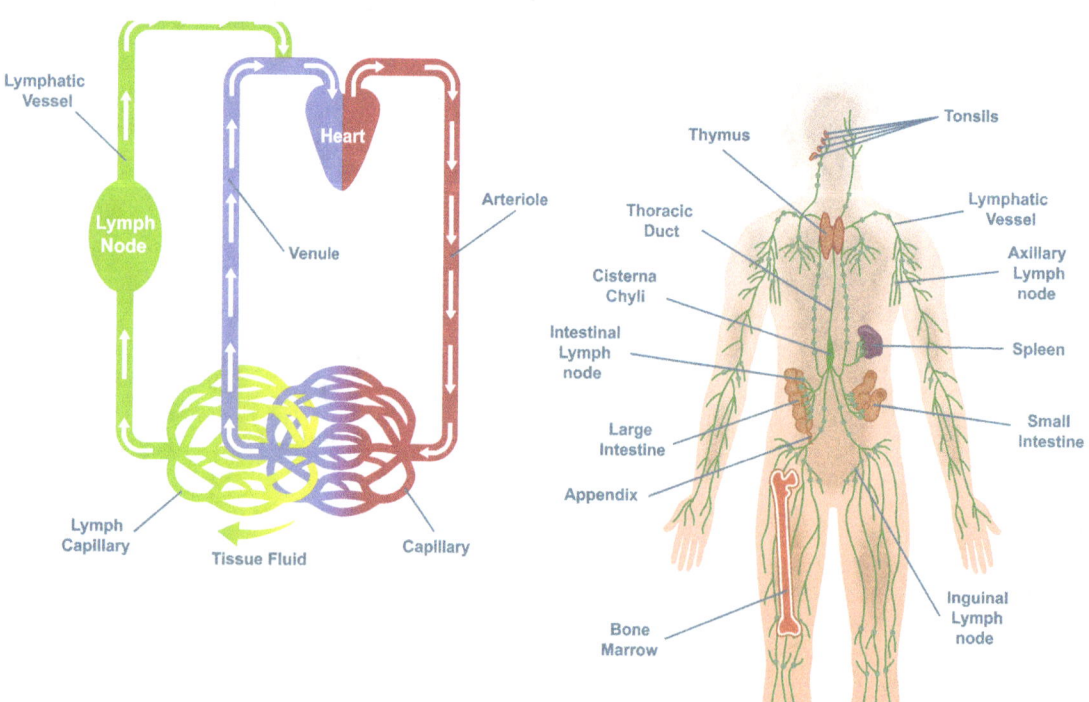

The lymphatic system

Haemostasis and thrombosis

Haemostasis is the process by which the body stops bleeding. It involves a series of steps to form a blood clot, which seals the damaged blood vessel and prevents further blood loss.

When a blood vessel is injured, it constricts to reduce blood flow to the damaged area. Platelets stick to the injured vessel wall and build up to form a platelet plug. A series of biochemical reactions, involving clotting factors, leads to the formation of a fibrin clot. Strands of **fibrin** (a protein) trap blood cells and platelets, which solidifies the clot.

Thrombosis is the formation of a blood clot inside a blood vessel. While haemostasis is a normal physiological process, thrombosis can be a **pathological** condition which can lead to serious health problems, such as heart attack, stroke, and pulmonary embolism.

Thrombosis occurs when the blood clotting process is activated inappropriately or when the body's natural anticoagulant mechanisms are impaired. This can lead to the formation of a blood clot (**thrombus**), that can block blood flow to vital organs.

- An **arterial thrombosis** occurs in the arteries and can lead to a heart attack or stroke.
- A **venous thrombosis** occurs in the veins and can lead to deep vein thrombosis (DVT) or **pulmonary embolism**.

An embolism occurs when part of the thrombus breaks off and travels through the bloodstream.

- If it blocks an artery in the lungs, then this is known as a **pulmonary embolism**.
- If it blocks an artery in the brain, it is a **cerebral embolism** and could cause a stroke.

The formation of blood clots

Deep vein thrombosis and an embolism

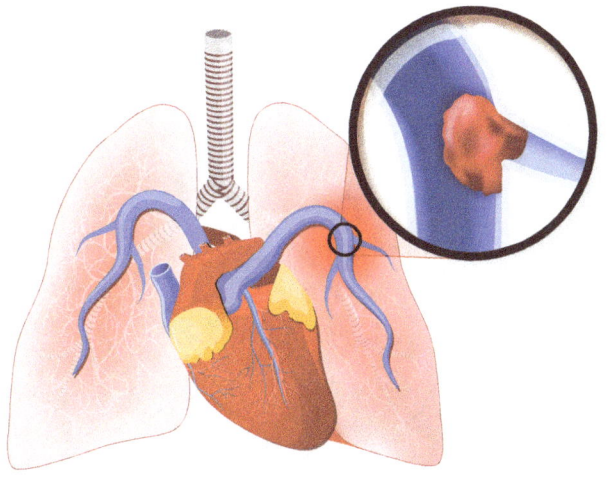

A pulmonary embolism

Recap questions

1. What is the main function of leukocytes?
2. What is lymphocytosis?
3. Which type of white blood cell does HIV primarily target?
4. What is the final stage of HIV infection?
5. What is leukaemia?
6. What is the primary characteristic of Acute Myelogenous Leukaemia (AML)?
7. What type of cells are affected in Chronic Myelomonocytic Leukaemia (CMML)?
8. What is the primary function of bone marrow?
9. What are the two main types of lymphoma?
10. What is a) haemostasis, b) thrombosis?
11. What is an embolism?
12. Name two risk factors for thrombosis.

There are certain risk factors that increase the chance of thrombosis:

- age
- inherited blood clotting disorders
- smoking
- obesity
- sedentary lifestyle
- certain medical conditions (heart disease, diabetes)
- certain medications (birth control pills, hormone replacement therapy).

Transmissible infections by blood transfusion

A blood transfusion is a life-saving medical procedure that involves transferring blood or blood products from one person to another. While it is a safe and effective treatment, there is always a risk of transmitting infectious diseases.

Clinical use of blood products

Blood products are used in a variety of clinical settings, including:

- **Surgery:** To replace blood loss during major surgeries.
- **Intensive Care:** To treat patients with severe bleeding or anaemia.
- **Cancer Treatment:** To replace blood cells destroyed by chemotherapy or radiation therapy.

Screening of blood products

To minimise the risk of transmitting infections, blood products are rigorously screened for a variety of diseases. Some of the most common tests include:

- **HIV-related disease:** Blood is tested for HIV antibodies to identify individuals infected with the virus.
- **Hepatitis:** Tests are conducted to detect hepatitis B and C viruses, which can cause liver damage.
- **Human parvovirus B19:** This virus can cause severe anaemia in individuals with certain blood disorders.
- **Malaria:** Blood donations from individuals who have recently travelled to malaria-endemic regions are carefully screened.

By screening blood products for these and other infectious agents, blood banks can significantly reduce the risk of transmitting diseases through transfusion.

Recap questions

1. What is a blood transfusion?
2. Name one clinical setting where blood products are used.
3. What is the purpose of screening blood products?
4. Name one infectious disease that blood products are screened for.

Find out more

www.eboru.com/BTEC-HSC-links

Rhesus disease.

Vaccinations.

Meningitis.

> **Apply your understanding**
>
> Takunda is a 28-year-old woman, who is pregnant with her first child. During her routine antenatal check-up, blood tests reveal that she is RhD-negative, while her partner is RhD-positive. Her doctor explains the potential risks associated with RhD incompatibility and the importance of receiving anti-D immunoglobulin injections.
>
> 1. What is rhesus disease, and how does it occur?
> 2. Why is Takunda's baby at risk of developing Rhesus disease?
> 3. How can anti-D immunoglobulin injections help prevent Rhesus disease?
> 4. What are the potential consequences of Rhesus disease for the baby?

Activity

Look at the following table that summarises sickle cell anaemia.

Disease/problem	About the disease/problem	Symptoms	Treatment
Sickle cell anaemia	Anaemia is an inherited disorder which causes red blood cells to become misshapen and rigid, resembling sickles (crescent-shaped).	These abnormal red cells can block blood vessels, leading to pain sickle cell crises and organ damage.	There is no cure for sickle cell anaemia, but treatments are available to help manage the symptoms and complications of the disease. These treatments include medications to relieve pain, prevent infections, and reduce the number of sickle cell crises. In some cases, blood transfusions or bone marrow transplants may be necessary.

Create your own table to summarise the following: HND, HIV/AIDS, leukaemia, non-Hodgkin lymphoma, thrombosis.

End of Learning Aim B Practice Activity

- Design and produce a scientific poster describing the body's defence mechanisms against infection and the factors that contribute to disease development in humans.

See fourwaves.com/blog/how-to-make-a-scientific-poster for guidance.

- Create an informative PowerPoint presentation that educates new healthcare workers about the transmission routes of different microorganisms and the associated risks of infection.

The PowerPoint should have:

- Clear and concise titles and bullet points.
- High-quality images or diagrams to illustrate key concepts.
- Simple and easy-to-understand language.
- Professional design and layout.
- A concise summary slide highlighting key takeaways.
- Conduct research and produce a scientific report discussing the effectiveness of humoral immunity.
- Can you explain how effective you think it is? Can you analyse the factors that can influence the effectiveness?

References: Include a complete list of all cited sources using a standard referencing format e.g. Harvard.

This practice task will help you prepare for the following assessment criteria:

B.P2 Describe the nonspecific defence methods of the human body.

B.P3 Describe how the immune system is involved in protecting the human body from harmful microorganisms.

B.M2 Compare the transmission routes of microbes involved in human diseases and relate them to specific infections.

B.D2 Evaluate the effectiveness of nonspecific defences and the immune system in helping the body defend itself against infections.

Learning Aim C: Understand the factors that can influence the development of diseases and infections

The development of diseases and infections involves various factors, both internal and external. These factors can include genetic predisposition, lifestyle choices, environmental exposures, and the presence of infectious agents.

C1 Nutritional deficiency diseases

Progressive nature of deficiency disease

Nutritional deficiency diseases develop as a result of a chronic lack of essential nutrients. These nutrients, including micronutrients like vitamins and minerals, and macronutrients like proteins and carbohydrates, are vital for optimal bodily function. When these nutrients are consistently absent from the diet, the body's systems begin to malfunction, leading to a range of health problems. The progressive nature of these diseases means that symptoms may not appear immediately, but rather develop gradually as the deficiency worsens. Early stages might involve subtle changes like fatigue or weakened immunity, while more severe deficiencies can lead to significant organ damage and life-threatening conditions.

Reversing conditions

With a timely diagnosis and appropriate dietary intervention, many of these conditions can be significantly improved or even cured. The body can regain the necessary nutrients to restore its health by taking specific vitamins and minerals, and by incorporating nutrient-rich foods into the diet.

However, the extent to which a deficiency can be reversed depends on the severity and duration of the nutrient deficiency, as well as the individual's overall health. In some cases of severe malnutrition some of the damage caused by prolonged nutrient deficiency may be irreversible.

Effect of a nutritional deficiency on the body

The actual effect of a nutritional deficiency will depend on which nutrients are missing from the diet. See the table below for details.

Nutrient	What it's used for	Effects of nutritional deficiency
Vitamin D	Calcium absorption and bone health	Deficiency can lead to rickets in children and osteomalacia in adults, characterised by weak and soft bones.
Vitamin B12	Nerve function and red blood cell production	Deficiency can cause anaemia, nerve damage, and cognitive impairment.
Folic acid	Cell growth and development. It is recommended that pregnant women take it for the first 12 weeks of pregnancy.	Deficiency can lead to anaemia, birth defects, and increased risk of certain cancers.
Iron	Iron is a key component of haemoglobin, the protein in red blood cells that carries oxygen	Deficiency can cause anaemia leading to fatigue, weakness, shortness of breath, and impaired cognitive function.
Protein	Essential for tissue growth and repair.	Severe protein deficiency, such as **kwashiorkor**, can lead to muscle wasting, oedema, stunted growth, and weakened immunity.
Water	Essential for various bodily functions, including temperature regulation, digestion, and nutrient transport.	Dehydration can cause thirst, fatigue, dizziness, headache, and, in severe cases, kidney failure and shock.

Kwashiorkor is a severe form of malnutrition caused by a deficiency of protein in the diet. It is most commonly seen in children, especially in developing countries where food insecurity is prevalent. It causes swelling in the abdomen due to fluid retention. If untreated it can lead to long lasting effects including slow growth, muscle wasting, enlarged liver and increased susceptibility to infections.

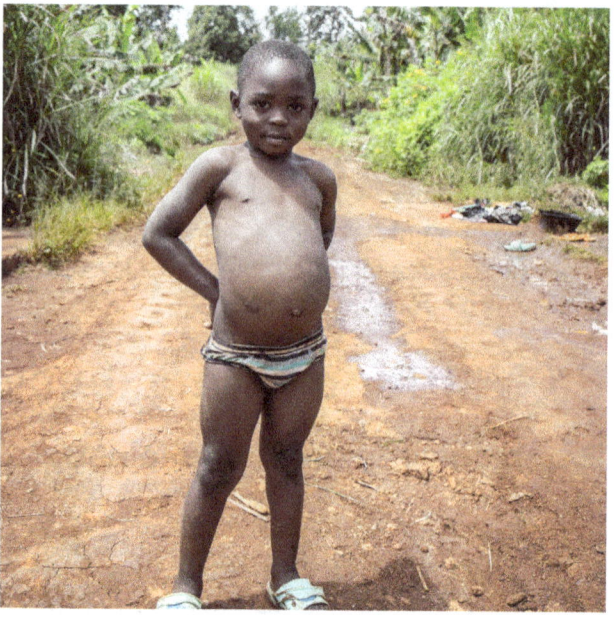

A child with kwashiorkor

Recap questions

1. What are the two main categories of nutrients that are essential for optimal bodily function?
2. Name two health problems associated with a deficiency in nutrients.
3. What are some examples of micronutrients?
4. What are some examples of macronutrients?
5. What are the potential long-term effects of nutrient deficiencies?
6. Can nutritional deficiencies be reversed?

Activity

1. Describe the relationship between vitamin D and calcium absorption.
2. Discuss the factors that influence the reversibility of a nutritional deficiency.

Apply your understanding

Hinna is a 31-year-old woman, is in her second trimester of pregnancy. She has been experiencing fatigue, shortness of breath, and a general feeling of weakness. During a routine prenatal check-up, her doctor orders a complete blood count (CBC) which reveals she has iron-deficiency anaemia.

2. What are the potential causes of iron-deficiency anaemia in pregnancy?
3. Why is iron deficiency a particular concern during pregnancy?
4. What are the potential consequences of untreated iron-deficiency anaemia in pregnancy for both the mother and the foetus?
5. Describe the typical treatment approaches for iron-deficiency anaemia in pregnancy.

C2 Chronic dietary disease

Chronic dietary diseases are a growing global health concern. They arise from poor dietary habits, such as excessive consumption of processed foods, sugary drinks, and unhealthy fats, combined with sedentary lifestyles. These diseases are often characterised by a slow onset and progressive nature, with symptoms developing over years or even decades.

Dietary habits

The consumption of diets high in sugar, refined carbohydrates, and saturated fats has been strongly linked to the development of various chronic diseases. These dietary patterns can lead to significant health problems.

Diets high in sugar lead to weight gain and obesity, which are risk factors for numerous health issues, including heart disease, type 2 diabetes, and certain cancers. They also increase the risk of tooth decay, as sugar provides a food source for bacteria in the mouth, leading to tooth decay and gum disease.

Diets high in refined carbohydrates: Refined carbohydrates, such as white bread and pasta, are rapidly digested, leading to spikes in blood sugar levels. This can contribute to insulin resistance and the development of type 2 diabetes. A diet high in refined carbohydrates can also disrupt the balance of gut bacteria,

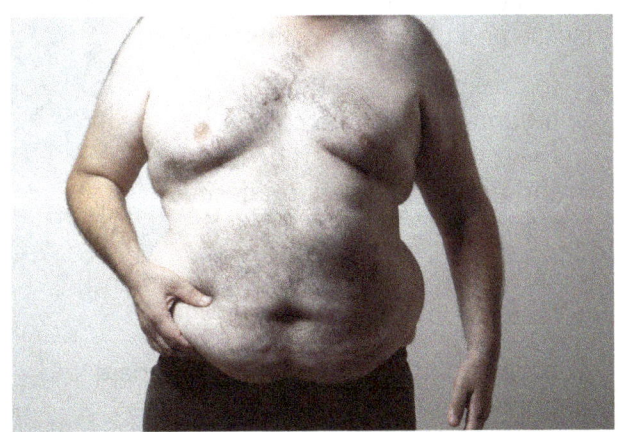

leading to digestive problems such as constipation and irritable bowel syndrome.

Diets high in saturated fats: Saturated fats raise levels of LDL cholesterol, the 'bad' cholesterol, which can clog arteries and increase the risk of heart attack and stroke. High-fat diets can also contribute to weight gain and obesity.

Disease linked to diet

Diet plays a significant role in the development of various **chronic diseases**. In this section you will learn about some of the diseases linked to dietary habits.

Type 2 diabetes

Type 2 diabetes is a chronic condition that affects how your body regulates blood sugar (glucose). It's the most common type of diabetes and is often associated with lifestyle factors like being overweight or obese and lack of physical activity. A diet high in sugar, refined carbohydrates, and unhealthy fats can contribute to the development of type 2 diabetes.

In type 2 diabetes, your body doesn't use insulin properly. Insulin is a hormone produced by the pancreas that helps move glucose from your blood into your cells for energy. When you have insulin resistance, your cells don't respond effectively to insulin, so glucose builds up in your blood instead of entering your cells.

If left unmanaged, type 2 diabetes can lead to serious health complications, including:

- Heart disease and stroke.
- Kidney disease.
- Nerve damage (neuropathy).
- Eye problems (retinopathy).
- Foot problems.
- Weakened immune system.

Treatment for type 2 diabetes focuses on managing blood sugar levels and preventing complications. It may involve lifestyle changes like healthy eating, regular exercise, and maintaining a healthy weight. Some people many need medications to help regulate blood sugar.

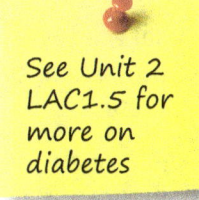

See Unit 2 LAC1.5 for more on diabetes

Inflammatory Bowel Disease (IBD)

Inflammatory bowel disease (**IBD**) is a term for a group of disorders that cause chronic inflammation in the gastrointestinal (GI) tract. The two main types of IBD are **Crohn's disease** and **ulcerative colitis**.

- In Crohn's disease there is inflammation in the colon, but the inflammation can be present throughout the entire digestive tract.
- Ulcerative colitis affects the colon and rectum.

Symptoms of IBD include abdominal pain and cramping, diarrhoea (may contain blood or mucus), rectal bleeding, fatigue and weight loss

There is no cure for IBD. Dietary changes are recommended as a diet high in processed foods, red meat, and saturated fats has been linked to increased inflammation in the gut, which can trigger or worsen IBD. In contrast, a diet rich in fruits, vegetables, and fibre can have a protective effect. Some people may need anti-inflammatory drugs to help manage the symptoms.

Cardiovascular diseases

Diets high in saturated fats, cholesterol, sodium, and added sugars can increase the risk of cardiovascular diseases, including heart disease and stroke. These dietary factors can contribute

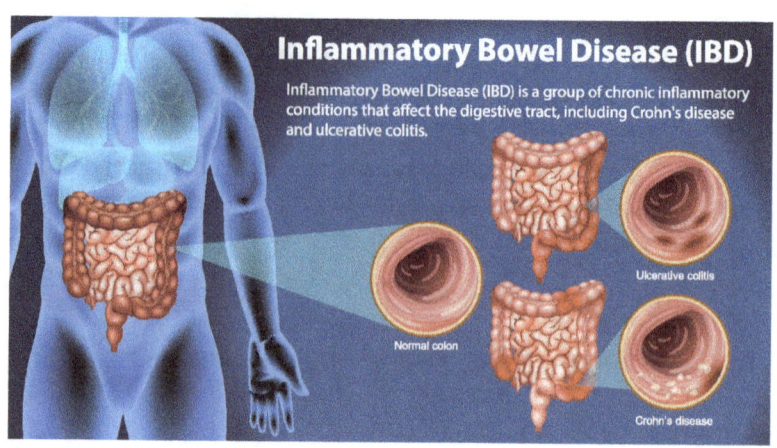

to high blood pressure, high cholesterol, and atherosclerosis (a condition where plaque builds up in the arteries).

Obesity

A diet high in calories, particularly from unhealthy sources like sugary drinks, processed foods, and fast food, can lead to weight gain and obesity. Obesity is a major risk factor for numerous health problems, including heart disease, stroke, type 2 diabetes, and certain types of cancer.

Activity

1. Describe the potential impact of obesity on the development of chronic diseases.
2. Discuss the role of dietary interventions in the management of type 2 diabetes.
3. Discuss the relationship between dietary choices and the development of cardiovascular disease.

Recap questions

1. How can diets high in sugar contribute to weight gain?
2. What are refined carbohydrates?
3. What type of cholesterol is raised by the consumption of saturated fats?
4. What is insulin, and what is its function?
5. What are two lifestyle factors that can contribute to the development of type 2 diabetes?
6. Name one potential long-term complication of uncontrolled type 2 diabetes.
7. What are the two main types of Inflammatory Bowel Disease (IBD)?
8. Which part of the gastrointestinal tract does Crohn's disease typically affect?
9. Which part of the gastrointestinal tract does ulcerative colitis typically affect?
10. What is one dietary recommendation for people with IBD?
11. What are two health conditions that can be increased by a diet high in saturated fats?
12. What is one major risk factor for numerous health problems, including heart disease and stroke?

> **Apply your understanding**
>
> Solomon is a 63-year-old man. He has recently been diagnosed with type 2 diabetes and high cholesterol. Solomon has a sedentary lifestyle, enjoys large portions of processed foods, and frequently indulges in sugary drinks and red meat. Solomon is concerned about his health and is seeking guidance on how to manage his conditions.
>
> 1. Explain the link between Solomon's lifestyle choices and his health diagnoses.
> 2. What are the potential long-term health consequences if Solomon continues with his current lifestyle?
> 3. Describe three key lifestyle modifications Solomon could implement to improve his health.
> 4. Why is it important for Solomon to monitor his blood sugar levels regularly?
> 5. What are some potential dietary changes Solomon could make to lower his cholesterol levels?

C3 Diseases due to environmental factors

Pollutants

Environmental pollution, particularly air and water pollution, can have significant health consequences. Exposure to harmful pollutants can lead to a variety of acute and chronic diseases.

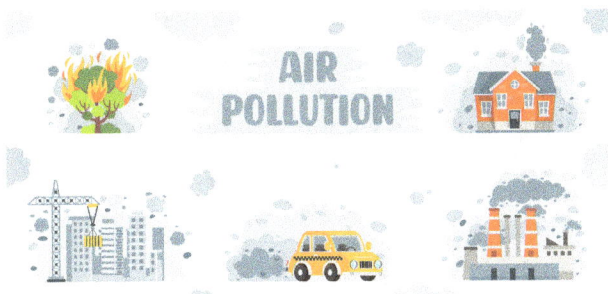

Air pollution

Air pollution, caused by emissions from vehicles and industrial processes can lead to respiratory and cardiovascular problems. Some of the key pollutants and their effects include:

- **Particulate matter** refers to tiny solid or liquid particles suspended in the air. Fine particulate matter (like asbestos fibres) can penetrate deep into the lungs, causing respiratory infections, lung inflammation, and heart disease.
- **Nitrogen dioxide (NO_2)** can irritate the respiratory tract, leading to respiratory infections and asthma.
- **Sulphur dioxide (SO_2)** can cause respiratory problems, particularly in individuals with asthma.

Water pollution

Water pollution can result from industrial waste, agricultural runoff, and sewage. It can contaminate drinking water sources and aquatic ecosystems. Some water pollutants and their health effects include:

- **Bacteria and viruses:** Untreated sewage can contaminate water leading to the transmission of waterborne diseases, such as cholera, typhoid fever, and hepatitis A.
- **Heavy metals:** these can leak into the water supplies from industrial waste. Exposure to heavy metals like lead, mercury, and arsenic can lead to neurological disorders, kidney damage, and cancer.
- **Pesticides and herbicides:** These chemicals can often get washed into the waterways from agricultural (farming) land. They contaminate water sources and pose risks to human health, including cancer, reproductive problems, and neurological disorders.

> **Recap questions**
>
> 1. What are some of the key air pollutants and their effects on human health?
> 2. What are some of the water pollutants and their effects on human health?
> 3. What are some waterborne diseases that can be transmitted through contaminated water?

Radiation and ultraviolet light (UVA and UVB)

Radiation refers to any part of the electromagnetic spectrum. There are two broad types of radiation:

- Ionising radiation
- Non-ionising radiation.

Both types can significantly increase the risk of developing cancer.

Ionising radiation

Ionising radiation is the highest energy part of the spectrum (X-rays, gamma rays, and alpha and beta particles). This type of radiation has enough energy to strip electrons from atoms, ionising them. This can **damage DNA**, the genetic material of cells. If DNA damage is severe enough it can lead to uncontrolled cell growth and cancer. Ionising radiation is what people often mean when they refer to 'radiation'. We are exposed to sources of ionising radiation throughout our lives:

- **Medical procedures:** X-rays, CT scans, and radiation therapy can expose individuals to ionising radiation.
- **Natural sources:** Radon gas, a naturally occurring radioactive gas, can accumulate in homes and increase the risk of lung cancer. Very low levels of gamma rays are naturally emitted from the earth and rocks, and very low levels of ionising radiation from space pass through people travelling on aircraft at high altitudes.

Non-ionising radiation

Non-ionising radiation is the rest of the electromagnetic spectrum, and includes light, microwaves and radio waves.

Ultraviolet (UV) radiation from the sun does not have enough energy to ionise atoms but it can still damage DNA and increase the risk of skin cancer. There are two types of UV radiation:

- **UVA:** This type of radiation can contribute to premature aging of the skin and may also increase the risk of skin cancer.
- **UVB:** This type of radiation is the primary cause of sunburn and can damage DNA, leading to skin cancer, including melanoma.

> **Ionising** – When an atom loses or gains an electron and becomes positively or negatively charged.

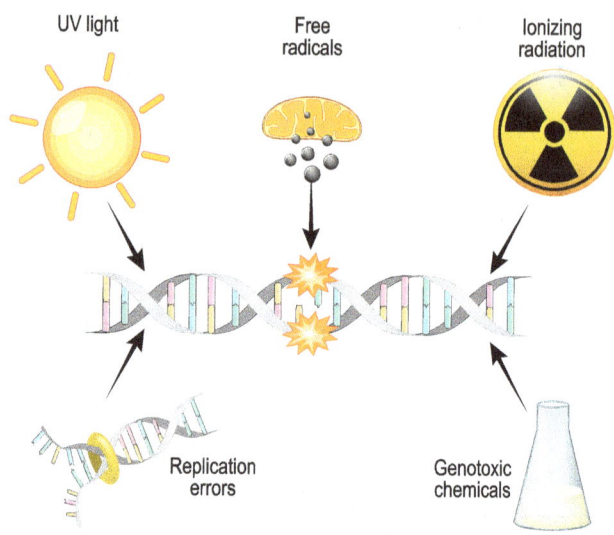

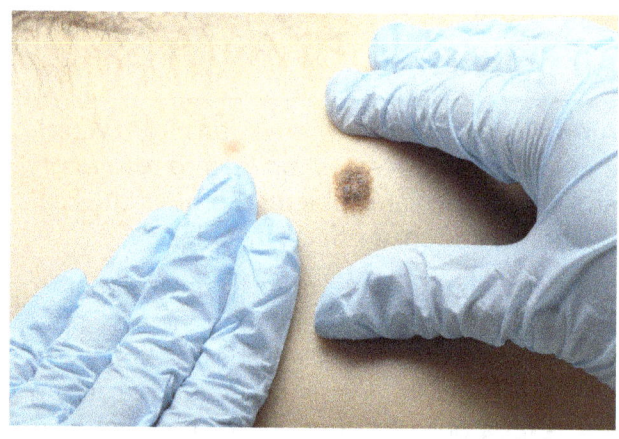

Examining a mole for the presence of melanoma

Recap questions

1. How does ionising radiation damage cells?
2. Name one natural source of ionising radiation.
3. What type of radiation is the main cause of sunburn?
4. How does non-ionising radiation, specifically UV radiation, increase the risk of cancer?

Diseases linked to environmental conditions

Environmental conditions play a significant role in the transmission and spread of diseases. Factors such as sanitation, pesticide use, and overcrowding can significantly impact public health.

Sanitation

Poor sanitation is a major contributor to the spread of infectious diseases. Inadequate sanitation facilities, such as poor sewage disposal and contaminated water sources, can lead to the transmission of waterborne diseases like cholera, typhoid, and dysentery. These diseases can cause severe illness and even death, particularly in vulnerable populations, such as children and the elderly.

Pesticides

Pesticides are widely used to control pests and diseases in agriculture. However, exposure to pesticides can have adverse health effects, including:

- **Acute poisoning**: Acute pesticide poisoning can cause a range of symptoms, such as nausea, vomiting, and respiratory problems.
- **Chronic health effects**: Long-term exposure to pesticides has been linked to various chronic health conditions, including cancer, neurological disorders, and reproductive problems.

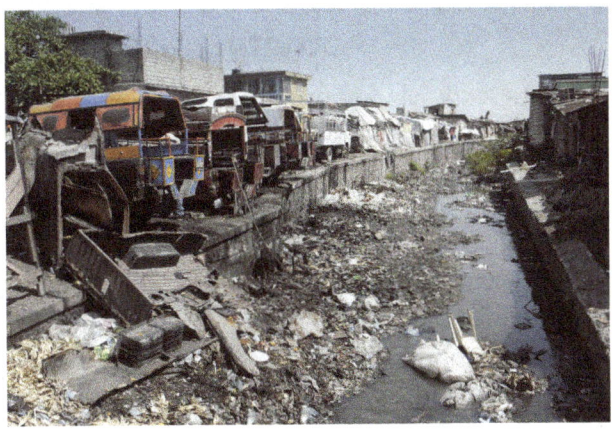

- **Environmental contamination**: Pesticides can contaminate water bodies and soil, affecting ecosystems and human health.

Overcrowding

Overcrowded living conditions can facilitate the spread of infectious diseases. In densely populated areas, respiratory diseases like tuberculosis (TB) and influenza can easily spread through airborne transmission. Overcrowding can also lead to poor sanitation and inadequate access to clean water, further increasing the risk of disease transmission.

Recap questions

1. What is the primary way that poor sanitation contributes to the spread of disease?
2. Name one waterborne disease that can spread due to inadequate sanitation.
3. What is one potential acute health effect of pesticide exposure?

Apply your understanding

Mr Sharma is a 68-year-old man. He has recently returned from a month-long visit to his family in India. While visiting, he stayed in a crowded household with multiple generations living under one roof, including young children. He noticed that ventilation in the home was poor, with limited windows which were often closed due to dust and noise.

During his visit, he spent considerable time indoors, sharing meals and spending evenings in close contact with family members.

Upon his return, Mr Sharma developed a persistent cough and began experiencing night sweats. He is now concerned about his health and seeks medical attention.

1. Based on the case study, identify potential risk factors for TB transmission.
2. How could overcrowding in Mr Sharma's family's home have increased his risk of TB infection?
3. Explain the role of ventilation in the transmission of TB.
4. Why is it important to consider travel history in diagnosing potential infectious diseases?

Activity

Create a knowledge organiser for this topic.

A knowledge organiser is a concise, visually appealing document that summarises key information on a specific topic. Knowledge organisers contain essential facts, concepts, vocabulary, and key ideas. They often use diagrams, mind maps, timelines, or other visual elements to make information more engaging and easier to remember.

Activity

1. Briefly explain how overcrowding can increase the risk of transmitting airborne diseases.

2. Describe two ways in which poor sanitation can contribute to the spread of infectious diseases.

3. Discuss the relationship between UV radiation and skin cancer, including the different types of UV radiation and their associated risks.

4. Explain the role of two environmental factors in the transmission of infectious diseases.

Find out more

www.eboru.com/BTEC-HSC-links

Heart disease.

Overcrowding and poor sanitation: Inside the biggest slum in Africa

Skin cancer.

End of Learning Aim Practice Activity

Part A

Produce a mind map that:

- Discusses nutritional deficiencies and associated diseases.
- Explores the link between unhealthy dietary and chronic diseases.

You could use Canva to help you produce a mind map.

www.canva.com/graphs/mind-maps/

Part B

- Produce a scientific poster about the impact of environmental factors on human health and disease.

See fourwaves.com/blog/how-to-make-a-scientific-poster/ for guidance on making a scientific poster.

- Investigate the progressive nature of nutritional deficiency diseases, exploring their development, impact on the human body, and potential for reversal.

Task:

- Select one nutritional deficiency disease.
- Research and describe the stages of the selected disease. Include the physiological and biochemical changes that occur at each stage.
- Analyse the impact of the selected disease on different bodily systems. How do they impact overall health and quality of life?

References: Include a complete list of all cited sources using a standard referencing format e.g. Harvard.

This practice task will help you prepare for the following assessment criteria:

C.P4 Describe human and environmental conditions that can lead to the development of diseases and infections.

C.M3 Assess the impact of human and environmental conditions on the human body.

C.D3 Analyse how diseases progress over time, and the effects this may have on affected individuals.

Learning Aim D: Investigate the impact of diseases and their treatment in a global context

Disease has had a profound impact on human history - shaping societies, economies, and individual lives. As seen recently with COVID-19, the emergence and spread of diseases can devastate communities and strain healthcare systems. The treatment of diseases, from ancient remedies to modern medicine, has evolved significantly, offering hope and improving quality of life for millions around the globe. However, challenges such as antibiotic resistance, emerging infectious diseases, and disparities in healthcare access continue to pose significant threats to global health.

D1 Epidemiology

Epidemiology

Epidemiology is the study of how often diseases occur in different groups of people and why. Epidemiologists play a vital role in public health by investigating the patterns and causes of disease. By understanding how diseases spread and who they affect, public health measures can be put in place to prevent them.

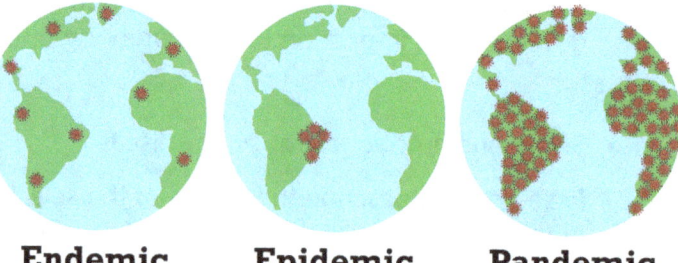

Endemic   **Epidemic**   **Pandemic**

Diseases can be classified in many different ways – the type of pathogen involved, the part of the body it impacts, or the symptoms it produces. Another way is by looking at how they spread throughout populations. The spread of infectious diseases can be classified into different categories based on their geographic scope and impact:

Endemic diseases

Endemic diseases are those that are constantly present at a low level in a particular geographic area. They are considered 'normal' for that region. An example is chickenpox.

- **Chickenpox** is a highly contagious disease that is caused by the varicella-zoster virus. It is most common in children. Symptoms of chickenpox include fever, headache, loss of appetite, and a rash of itchy, fluid-filled blisters. Chickenpox is usually not a serious illness, but it can be dangerous for pregnant women, newborns and people with weakened immune systems.

  Chickenpox is an endemic disease in many countries, including the UK. In the case of chickenpox, this means that there are always some people in the population who are infected with the virus that causes it. While outbreaks may occur periodically, the virus is consistently present in the population.

Epidemic diseases

An **epidemic** occurs when a disease spreads rapidly and affects a significant number of people in a specific geographic area within a short period. Both flu (influenza) and measles can be considered epidemic diseases.

- During **flu seasons** (autumn and winter) the virus spreads rapidly, leading to a surge in

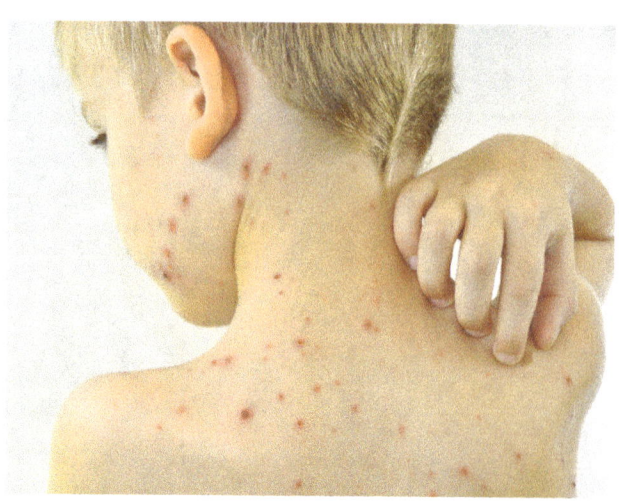

Chickenpox

cases. For vulnerable people (the elderly, those with compromised immune systems) the best way to protect yourself from the flu is to get an annual flu vaccine.

- **Measles** is a highly contagious viral disease that can have serious consequences. Measles can cause a range of symptoms, including high fever, cough, runny nose, and a distinctive rash. It can also lead to serious complications like pneumonia and encephalitis. Measles is a significant cause of death in children in developing countries.

The measles vaccine is highly effective but there has been a downturn in the number of people vaccinated against measles in recent years, particularly since the beginning of the COVID-19 pandemic. This decline in vaccination rates is a significant concern as it increases the risk of measles outbreaks.

> Compromised immune systems – A state in which the body's ability to fight off infections and diseases is weakened. This could be due to cancer treatment or conditions like HIV.
>
> Pneumonia – An infection that inflames the air sacs in one or both lungs, which may fill with fluid.
>
> Encephalitis – An inflammation of the brain, often caused by viral infections.

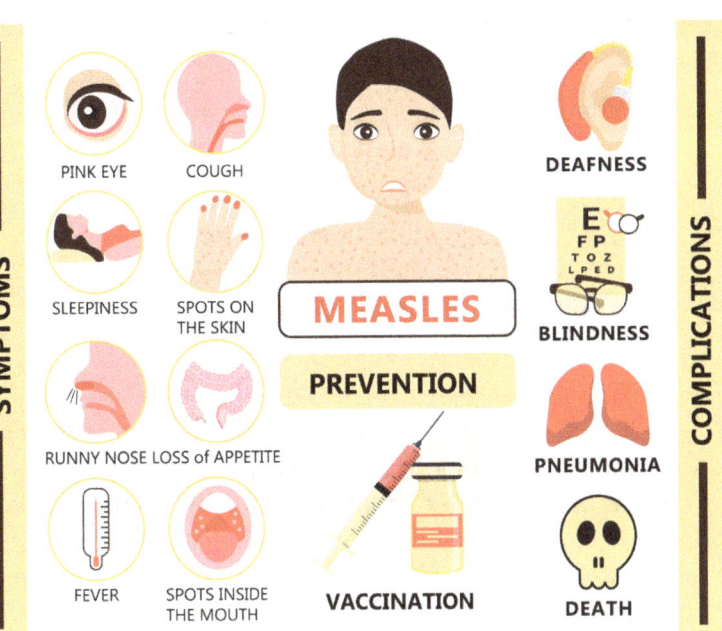

Pandemic diseases

A pandemic is defined as an epidemic that has spread over multiple countries or continents, affecting a large number of people.

COVID-19, a respiratory illness caused by the SARS-CoV-2 virus, was declared a pandemic in 2020 due to its rapid global spread and severe impact on public health. The COVID-19 pandemic has had a significant impact globally, causing widespread illness, death, and economic disruption.

Changes in disease classification

The **classification of a disease can change over time** due to various factors, including changes in public health measures, the emergence of new strains, and increased global travel. For example, a disease that was once epidemic might become endemic if it establishes itself within a population. Or an epidemic can easily become a pandemic if people travelling between countries take the pathogen with them.

- The Spanish Flu of 1918 was a flu pandemic that killed millions. It was thought to be first identified in the USA in 1918 and quickly spread around the world due to global travel associated with World War 1.

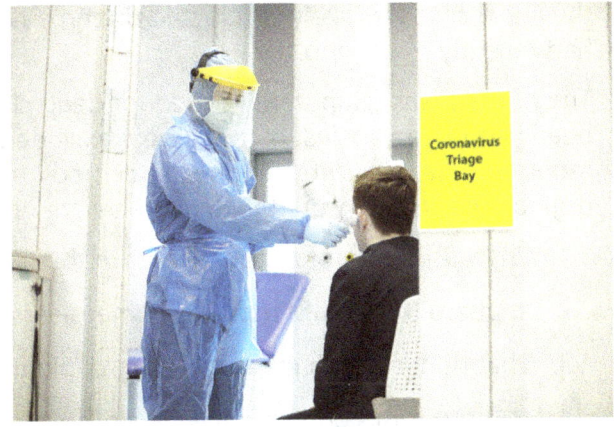

The COVID-19 pandemic had a significant global impact

- Historically, malaria has caused widespread epidemics. Thanks to public health interventions such as mosquito control and the use of antimalarial drugs, malaria has been largely eradicated in many parts of the world. The disease remains endemic in certain regions, particularly in tropical and subtropical areas. If an outbreak occurred outside its typical endemic areas, then it could be classed as an epidemic due to a sudden increase in cases beyond the normal levels.

Recap questions

1. What is epidemiology?
2. What are endemic diseases?
3. What are epidemic diseases?
4. What is a pandemic?
5. What are the symptoms of chickenpox?
6. How can the spread of infectious diseases be classified?
7. What are some factors that can lead to changes in the classification of a disease?
8. What are some public health measures that can be used to prevent the spread of disease?

Activity

1. Explain how a decline in measles vaccination rates can increase the risk of outbreaks.
2. Describe the public health measures that can be taken to prevent the spread of an infectious disease outbreak in a school setting.
3. Discuss the importance of epidemiology in understanding and controlling the spread of infectious diseases. Provide specific examples to illustrate your points.

Apply your understanding

A popular nursery in a small town experienced an unexpected measles outbreak in spring. The first case was identified in a 3-year-old child who developed with a high fever, cough, and a distinctive red rash. Within a week, several other children in the nursery began to show similar symptoms.

The local health authorities were immediately notified. An investigation was launched to determine the source of the outbreak and to implement control measures. It was discovered that the initial case was likely contracted during a family trip to a nearby town where measles cases had recently been reported.

The nursery was temporarily closed for deep cleaning and disinfection. All children who had not been vaccinated against measles were excluded from the nursery until two weeks after the last reported case. Public health officials carried out an immunisation campaign in the community, urging parents to ensure their children were up to date on their measles vaccinations.

1. Why was the outbreak of measles in the nursery a concern?
2. What are the main symptoms of measles?
3. What public health measures were implemented to control the outbreak?
4. How could this outbreak have been prevented?

D2 Factors in controlling a global disease outbreak

Role of authorities

In 2020 COVID-19 was declared a global pandemic. Many steps were put in place to try to control the spread and to minimise the impact on healthcare services. A global disease outbreak, like COVID-19 requires a coordinated and multi-faceted response from various authorities:

- **Governments:** Governments are responsible for implementing public health measures, such as quarantine, isolation, and social distancing. They allocate resources (money, personnel, equipment and facilities) for research, vaccine development, and healthcare infrastructure. They are responsible for providing clear and timely information to the public about the outbreak, its risks, and recommended precautions.

- **Non-Governmental Organisations (NGOs):** NGOs often play a vital role in providing humanitarian aid, supporting healthcare workers, and educating the public. Examples of NGOs involved in pandemics include Médecins Sans Frontières/Doctors Without Borders (MSF), Oxfam International and Save the Children.

- **Scientists, including epidemiologists:** Scientists, particularly epidemiologists, are essential for tracking the spread of the disease, identifying risk factors, and developing effective control strategies. They also contribute to the development of vaccines and treatments.

- **World Health Organisation (WHO):** The WHO plays a vital role in coordinating the global response to outbreaks. The WHO provides leadership, coordinates international response efforts, and shares information and expertise across countries. It provides guidance to countries, allocates resources (including financial assistance and medical supplies), and monitors the situation to prevent the spread of disease. The WHO also develop and maintain global surveillance systems to detect and report any outbreaks promptly.

Factors to consider in any outbreak

Several factors need to be considered when responding to a disease outbreak:

- **Cost:** The financial cost of an outbreak can be substantial, including expenses for healthcare, research, and public health measures. During COVID-19 hospitals desperately needed to buy more PPE, money was needed for vaccine research and rolling out the vaccine programme, there was also the cost of COVID testing kits.

- **Availability of health personnel:** A sufficient number of healthcare workers, such as doctors and nurses, are essential to provide care to infected individuals and manage the outbreak. During the COVID-19 pandemic many retired doctors and nurses returned to the profession to ensure there was sufficient healthcare workers. Army medical personnel also contributed to caring for patients.

- **Drug availability and development:** The availability of effective drugs, including vaccines and antiviral medications, is crucial for treating and preventing the disease. In some cases, rapid drug development may be necessary. During the COVID-19 pandemic vaccine research scientists worked together on a global scale to ensure the rapid development of effective vaccines.

- **Location:** The location of the outbreak can influence the spread of the disease. Urban areas with high population density can facilitate rapid transmission of the disease, while remote areas may pose challenges for access to healthcare and resources.

- **Community agreement:** Public cooperation is essential for implementing control measures, such as vaccination campaigns and social distancing. Community engagement and education can help to increase compliance and reduce the spread of disease. During COVID-19, government briefings on the TV explained the importance of staying at home and social distancing.

- **Local customs and culture:** Cultural beliefs

and practices can influence people's attitudes towards disease and their willingness to adopt preventative measures. It is important to consider these factors when designing public health interventions.

For pandemics, additional resources and expertise may be required, including:

- **Experts in infectious disease:** These experts can provide guidance on disease transmission, prevention, and treatment.
- **Epidemiologists:** Epidemiologists can track the spread of the disease, identify high-risk populations, and evaluate the effectiveness of control measures.
- **WHO Risk Assessments:** The WHO can assess the global risk of a pandemic and provide recommendations to countries.

> **Recap questions**
> 1. What is the World Health Organisation (WHO)'s role in responding to a global disease outbreak?
> 2. What are some of the responsibilities of governments in responding to a global disease outbreak?
> 3. Why is the work of scientists, particularly epidemiologists, important during a pandemic?
> 4. What are some of the financial costs associated with a disease outbreak?
> 5. Why is the availability of health personnel so important during an outbreak?
> 6. How can local customs and culture influence the response to a disease outbreak?

D3 Consequences to society of a disease outbreak

Effects on an individual, on family, on communities, on societies

A disease outbreak can have far-reaching consequences for individuals, families, communities, and societies as a whole. As well as the obvious impact disease can have on physical health, disease outbreaks often lead to a decline in mental health too.

Individual consequences

The effect on **physical health** is the most obvious during any outbreak. Individuals may experience a range of symptoms, from mild to severe, depending on the nature of the disease. This can include fever, cough, respiratory distress, and other symptoms.

The fear and uncertainty associated with a disease outbreak can lead to anxiety, depression, and other **mental health** issues. Individuals may be required to isolate themselves to prevent the spread of the disease, leading to feelings of loneliness and **social isolation**.

Family consequences

Medical expenses, lost wages, and increased costs of living can put a significant **financial strain** on families. Caring for sick family members can be emotionally draining, leading to **stress** and burnout.

Disease outbreaks can also disrupt daily routines, schooling and family gatherings.

Community consequences

A surge in cases can overwhelm healthcare systems, leading to delays in treatment and increased mortality rates. Scheduled routine operations may have to be cancelled and postponed as healthcare staff are dealing with the outbreak.

Disease outbreaks can disrupt businesses, supply chains, and tourism, leading to economic losses. This could lead to smaller businesses closing down, leading to a loss of jobs in the community.

Fear and uncertainty during disease outbreaks can lead to social disruption, panic buying, and discrimination against affected individuals or communities. During the start of COVID-19 there was a toilet paper shortage due to people panic buying it in bulk.

Societal consequences

- **Global economic impact:** Pandemics can have a significant impact on the global economy, leading to job losses, reduced trade, and financial instability.

- **Political instability:** Disease outbreaks can exacerbate social and political tensions, leading to civil unrest and instability.

- **Long-term health consequences:** Even after the initial outbreak, the long-term health

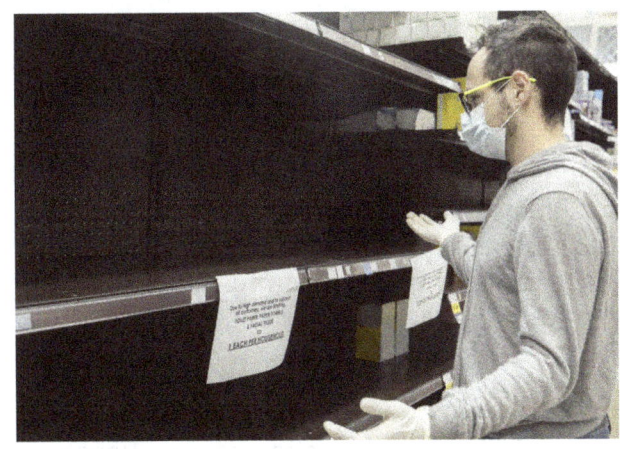

consequences, such as chronic illnesses and disabilities, can continue to affect individuals and societies. There are many people still suffering from the effects of long COVID.

Ethical considerations

Disease outbreaks, especially those that escalate into pandemics, present significant ethical challenges. There are many different factors to consider including the use of untested drugs, prioritisation of patients and exposing healthcare workers to infection.

Use of untried/unlicensed drugs

- **Potential benefits**: In a crisis, experimental drugs may offer the only hope for survival. Drugs will often bypass the usual stages in approval if there is sufficient evidence that they might be lifesaving.

- **Ethical concerns**: Using untested drugs raises concerns about potential side effects and long-term consequences. Informed consent is vital but may be difficult to obtain in emergency situations.

Methods of treatment

- **Prioritising patients**: Decisions about who receives limited resources, such as ventilators or ICU beds, can be difficult and emotionally charged. Ethically, healthcare staff may be having to make decisions about who they save and who dies.

- **Resource allocation**: Allocating resources fairly and equally can be challenging. If resources are limited, then a decision has to be made as to where they will be used. Resources include healthcare personnel, PPE, lifesaving drugs, vaccines etc.

Exposure of healthcare workers

Healthcare workers are at a **higher risk of infection** due to their direct contact with patients. While healthcare workers have a duty of care to service users, it is essential to balance this with their own safety and wellbeing. Employers should ensure there are adequate supplies of PPE to protect healthcare workers.

Recap questions

1. What is one potential impact of a disease outbreak on physical health?

2. How can a disease outbreak negatively impact an individual's mental health?

3. What are some of the financial consequences that a disease outbreak can have on families?

4. How can a disease outbreak disrupt a community?

5. What are the potential benefits of using untested drugs during a disease outbreak?

6. What are the ethical concerns related to using untested drugs?

Problems associated with using treatments regimes and ideas not familiar to a society

During a disease outbreak, it is vital to have community agreement to ensure that public health measures that are put in place to minimise the spread of the disease are adhered to. However, there are often some stumbling blocks to new and unfamiliar ideas.

Cultural beliefs and practices

Cultural beliefs and practices may influence people's willingness to accept medical interventions, such as vaccination or quarantine. Some religious beliefs may have concerns about certain vaccine components, leading to refusal or hesitancy. For example, some vaccines may contain traces of animal products, which can be a concern for individuals with dietary restrictions or religious objections to consuming certain animal products.

Mistrust of authorities

Misinformation and **mistrust of authorities** can hinder public health efforts and lead to non-compliance with preventive measures. The rise in the spread of misinformation and conspiracy theories about vaccines through social media and other channels can lead to vaccine hesitancy.

Language barriers

Language barriers can prevent communication and understanding of health information, leading to non-compliance with treatment programmes. Governments should ensure the information is widely available in a variety of languages.

Risks of antibiotic resistance

Antibiotics are drugs that are used to kill bacteria and stop bacterial infections. Antibiotics were developed in the 1940s and have saved millions of lives. Prior to their use, many people died every year from what are now treatable diseases. However, in recent years antibiotics are becoming less effective in the fight against bacterial disease, and we are seeing a huge increase in the number of bacteria that are **antibiotic resistant**.

The overuse and misuse of antibiotics can contribute to the development of antibiotic-resistant bacteria, making infections more difficult to treat. Antibiotics are frequently used in intensive farming to minimise the risk of disease spreading throughout populations of animals. This overuse of antibiotics has led to strains of bacteria mutating to become resistant to the antibiotics.

In humans, misusing antibiotics, such as not completing the full course of treatment, can also contribute to antibiotic resistance. If you don't finish the full course of treatment, then some bacteria are left in the body, and they can mutate to become resistant.

Antibiotic resistance is a global problem that can lead to serious infections that are difficult to treat. We will start to see an increase in deaths from bacterial diseases that were once treatable with antibiotics. Scientists are continually working to find new antibiotics, but the bacteria are mutating and evolving at a faster rate than our production of new drugs.

> Intensive farming – An agricultural system that prioritises maximising output from a given piece of land. This can be through the use of fertilisers or pesticides, or by raising large numbers of animals in confined spaces.

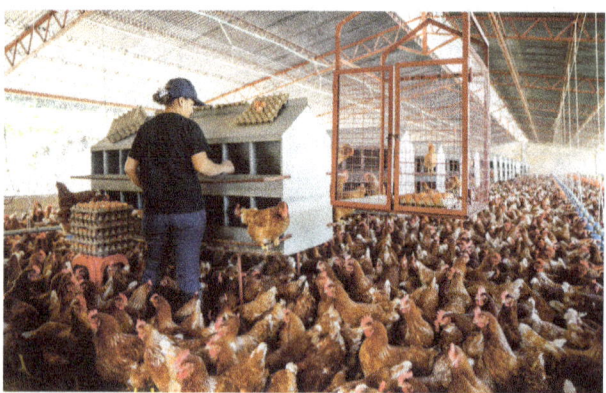

Activity

1. Define antibiotic resistance.
2. What is vaccine hesitancy?
3. Explain how cultural beliefs can impact public health responses to a disease outbreak.
4. Describe the ethical challenges associated with resource allocation during a pandemic.
5. Discuss the importance of community engagement in controlling the spread of an infectious disease.

Activity

Create a mind map to show the factors to consider in an outbreak. You could draw your own or use a website like Canva to help you.

www.canva.com/graphs/mind-maps

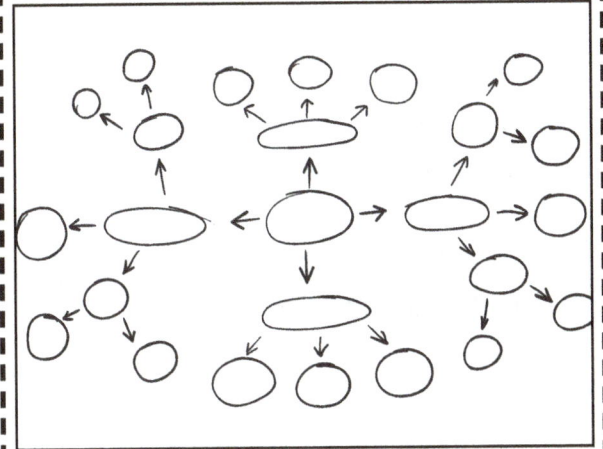

Recap questions

1. How can cultural beliefs and practices influence the acceptance of public health measures?
2. How can misinformation and distrust of authorities limit public health efforts?
3. What are the potential consequences of language barriers during a disease outbreak?
4. What steps can governments take to address language barriers during a disease outbreak?
5. What are antibiotics and how do they work?
6. What are two main factors that contribute to the development of antibiotic resistance?
7. How does the overuse of antibiotics in animal agriculture contribute to antibiotic resistance?
8. What are the potential consequences of antibiotic resistance for human health?

Find out more

www.eboru.com/BTEC-HSC-links

Timeline of WHO's response to COVID-19

Coronavirus: First British death - BBC News

Apply your understanding

Shipford is a small city with a diverse population and many different languages spoken. It has recently experienced a concerning increase in cases of measles. Despite the availability of a safe and effective measles vaccine, vaccine uptake is far below the national average.

1. Based on the case study, identify three key factors that might contribute to vaccine hesitancy in Shipford.
2. How might misinformation and distrust in authorities have influenced vaccine hesitancy in this community?
3. How could public health officials address the cultural beliefs that may have contributed to vaccine hesitancy in Shipford?
4. What strategies could be implemented to improve access to vaccination services and increase vaccine uptake in communities like Shipford?

End of Learning Aim Practice Activity

- Produce an infographic which defines and differentiates between endemic diseases, epidemic diseases and pandemic diseases. It should include an example of each classification.

- Produce a mind map that shows the role of epidemiologists in controlling the outbreak of disease.

You could use Canva to help you produce a mind map.

- Evaluate the importance of different authorities in controlling disease.

- Conduct a case study of a specific disease outbreak to analyse the response of public health authorities and its impact on the outcome.

- What factors do you think contribute to outbreaks of diseases becoming more global?

The websites might help you. You can find the links on www.eboru.com/BTEC-HSC-links

https://piktochart.com/infographic-maker/

www.canva.com/graphs/mind-maps/

https://www.gov.uk/government/publications/national-measles-guidelines

https://www.gov.uk/government/publications/health-protection-in-schools-and-other-childcare-facilities/managing-outbreaks-and-incidents

https://www.ons.gov.uk/peoplepopulationandcommunity/healthandsocialcare/conditionsanddiseases

This practice task will help you prepare for the following assessment criteria:

D.P5 Explain the characteristics of the classifications of outbreaks and a disease associated with each classification.

D.P6 Describe the role of authorities in controlling the outbreak of disease.

D.M4 Assess the effectiveness of authorities in controlling the outbreak of diseases and managing the impact on society.

D.D4 Evaluate the reasons for and consequences of outbreaks of diseases becoming more global.

Photo credits

Page 30: The Eatwell Guide is subject to Crown copyright protection, which is covered by an Open Government Licence. Source: OHID in association with the Welsh government, Food Standards Scotland and the Food Standards Agency in Northern Ireland.

Page 7: 0-4 Growth Charts © 2009 Department of Health. Reproduced with permission of Royal College of Paediatrics and Child Health. These charts were developed by RCPCH / WHO / Department of Health.

The rest of the photo credits can be found here:

www.eboru.com/BTEC-AAQ-HSC-photo-credits

Index

A

abdomen, 75, 111, 121, 320
abortions, 210
access to services, 35–36, 154, 161, 163
acquired brain injuries, 105, 107–8
acquired brain injury, 90, 105–8, 115
activities, high-impact, 223
acute care, 229, 248
Acute Myelogenous Leukaemia (AML), 314–15
adaptive immune system, 86, 298
ADH, 70, 80–81
adipose tissue, 62–63
adolescence, 10, 12–15, 42–43, 45, 80, 227, 244
adrenal cortex, 82
adrenal glands, 78, 81–82, 113
adrenaline, 78, 81–82
adulthood, 10–11, 13–15, 18, 20–23, 42, 44, 46, 56, 131, 227, 244
aerobic respiration, 66–67
aerosols, 306–7
aims of public health policy, 173
Ainsworth's Theory of Attachment, 5–7
air pollution, 36, 98, 190, 199, 208–9, 211, 323
alcohol, 31–33, 42–43, 49, 159, 190, 199, 208, 215, 265, 291, 295
alcohol consumption, 16, 31, 109–10
  excessive, 110, 113
alcohol misuse, 32, 209, 211, 218
aldosterone, 82
alimentary canal, 88–89
alveoli, 62, 74–75, 94, 96
Alzheimer's disease, 102, 104
amino acids, 61, 81
AML (Acute Myelogenous Leukaemia), 314–15
amnesia, 44–45, 106
anabolism, 66–68
anaemia, 28, 30, 111–12, 312, 316–17, 319
anaerobic respiration, 67–68, 114
angina, 44–45, 90–91
antagonistic pairs, 84
antibiotic resistance, 287, 328, 334–35
antibiotics, 27, 287, 291, 295, 334–35
antibodies, 46, 73, 86, 114, 285, 298–99, 301, 303, 311–12
antibody-mediated immune system, 298
antidiuretic hormone, 70, 80
Antigen Presenting Cells (APCs), 299
antigens, 86, 284–85, 298–99, 301–2
antiseptics, 291
anxiety, 33, 35–36, 38, 43–44, 98, 100, 103, 107, 124, 129, 241, 243, 247
anxiety and depression, 36, 38, 98
aorta, 71–72
APCs (Antigen Presenting Cells). See Antigen Presenting Cells (APCs)
areolar, 62
areolar tissue, 63
armpit hair, 11
arteries, 18, 25, 62–63, 71–73, 90, 96, 99, 101–2, 108, 315, 322
asexual reproduction, 288
asthma, 36–37, 90, 98–99, 104, 114–15, 179, 208–9, 323
asthma attack, 98, 115
atherosclerosis, 44–45, 90–91, 93, 96–97, 99, 101–2, 108, 322
athlete's foot, 310
ATP, 61, 66–67
attachment, 4–7, 12, 15, 284–85
autism, 13, 41, 161–62, 184–85
autonomic nervous system, 65, 77–78
autonomy, 12–13, 119, 122, 131–32, 163, 165, 223–25, 238–39
axon, 64

B

bacilli, 286
bacteria, 284, 286–88, 291, 293, 297–300, 305–6, 308–9, 311, 321, 323, 334
bacteria and viruses, 298, 305, 323
bacterial cells, 284, 286–87
bacterial infections, 41, 86, 287, 291, 309, 313, 334
bacterial reproduction, 286–87
bacteriophage, 284–85, 296
Basal Metabolic Rate (BMR), 67–68
B-cells, 298–99, 304
behaviour change, 222–23, 225–26
biases, 155–56, 164, 166, 189, 262
binary fission, 286–87
bladder, 25–27, 64, 78, 104
blood, deoxygenated, 71–72
blood capillaries, 62–63, 75
blood cells, 313–14, 316
blood clots, 44, 90–92, 108, 112, 315
blood glucose regulation, 70, 82
blood infections, 311
blood pressure, 25, 42, 47, 76, 78, 80–82, 90–91, 96, 108, 220
blood stem cells, 313
blood sugar levels, 47, 70, 99–100, 102, 113–14, 131, 321, 323
blood tests, 47–48, 276, 317
blood transfusions, 312, 316–17
blood vessels, 25, 63–64, 69, 71–73, 86, 90, 92, 101–2, 106, 108, 311, 315, 317
BMR. See Basal Metabolic Rate
body composition, 68
body fat, 8, 16, 30
body language, 127, 129
body temperature, 67, 69, 76, 78, 290, 309
bone marrow, 63, 86, 313–15
bones, 20–21, 30–31, 62–63, 76, 80, 83–86, 110–

11, 113, 313–14
bowel cancer, 47, 109–13, 115, 159, 183
Bowlby's attachment theory, 5
brain, 4–5, 13–14, 19, 21, 25–26, 44, 63–65, 69–70, 76–77, 79, 91–93, 96–98, 102–8, 110, 112–15, 158–59
brain activity, 66
brain and spinal cord, 41, 64–65, 76, 309
brain cells, 18, 21, 92, 102
brain damage, 92, 106, 109, 309, 312
  initial, 93
brain function, 19
brain injury, 43, 105–9, 114
brainstem, 76, 78, 108
brain tissue, 92, 106
BRCA genes, 109–10
breaching confidentiality, 134
breast cancer, 25, 29, 47, 109–10, 113, 115, 183
breast cancer screening, 183
bronchi, 74, 94, 96
bronchioles, 74, 94, 96
BSL, 129–30, 132

C
calcium, 33, 63, 90
calories, 16–17, 30, 68, 96, 322
cancer, 24–26, 31–32, 36–39, 45, 47, 109–13, 186, 215, 219, 308, 313–14, 319, 321–25
cancer cells, 86, 110–11, 113
cancer screening, 47
cancer treatment, 316, 329
Candida, 310
candidiasis, 310–11
capsid, 284–85
carbohydrates, 29, 66, 88, 290, 319
carbon dioxide, 60, 67, 71, 74–75
cardiac cycle, 71–73
cardiac muscle, 64–65
cardiovascular disease, 19–20, 25, 28–29, 31, 36, 38, 44–45, 96–97, 102, 108, 207, 322
cardiovascular system, 71, 73, 91, 93, 96–97, 99, 102, 104, 108–9, 111–13, 115
Care Act, 122, 145, 149, 174, 185, 192, 194, 203–4, 249–50
Care Certificate, 261–62
Care Certificate Standards, 261
care plans, 120, 125–27, 146, 233, 250, 273, 276
Care Quality Commission. See CQC
care services, domiciliary, 142, 145–47, 230
care values, 118–21
cartilage, 16, 62, 74, 83–85, 114
cartilaginous joints, 84–85
catabolism, 66–67, 114
cell-mediated immunity, 298–99
cell membranes, 60–61, 286–87, 293
cell organelles, 60
cells
  abnormal, 109, 112, 313
  epithelial, 62

  neuroglial, 65, 68
central nervous system (CNS), 64–65, 76–78, 108
cerebellum, 76–78, 107
cerebrum, 76–78
CHD (Coronary heart disease), 59, 90–91, 97, 115
chemotherapy, 29, 126, 225, 314, 316
chickenpox, 303, 328, 330
Childcare Act, 250
child health, 179, 210
Children and Families Act, 250
children and young people, 50, 143
cholesterol, 47, 90, 321–22
chromosomes, 24–25, 60–61
chronic dietary diseases, 321
chronic diseases, 321–23, 327
chronic health conditions, 20, 325
Chronic Myelomonocytic Leukaemia (CMML), 314–15
chronic obstructive pulmonary disorder, 38, 90, 94
chronic obstructive pulmonary disorder. See COPD
cigarettes, 42, 112, 179, 188, 207
circulatory system, 85–86, 88
climate change, 187, 190
clinical trials, 302
CMML. See Chronic Myelomonocytic Leukaemia
CNS. See central nervous system
cognitive decline, 21, 102–4, 110, 113
collagen, 20, 61, 63
colon, 88, 322
community health, 141, 151
community health services, 144, 150–51, 229–30
compassion, 117, 120–21, 135, 175, 194
competency, 119–21, 124
conditions
  chronic, 99, 321
  existing, 47, 278
  recessive, 27–28
  smoking-related, 207
  workplace, 37
confidentiality, 132–34, 136, 143, 177, 226, 239, 267–68, 273
conjunctivitis, 40–41
consent, 22, 133–34, 249, 256, 260
continuous professional development. See CPD
contraception, 187, 210–11
COPD (Chronic obstructive pulmonary disorder), 38, 59, 90, 94–97, 170, 207–8, 266
coronary arteries, 44, 90
coronary heart disease. See CHD
COSHH, 137, 250–51
coughing, 27, 94, 98, 103–4, 112, 297, 305–6
COVID-19, 167–69, 173, 177, 182–85, 188, 191–93, 200, 266, 305–6, 328–29, 331, 333, 335
COVID-19 vaccines, 184, 186, 302
CPD (continuous professional development), 119, 142–43, 194, 202
CQC (Care Quality Commission), 142, 144–45,

149, 156, 164, 178, 249–51, 258–62, 270–71, 274, 281
Crohn's disease, 111, 322
cultural beliefs, 177, 331, 335
cultural competence, 164, 238–39
cultural differences, 15, 167, 267
cystic fibrosis, 27–29, 157

D

data breach, 134, 145, 148, 279
data protection officer (DPO), 145, 148
DBS (Disclosure and Barring Service), 146, 148, 261–64, 281
deep vein thrombosis (DVT), 315
dehydration, 28, 80, 100–101, 309, 319
dementia, 21, 44–45, 48, 102–4, 129–31, 137, 139, 176, 179, 238, 254, 256, 261
demographic data, 176–77, 200, 205–6, 226
dendrites, 64–65
Department of Health and Social Care, 141–42, 149, 174, 178, 183, 196, 201, 202, 219
deprived areas, 34–37, 213, 216–17, 224, 265
designated safeguarding leads (DSLs), 138
determinants of health, 158–60, 209, 216
diabetes, 30–32, 37–38, 44–45, 47, 49, 99–102, 104, 113, 159, 177, 179, 195, 205, 207, 321–23
diabetic retinopathy, 100–102
diaphragm, 74–75, 108
diet, 16, 33, 46, 55, 111, 113, 159–60, 172, 177, 207, 319–22
  unhealthy, 30, 199
dietician, 28, 55
diets high in sugar, 321–22
digestion, 63–65, 76–78, 88–89, 319
digestive system, 71, 78, 86–89, 91, 96, 102, 104, 112, 115
digital communication, 127, 130–32
digital records, 277–79
digital technology, 130, 132, 153, 277
dignity, 117–18, 120–22, 128, 135, 137, 163, 165, 230, 238–39, 241, 260–61, 267
Director of Public Health, 204
disabilities, 27, 36, 54–55, 148, 152, 161, 187, 217–18, 241–42, 250, 255–56
Disclosure and Barring Service. *See* DBS
discrimination, 35–36, 38, 147–48, 161–67, 170, 213, 216–17, 224, 226, 236–39, 255, 262–63, 265
disease outbreaks, 190, 331–36
diseases
  autoimmune, 313
  coronary artery, 96
  inflammatory, 96
  lung, 28
  non-communicable, 179
  progressive, 21
  smoking-related, 188
  transmitting, 316

disease transmission, 292, 305–7, 325, 332
disengagement theory, 22–23
disinfectants, 291, 295
disorders
  autoimmune, 99
  foetal alcohol spectrum, 31
diversity and inclusion, 116, 158, 162, 164–65, 170, 185
DNA, 24, 60–61, 82, 284–87, 291
domiciliary care, 142, 145–47, 230
DPO (data protection officer), 145, 148
drug use, 42, 45, 49, 208
DSLs (designated safeguarding leads), 138
duty of candour, 175, 249, 258–59, 261
DVT (deep vein thrombosis), 315
dysphasia, 92, 114–15

E

ear infections, 40, 45, 309
early adulthood, 13–15, 17, 21, 45, 136, 244
early childhood, 3, 8–10, 13, 27, 40, 43, 98
economic conditions, 186
effective communication, 119, 128, 140, 264
elastin, 20–21, 63
elective care, 150
electronic patient records (EPR), 125–27, 154–55, 277–78
embolism, 315
emergency care, 150, 229
emphysema, 32, 42, 49, 90, 94–95
endemic diseases, 328, 330, 336
endocrine system, 79–82, 87, 89, 102
end-of-life care, 152, 169, 231
environmental conditions, 290, 325, 327
environmental factors, 38–39, 98–99, 109–10, 112–13, 170, 187, 190, 205, 213, 323, 326–27
environmental health impact assessment, 190, 193
enzymes, 61, 67, 88–89, 284–85, 297
epidemic, 301, 328–29
epidemic diseases, 328, 330, 336
epidemiologists, 328, 331–32, 336
epidemiology, 176–77, 205, 283, 301, 303, 328, 330
epithelial tissue, 62–63
EPR. *See* electronic patient records
Equality Act, 36, 118, 122, 147, 161, 165–66, 213, 255–56, 262
erythrocytic diseases, 312–13
eukaryotic organisms, 289
exercise, 27, 30–32, 34, 53–54, 98, 159–60, 166, 187–89, 212, 215, 220, 223, 227

F

Faculty of Public Health, 178–80, 202–3
Families Act, 250
fats, 19–20, 29, 63, 66, 68, 87–88, 207
  unhealthy, 321

female reproductive systems, 87–89, 102, 210–11
female sex hormones, 11, 89
fertility, 10, 13–14, 16–17, 210–11
fibrous joints, 84–85
fine motor skills, 3–5, 8, 92, 106
flu, 40, 46, 183, 328–29
fungal infections, 306, 310
fungi, 85, 100, 284, 287–89, 308, 310

G

gallbladder, 88–89
gametocytes, 288–89
gas exchange, 63, 74–75, 96
GDPR, 122, 134, 145
gender, 20, 35–36, 68, 148, 162, 177, 187, 205, 213, 237, 262
General Medical Council. *See* GMC
General Practice. *See* GP
genes, faulty, 26–28
genetic disorder, 26, 28–29, 235
genetic factors, 24, 30, 98, 109–10, 112, 115
genetic material, 60, 284–87, 302, 324
genetic predisposition, 24–26, 99, 109–10, 112, 319
GERD, 96–97
glands, sweat, 62
glial cells, 65
glucagon, 70, 80–82
glucose, 60, 62, 66–67, 70, 78, 80–81, 321
glycogen, 67, 70, 78, 80–81
GMC (General Medical Council), 143–44, 149, 270
GP (General Practice), 42, 47–48, 51–52, 150, 157, 210, 213, 233, 237, 240, 276–77
gross motor skills, 3–5, 7–10

H

haemoglobin, 28, 73, 75, 311–12, 319
haemolytic diseases of the newborn. *See* HDN
haemorrhagic strokes, 92, 108–9, 115
haemostasis, 315
Havighurst, 22
HCPC, 143, 270
HDN (Haemolytic Diseases of the Newborn), 312–13
Health Act, 146
Health and Care Act, 185, 192, 194, 203–4
Health and Care Plans, 250
Health and Safety Executive, 251–54
Health and Social Care Act, 143–44, 192, 196, 204, 249, 260–61, 274
health and social care practice, 116–17, 140, 165
health and social care services, 141–44, 149, 154, 156–57, 164–65, 175, 177, 179, 228–29, 246, 248, 250–53, 258–59, 267–71, 273–75
Health Belief Model of behaviour change, 221, 225
health campaigns, 207, 221, 223
healthcare assistants, 175

health conditions, 22, 24, 26, 38–40, 42–45, 47–51, 159–60, 169, 172, 199, 214–15, 235–37, 244, 246
health education, 49, 52, 54–55, 172, 198–204, 206, 209–10, 214, 217–19, 221, 223–25
health education campaigns, 50, 198, 202, 204, 219–22, 224–27
Health Impact Assessments (HIA), 190–91
health inequalities, 34–39, 159, 168, 173, 191, 200, 205, 207, 210, 216–18, 224–25
health issues, 43–44, 46, 185, 188, 198, 201, 205, 208–9, 211, 214, 217–19, 223, 225, 227
health officials, 304
health promotion, 49–50, 199
health screening, 48, 51
health services, 35, 131, 173, 175–76, 187, 189, 204, 213–14, 217, 277
health status, 158–60, 162–63, 170, 200
health visitors, 46, 50–51, 151, 153, 210, 264
healthy balanced diet, 29, 33, 37, 212
healthy weight, 29, 31, 227, 321
heart attack, 18, 25, 90–91, 93, 96, 99, 101–2, 216, 219–20, 315, 321
heart disease, 24–25, 30–32, 44–45, 47, 49, 101–2, 104, 159, 316, 321–23, 326
heart failure, 30, 90–91, 93, 96, 99, 111–12, 245
heart muscle, 18, 72, 90–91, 93
heart rate, 65, 76–78, 95–96, 98, 278
hepatitis, 46, 208, 303, 316, 323
herd immunity, 46, 183, 185, 301, 303–4
HIA (Health Impact Assessments), 190–91
high blood pressure, 18–19, 90, 92–93, 99, 101–2, 104, 108, 115, 205, 208, 220
HIV (Human immunodeficiency virus), 179, 185, 208, 210, 284, 305–6, 308–9, 311, 313, 315, 329
holistic health, 58, 211, 218, 223, 225, 236
homeostasis, 67–69, 114
horizontal gene transfer, 287
hormones, 10, 13–14, 16, 61, 65, 67–68, 70–71, 79–82, 87–89, 99, 109
hospice care, 231
HPV vaccine, 46
human growth and development, 1–22
human immunodeficiency virus. *See* HIV
Human Rights Act, 122, 136, 138, 149, 255, 257
humoral immunity, 298–99, 301, 318
Huntington's Disease, 26, 28–29
hypertension, 18–19, 28, 31–32, 45, 47, 90, 121, 130, 219–20
hypothalamus, 69–70, 79–82, 114

I

IBD (Inflammatory Bowel Disease), 111, 322
ICP, 154, 202, 246
ICSs. *See* Integrated Care Systems
immune cells, 71, 86, 102, 299–300, 308, 313
immune response, 21, 65, 86, 89, 98, 285, 299, 301–3

immune system, 20–21, 45–46, 73, 85–86, 88–89, 99, 102, 298–99, 301, 303, 308, 311–13, 318
impact assessments, 190–91, 193
impact of health conditions, 235–36
improving health outcomes, 162, 165
inclusion, 36, 116, 158, 162–65, 167, 170, 185, 237–38
inclusive practice, 123, 163, 165
independence, 13, 15, 22, 27, 51, 53, 117, 120–23, 130–32, 137, 152, 244, 249
infants, 3–8, 10, 41, 46, 51, 136, 172, 244
infectious diseases, 159, 161, 167, 174–75, 178, 180, 199, 216–17, 283–84, 292–94, 301, 303–4, 306–8, 325–26, 330
inflammation, 20, 25, 36, 38, 41, 44, 86, 95–96, 98, 300–301, 304, 322, 329
inflammatory bowel disease. *See* IBD
influenza, 303, 305–8, 311, 325, 328
information, sensitive, 133–34
Information Act, 145, 274
insulin, 70, 80–82, 99–102, 321–22
insulin resistance, 100–101, 321
integrated care, 192, 195–97, 202, 233, 246
Integrated Care Boards, 154, 182, 185, 196, 202, 211, 247
integrated care model, 197
Integrated Care Partnerships, 154–55, 185, 246–47
Integrated Care Services, 203
Integrated Care Systems, 56, 154–55, 157, 192, 194, 196, 202–3, 246–47
intercostal muscles, 75, 108
intersectionality, 162–63, 167
intestines, 62, 64, 75, 87–89
intimate relationships, 5, 12, 14
iron-deficiency anaemia, 320
ischaemic stroke, 92–93, 108

J

joints, 44, 62, 83–85
Joint Strategic Needs Assessments (JSNAs), 191, 194

K

kidney disease, 321
kidneys, 62, 70, 79–82, 101
kwashiorkor, 319–20

L

lactation, 14
lactic acid, 67
larynx, 11, 74
late adulthood, 18–19, 23
learning disabilities, 35, 39, 50–51, 129, 153, 185, 189, 229–30, 236, 261, 265
LEDCs. *See* less economically developed countries
less economically developed countries (LEDCs), 167

leukaemia, 313–15, 317
leukocytes, 73, 86, 114, 299, 301, 311, 313, 315
libido, 16–17
life expectancy, 34–35, 39, 173, 181, 187, 205, 209, 221
life stages, 1–58, 136, 228–30, 232–48
lifestyle choices, 12, 43, 45, 47, 49, 199–200, 210, 221, 236, 297, 319
lifestyle factors, 16, 28–30, 33, 52, 58, 99, 109–13, 225, 321–22
liver, 20, 33, 67, 70–71, 75, 78, 80–81, 88, 91, 110–11, 113
local authorities, 145, 148, 154, 188–89, 191–92, 194, 196, 201–4, 220, 223, 249, 253, 274
local services, 204, 229, 240, 246
long-term health conditions, 20, 195, 235–37, 277
lung cancer, 32, 42, 49, 109, 112–13, 115, 183, 199, 208, 324
lungs, 27, 32, 37–38, 62–63, 71–75, 90–91, 94–96, 98–99, 103, 108–13, 309, 311, 315
Lyme disease, 292, 306
lymphatic system, 85–89, 110, 314
lymphatic vessels, 86–88
lymphocytes, 86, 313–14
lymphocytosis, 313, 315
lymphoma, 314–15

M

macrophages, 86, 298–301
malaria, 288, 292, 294, 306, 310, 316, 329
malpractice, 120, 133, 167
Marmot Review, 187, 189, 193
MDT. *See* multi-disciplinary team
measles, 46, 172, 183, 199, 303–5, 328–30, 335
MEDCs (More economically developed countries), 167
melanoma, 324
memory B-cells, 298–99, 301
meningitis, 28, 40–41, 46, 105, 311, 316
meningococcal meningitis, 309
menopause, 16, 18, 20, 109, 210
Mental Capacity Act, 147, 256–57
Mental Health Act, 35, 146, 256
mental health services, 141–42, 144–47, 150–51, 194, 225, 280
merozoites, 289
metabolism, 17, 66, 79, 89, 106–7
metastasis, 110–11, 113
microbiology, 283–96
microorganisms, 63, 65, 73, 95, 283–85, 290–91, 293, 295–98, 308–11, 318
middle adulthood, 16–18, 43, 244
midwife, 33, 48, 51, 56
Midwifery Council, 149, 270
minerals, 29, 290, 319
miscarriage, 101–2
misinformation, 184–85, 334–35
mitochondria, 60–61, 66
mitosis, 67

MMR vaccine, 46, 183–84, 186
models of behaviour change, 223, 226
monocytes, 314
mortality rates, 167–69, 217
mosquitoes, 290, 292, 305–7
motility, 13–14
motor neurones, 64–65, 68
mRNA, 60–61, 302
mucous membranes, 74–75, 86, 290, 297–98, 305
mucus, 27, 74, 94–95, 297, 322
multi-disciplinary team (MDT), 28, 40, 56–58, 119, 128, 131–32, 150, 153, 204, 231
muscle contractions, 61, 65–67
muscles, 3, 63–65, 67–68, 70–71, 76, 78, 80–81, 83–84, 93, 95–96, 103–4, 108–9, 319–20
muscle tissue, 11, 63, 65, 67
muscle weakness, 92, 96–97, 106–8, 114
musculoskeletal system, 52, 59, 83, 85–86, 93, 96–97, 108–9, 111, 113, 115
mutations, 26–28, 109–10, 112
myeloid cells, 314

N
National Health Service. See NHS
National Health Service Act, 172
National Institute for Health and Care, 178
NEET, 188
negative feedback, 69–70
neglect, 127, 137–38, 209, 211, 265, 267, 280
nerve damage, 101, 107, 319, 321
nervous system, 59, 64–65, 68, 76–78, 83, 88, 93, 102, 104, 108–9, 115
neurodiversity, 161–62
neuroglia, 64–65, 68
neurologist, 158
neurones, 15, 18–19, 21, 64–65, 67, 76, 103
neuropathy, 101–2, 321
neutrophils, 86, 298, 300
NGOs, 331
NHS (National Health Service), 37–38, 47–50, 56, 117–18, 141, 145–46, 149, 172, 174–75, 181–82, 186–87, 191–92, 194–96, 201–3, 207–8, 215, 219, 246, 256–58, 274
NHS and social care services, 203
NHS Core Values, 117–18
NHS England, 120, 141, 149, 154, 178, 189, 201–2, 246, 277
NHS health services, 147
NHS organisations, 154, 196, 220, 246
NHS services, 47, 51, 117, 142, 154–55, 159, 178, 192
NICE, 141
non-traumatic brain injuries, 105–6
norovirus, 294, 307
nucleus, 60–61, 73, 286–87
Nursing and Midwifery Council, 149, 270
nutritional deficiencies, 319–20, 327
nutritional deficiency diseases, 319, 327

O
obesity, 30–32, 37, 44–45, 159, 161, 188, 192–93, 197, 201, 207, 225, 227, 321–22
obesity strategy, 194–95, 197
oesophagus, 88, 96–97
oestrogen, 10–11, 13–14, 20, 25, 80, 87, 109–10
Office for Health Improvement and Disparities. See OHID
OHID (Office for Health Improvement and Disparities), 174–75, 178, 266, 336
oral health, 32, 44, 49
oral thrush, 310
organelles, 60
organic compounds, 290
organisations, third-sector, 192
osmoregulation, 70, 80–82
osteoporosis, 20–21, 23, 30–31, 44, 97
othering, 166
ovaries, 11, 13, 16, 80–81, 87
ovulation, 10–11, 13, 87

P
palliative care, 148, 152, 231
pancreas, 70, 75, 80–82, 88–89, 99–100, 102, 114, 321
pandemics, 167–70, 181, 185–86, 191, 266, 329–33, 335
paralysis, 92–93, 106–8, 196
parasympathetic nervous systems, 78
pathogens, 62–63, 65, 73, 85–86, 89, 95, 98–99, 290, 292–93, 297–99, 301–3, 305–7, 311, 313, 328–29
penis, 11, 27, 87
perimenopause, 16–18
peripheral nervous system. See PNS
personal care, 56, 152–53, 235, 259
personalisation, 174, 176–77
personalised care, 56, 278
personal protective equipment. See PPE
person-centred approach, 57, 120, 144, 147–48, 163, 224, 232–34
person-centred care, 57, 127–28, 132, 140, 234, 244–45, 249, 260, 280
pesticides, 323, 325, 334
phagocytes, 114, 298–99
phagocytosis, 298–301
physical activity, 16, 31, 96–97, 160–61, 199, 235, 321
physical barriers, 86, 217, 293–94, 297
physiotherapist, 26–27, 53, 58, 121, 150, 270
pincer grip, 4–5
pituitary gland, 10, 79, 87
placenta, 306, 312
plasma, 62, 73, 311–12
plasmodium, 288, 294
platelets, 62, 73, 311–13, 315
pneumonia, 45, 93, 95, 98–99, 104, 112, 159, 304, 308, 329

PNS (peripheral nervous system), 52, 64–65, 76–79, 108
policies, safeguarding, 137–38, 146, 268
policies and procedures, 122, 133, 137–38, 239, 267–68, 279
pollution, 36, 94, 190, 200, 208
positive risks, 137
power of attorney, 147–48
PPE (personal protective equipment), 253–54, 294, 331, 333
pregnancy, 11, 14, 31–34, 36, 51, 56, 101–2, 173, 175, 177, 204, 312, 319–20
primary care services, 52, 56, 150, 153, 219, 229
processed food, 159, 321–23
Professional Standards Authority, 144, 149
progesterone, 10–11, 25, 80, 87
prostate, 25, 27
prostate cancer, 25–26
protected characteristics, 118, 147, 149, 161, 166, 213, 255, 257, 262–63
protective factors, 265–66
proteins, 21, 24, 29, 33, 60–61, 63, 66, 73, 86, 88, 310–12, 315, 319–20
protein synthesis, 60–61, 66, 80, 82
protozoa, 284, 288–89, 308, 310
psychiatrists, 52, 55–56
psychologists, 55, 150, 181
puberty, 10–12, 14, 28, 43, 244
public health aims, 180
public health experts, 307
public health initiatives, 178
public health issues, 192, 196, 202, 206
public health policy, 171–73, 178–81, 183–84, 190, 192–93, 208
public health practitioners, 206, 218
public health responses, 335
public health schemes, 210
public health strategy, 292
public health surveillance, 191
Public Health Wales, 191
pulmonary artery, 71–72, 96
pulmonary embolism, 112, 315
pulmonary hypertension, 96–97

Q

quality of care, 117–19, 121, 124, 142, 146, 165, 213, 270
questionnaires, 225–26

R

rabies, 303, 305–6
Race Equality Framework for NHS England, 189
radiation, 109, 291, 295, 324
receptors, sensory, 64–65
record keeping, 135, 228, 239, 273–74
red blood cells, 28, 62, 73, 75, 111–12, 289, 311–13, 317, 319
reducing health inequalities, 173, 192
reflexes, 76

refugee, 161–62, 168, 170
regulatory bodies, 143, 145, 149, 270–71, 302
reproductive health, 210
respiratory infections, 93, 98, 104, 323
retrovirus, 284, 308
RhD, 312
rhesus disease, 312, 316–17
ribosomes, 60–61, 286
RIDDOR, 253–54
rights of individuals, 226, 238, 255, 263
risk assessment, 178, 251–54, 263
RNA, 61, 284–86, 308

S

safeguarding, 120, 138–39, 145–46, 177, 239, 249–50, 258, 260, 267–68, 274
salivary glands, 88
salmonella, 306–7, 309
saturated fats, 321–22
schemas, 4–5
SDGs (Sustainable Development Goals), 179, 203
secondary care, 52, 150
secondary sexual characteristics, 10–11, 13–14, 80
self-concept, 9, 11–14
self-esteem, 11–12, 15, 236, 243
sense of humour, 123–25
sensory impairments, 107, 240
sensory neurones, 64–65, 68
sex hormones, 10–11
sexual health, 43, 49, 187, 204, 210–11
sexual health clinics, 151, 192, 194, 210, 225
sexual intercourse, 43, 87
sexually transmitted infections. See STIs
sexual orientation, 36, 118, 161, 213, 217–18, 237, 255–56, 262
sickle cell anaemia, 28–29, 312–13, 317
sickle cell crises, 312, 317
sickle cell gene, 28
skeleton, 62–63, 83
Skills for Care values, 118–19
skin cancer, 199, 324, 326
sleep apnoea, 99, 115
smart wearables, 277–78
smoking, 12, 16, 32–33, 42, 45, 49, 110, 112–13, 159, 207, 211–12, 221, 223
Social Care Act, 143–44, 192, 196, 204, 249, 260–61, 274
Social Care Institute, 142, 149, 249
social care practice, 116–40, 142, 165
social care services, 141–45, 149, 152, 154, 156–57, 175, 177, 179, 202–3, 228–29, 250–53, 258–59, 267–71, 273–75, 277–78
Social Cognitive Theory, 222
social media, 42–43, 136, 156, 184–85, 215, 334
social workers, 52, 54–55, 135, 139, 143–44, 195, 233, 270
somatic nervous system, 77
speech development problems, 40–41

sperm, 10, 14, 87, 211
sphygmomanometer, 47
spinal cord, 41, 64–65, 68, 76–77, 79, 158, 309
spirilla, 286
sporozoites, 288–89
Stages of Change Model, 222
standards of care, 121, 123, 135, 144, 260–61
stereotypes, 213, 226
stereotyping, 166, 213
STIs (sexually transmitted infections), 43, 151, 210, 305
streptococci, 286, 306, 309
strokes, 18, 21, 25, 31–32, 90–93, 96–97, 99, 101–2, 104–6, 108, 112, 114–15, 219–20, 315, 321–22
Sustainable Development Goals (SDGs), 179, 203
sympathetic nervous system, 78
synergistic muscles, 84
synovial joints, 84–85

T

TB. *See* tuberculosis
T-cells, 299, 301
telehealth and telemedicine, 277–79
telemedicine, 188, 277–79
tendons, 20, 38, 63, 83–85
tertiary care, 52, 151
testes, 10–11, 27, 80, 82, 87
thorax, 75
thrombosis, 92, 315–17
TIAs. *See* transient ischemic attacks
toxoplasmosis, 305–6
trachea, 62, 74–75, 83, 94, 96
transient ischemic attacks (TIAs), 102–4
transmission of infectious diseases, 307, 326
transtheoretical model, 222
traumatic brain injury, 105–7, 115
tsetse fly, 288–89
tuberculosis, 37, 306, 309, 325
tumours, 25, 32, 105, 112

U

UK government, 29, 32, 50, 169, 181, 188, 205, 207, 274
UK Health Security Agency, 174, 178, 191, 202
UKHSA (UK's Health Security Agency), 174, 178, 191, 202–3, 205, 210
UK's Health Security Agency. *See* UKHSA
ulcerative colitis, 111, 322
unconscious bias, 166
uterus, 11, 78, 80, 87, 89
UV radiation, 324, 326

V

vaccination rates, low, 304
vaccinations, 46, 50, 168, 172–73, 176, 179, 182–84, 188, 189, 191, 194, 199, 285, 291, 301–4, 331, 333–34
vaccine development, 179, 301–3, 331
vaccine hesitancy, 334–35
vaccines, 194, inactivated, 303
vaccine uptake, 335
vagina, 87, 89, 100, 306, 310
vascular dementia, 102–4
vectors, 292, 294, 305–7
viral infections, 40, 308–9, 311, 313, 329
virtual hospitals, 153, 231
virtual wards, 130–32, 153, 231–32
viruses, 40, 177, 182, 184–85, 188, 191–92, 284–85, 296, 298–99, 302, 304–5, 308–9, 313, 316, 328
vitamins, 29, 33, 210, 290, 319–20
vulnerable individuals, 139, 146–47, 228, 251, 254–59, 262–63, 265–73, 280, 282

W

Wales Health Impact Assessment Support Unit, 191
waterborne diseases, 323, 325
wellbeing of vulnerable individuals, 255, 267
whistleblowing, 133–34, 239, 268, 270
whistleblowing policies, 268
white blood cells, 62, 73, 86, 102, 114, 298–300, 311–15
WHO (World Health Organisation), 179, 182–83, 190–91, 194, 196–97, 201, 203–5, 207, 219–20, 227, 304, 331–32, 335
women's health hubs, 211
World Health Organisation. *See* WHO

www.ingramcontent.com/pod-product-compliance
Lightning Source LLC
Chambersburg PA
CBHW081102070526
44584CB00021B/3170